Foodborne Microorganisms and Their Toxins: Developing Methodology

ift Basic Symposium Series

Edited by
INSTITUTE OF FOOD TECHNOLOGISTS
221 N. LaSalle St.
Chicago, Illinois

Foodborne Microorganisms and Their Toxins:
Developing Methodology   *edited by Merle D.
Pierson and Norman J. Stern*

Foodborne Microorganisms and Their Toxins: Developing Methodology

edited by

Merle D. Pierson
Department of Food Science and Technology
Virginia Polytechnic Institute and State University
Blacksburg, Virginia

Norman J. Stern
United States Department of Agriculture
Agricultural Research Service
Russell Research Center
Athens, Georgia

Marcel Dekker, Inc.   New York and Basel

Library of Congress Cataloging-in-Publication Data

Foodborne microorganisms and their toxins.

(IFT basic symposium series)
Proceedings of a symposium held June 7-8, 1985,
sponsored by the Institute of Food Technologists and
the International Union of Food Science and Technology.
Includes bibliographies and index.
1. Food--Microbiology--Congresses. 2. Food--
Analysis--Congresses. 3. Microbial toxins--Analysis--
Congresses. I. Pierson, Merle D. II. Stern, Norman J.
III. Institute of Food Technologists. IV. International
Union of Food Science and Technology. V. Series.
[DNLM: 1. Bacterial Toxins--congresses. 2. Food
Contamination--congresses. 3. Food Microbiology--
congresses. QW 85 F6873 1985]

QR115.F665 1986   615.9'54   86-6411
ISBN 0-8247-7607-0

MARCEL DEKKER, INC.
270 Madison Avenue, New York, New York 10016

Current printing (last digit):
10 9 8 7 6 5 4 3 2 1

PRINTED IN THE UNITED STATES OF AMERICA

Preface

The Institute of Food Technologists (IFT) and the International Union of Food Science and Technology annually sponsor a two-day basic symposium that provides an in-depth analysis of an area of major importance in food science and technology. This book presents the Ninth Basic Symposium, "Foodborne Microorganisms and Their Toxins: Developing Methodology," which was held June 7–8, 1985, immediately prior to the 45th Annual IFT Meeting. Methods for analysis of foods for microorganisms and their metabolic products, as well as concepts in interpreting these data, are rapidly changing. This symposium was organized to provide an up-to-date analysis and discussion of these areas rather than simply another volume of methods. It is essential that food microbiologists and other food scientists review the current status of food microbiology so that they can deal more intelligently with microbiological problems and continue to provide the public with food that is wholesome, safe, and economical.

The classical observations of Louis Pasteur and others served as the basis for the development of food microbiology as a distinct and separate discipline. These early scientists first correlated certain illnesses with the presence of pathogens and toxins in foods. From this awareness it was only a short step to determining that proper processing and handling of foods could effectively prevent foodborne illness and food spoilage.

Microbiologists next began to study specific characteristics of spoilage, indicator, and pathogenic microorganisms. These studies included diagnostic criteria useful in the isolation of these organisms or toxins as well as

microscopic examination of bacterial isolates, biochemical tests, and production of specific metabolites. For example, isolates from seafood can be
microscopically examined to detect pleomorphic, curved, rodlike organisms
to determine the presence of *Vibrio* spp. A biochemical criterion used for
assessing the presence of coliform bacteria is the characteristic fermentation
of lactose with the production of acid and gas. An example of testing for a
specific toxin in food is the mouse bioassay for the botulinal neurotoxin.

An important motivation for the development of analytical food microbiology has been the role of industry and government in assuring food quality
and safety. Regulations, referenced methodologies, and industrial competition have played an integral part in the development of food microbiology.
Government agencies routinely monitor food processors and distributors and
thus continually strive for rapid, reproducible, and accurate techniques for
detection of microorganisms and microbial toxins in food.

In this volume, the authors share their thoughts regarding methodology,
regulatory criteria, and means for predicting shelf life for food products.
These areas have been, and continue to be, enormously important. Food
microbiology has undergone substantial change recently in analytical methods and their interpretations.Research in other than these traditional domains
has become increasingly important to food microbiology. New bacterial
detection systems are vying for the microbiologist's approval in the marketplace. Many of these systems have been developed from research modifications in other fields of study. The potential benefits include the more rapid
detection and quantitation of specific bacteria. However, the proven, traditional approaches may continue for some time to serve as the yardstick for
comparison.

Advances in both immunology and DNA hybridization techniques appear
to be shaking the very foundations of traditional food microbiology. Bor-
rowing from other disciplines is within the honorable tradition of our profes-
sion; however, the depth and the potential for changing food microbiology
have never been greater. Study of immune system physiology has led to the
development of hybridoma technology. This technology has fostered production of monoclonal antibodies, which are capable of serving as reagents
in rapid ELISA and other immunological assays for the detection of target
organisms. These reagents have also been used to identify specific virulence
determinants, which aid in discriminating pathogenic from innocuous microorganisms. In turn, use of these highly specific reagents will aid the food
processor in preventing adulterated foodstuffs from reaching the marketplace.
Application of DNA hybridization techniques also provides a means for
noncultural detection of bacteria and/or discrimination between virulent and
avirulent bacterial varieties. Undoubtedly, each of these biotechnological
approaches will have its specific strengths and weaknesses.

In addition to discussing developments in instrumental methods, biotechnology applications, and immunology techniques, advances in knowledge of specific microorganisms and their toxins are presented. As our colleagues from clinical microbiology laboratories are uncovering newly recognized enteropathogens, it becomes incumbent upon the food microbiologist to determine which foods may be at risk and how to alleviate the presence of the pathogenic organism and/or toxins, and to rapidly detect the causative agent in foodstuffs.

Dr. John Troller, as 1981–82 Chairman of the IFT Food Microbiology Division, provided the initial suggestion for a basic symposium on food microbiology. The subsequent development and success of the Ninth Basic Symposium was due to the expert assistance of Dr. Larry Beuchat, Chairman, and the IFT Basic Symposium Committee; Dr. Bernard Liska, 1984–85 IFT President; Calvert L. Willey, IFT Executive Director; John B. Klis, IFT Director of Publications; and the IFT staff who provided publicity, facility planning, and numerous other details essential to a successful meeting.

John Klis served as coordinator and Anna May Schenck, JFS Assistant Scientific Editor, as copyeditor for this symposium volume. This book was published as a result of their professional insight, patience, and persistence.

In particular, the contributing authors are gratefully recognized for making possible the symposium and this book. It is through the expertise of scientists such as these that food microbiology is experiencing essential growth and change.

Merle D. Pierson
Norman J. Stern

Contributors

O. Brian Allen, PH.D.   Department of Animal and Poultry Science, Department of Mathematics and Statistics, University of Guelph, Guelph, Ontario, Canada

Douglas L. Archer, Ph.D.   Center for Food Safety and Applied Nutrition, Food and Drug Administration, Washington, D.C.

R. W. Bennett, M. S.   Center for Food Safety and Applied Nutrition, Food and Drug Administration, Washington, D.C.

David L. Collins-Thompson, Ph.D.   Departments of Environment Biology/Food Science, University of Guelph, Guelph, Ontario, Canada

Carl S. Custer, M.S.   USDA Food Safety Inspection Service, Meat and Poultry Inspection Technical Service, Processed Products Inspection Division, Washington, D.C.

Michael P. Doyle, Ph.D.   Department of Food Microbiology and Toxicology, University of Wisconsin-Madison, Madison, Wisconsin

Phyllis Entis, M.Sc.   QA Laboratories Limited, Toronto, Ontario, Canada

Jeffrey M. Farber, Ph.D.   Microbiology Research Division, Health and Welfare Canada, Health Protection Branch, Sir Frederick G. Banting Research Centre, Tunney's Pasture, Ottawa, Ontario, Canada

Ruth Firstenberg-Eden, Ph.D.   Research and Development Microbiology, Bactomatic, Inc., Princeton, New Jersey

Renee A. Fitts, Ph.D.   Department of Applied Biological Sciences, Massachusetts Institute of Technology, Cambridge, Massachusetts

Peggy M. Foegeding, Ph.D.   Food Science Department, North Carolina State University, Raleigh, North Carolina

Richard A. Goldsby, Ph.D.   Biology Department, Amherst College, Amherst, Massachusetts

Paul A. Hartman, Ph.D.   Department of Microbiology, Iowa State University, Ames, Iowa

James M. Jay, Ph.D.   Department of Biological Sciences, Wayne State University, Detroit, Michigan

Charles W. Kaspar, M.S.   Department of Microbiology, Iowa State University, Ames, Iowa

Raymond L. Konger, B.S.   Department of Foods and Nutrition, Purdue University, West Lafayette, Indiana

Edward P. Larkin, Ph.D.   Division of Microbiology, CFSAN, Food and Drug Administration, Cincinnati, Ohio

Kathleen A. LaRocco, M.S.*   Packard Instrument Company, Downers Grove, Illinois

Kenneth J. Littel, M.S.   Packard Instrument Company, Downers Grove, Illinois

Joseph M. Madden, Ph.D.   Division of Microbiology, Food and Drug Administration, Washington, D.C.

Barbara A. McCardell, Ph.D.   Division of Microbiology, Food and Drug Administration, Washington, D.C.

David A. A. Mossel, Ph.D.   Faculty of Veterinary Medicine, The University of Utrecht, The Netherlands

Douglas L. Park, Ph.D.   Center for Food Safety and Applied Nutrition, Food and Drug Administration, Washington, D.C.

James P. Petzel, M.S.   Department of Microbiology, Iowa State University, Ames, Iowa

Merle D. Pierson, Ph.D.   Department of Food Science and Technology, Virginia Polytechnic Institute and State University, Blacksburg, Virginia

Albert E. Pohland, Ph.D.   Center for Food Safety and Applied Nutrition, Food and Drug Administration, Washington, D.C.

Current affiliation: Abbott Laboratories, North Chicago, Illinois

Samuel Schalkowsky, B.S.   Spiral System Instruments, Inc., Bethesda, Maryland

Anthony N. Sharpe, Ph.D.   Bureau of Microbial Hazards, Health Protection Branch, Health and Welfare Canada, Tunney's Pasture, Ottawa, Ontario, Canada

B. Swaminathan, Ph.D.   Department of Foods and Nutrition, Purdue University, West Lafayette, Indiana

Contents

Foodborne Microorganisms and Their Toxins: Developing Methodology

1

Developing Methodology for Foodborne Microorganisms— Fundamentals of Analytical Techniques

David A. A. Mossel

Faculty of Veterinary Medicine, The University
Utrecht, The Netherlands

PRECEPTS

The assurance of microbiological safety and quality of foods must rely on intervention (Meyer 1931; Dack 1956; Wilson 1933, 1973; Ingram and Roberts 1971; Mossel and Kampelmacher 1981; Kayser and Mossel 1984). This would, as the first priority, include identification of hazard points (Bauman 1974; Kayser and Mossel 1984) in manufacture, distribution, storage, and culinary preparation. Subsequently, measures must be designed to assure improved "Good Manufacturing and Distribution Practices." Such procedures should be elaborated and validated, guided by the examination of line samples and, to a lesser extent, assessment of the microbiological condition of end products. Analytical techniques to be used for this purpose should be (1) as simple and rapid as possible; (2) accurate and reproducible; and (3) economically feasible.

Three general principles have been adopted in the area of microbiological examination of foods. First and foremost, the fewest possible criteria are to be used. The indispensable ones are selected, guided by a careful study of

1

the microbial ecology of every specific commodity, paying attention to health risks as well as to the food's so-called spoilage association (Mossel 1983). Furthermore, reference ranges ("target values") should be available for comparison of the results of a given analysis. As is done in clinical medicine (Grasbeck and Alstrom 1981), such reference ranges should be derived from surveys on 'valid' specimens, i.e., originating from production or catering lines previously inspected and noted for using correct practices, but modified before samples are drawn if necessary (Mossel 1980). Finally and quite obviously, the methods used in assessing the conformity of production samples with reference values should be exactly the same as those used in determining reference values and rigorously standardized for that purpose. If this aspect of monitoring is neglected, a most embarrasing conflict of opinion can result between production and quality assurance departments of the same factory or, worse, between manufacturer and buyer or Government Inspection Services.

ANALYTICAL ESSENTIALS

Isolation and enumeration methods for specific groups of microorganisms in foods and drinking water invariably rely on. the use of selective culture media. This entails two types of problems that require the permanent attention of the food microbiologist.

Limitations of Selective Media and Their Control

In view of the extensive genetic variation observed in almost all niches of significance in food microbiology (Altherr and Kasweck 1982; Bensink and Botham 1983; Alcaide and Garay 1984) no selective medium will exclusively allow the growth of all the microorganisms for which it was designed. Even if the medium did initially accomplish this goal, there is no guarantee that it will continue to do so (Dijkmann, 1982). Consequently, most selective media are either insufficiently selective, or else are inhibitory to differing degrees for the group of organisms they are supposed to enumerate. Every formula, whether prepared in the laboratory or purchased commercially, therefore, represents a compromise. This is unavoidable, but can lead to workable situations, provided the performance of a medium is 'constant', i.e., not varying too much from lot to lot. Consequently, media must be checked for effectiveness both when purchased and in the course of time, when a given batch number is used for more than one or two weeks. Unfortunately, such monitoring is often abandoned when testing methods become too complicated, time consuming or expensive.

Rather than using conventional, fully quantitative techniques for monitoring performance of media, we found it useful to rely on the principle of constantly decreasing density of inoculation as practiced in spiral plating (Masters and Palmer 1981; Reusse 1982; Walsh et al. 1985). Sequential streaking of test strains with disposable plastic 1 μl loops over 21 lines on a standard Petri dish containing the medium under test, as illustrated in Fig. 1.1 and 1.2, is useful to attain this goal (Mossel et al. 1983a). In the few instances where a higher accuracy is required, the same loops can be used for making conventional spread drop plates (Corry 1982). Whichever technique is used, a medium is always challenged by a selection of test strains that should be recovered quantitatively and another series that should be completely or almost totally inhibited.

Effects and Remedying of Sublethal Damage

The use of selective media invariably entails the risk that sublethally damaged cells in the viable part of the population to be enumerated will not be included in counts. Virtually all foods in commerce will contain such damaged cells,

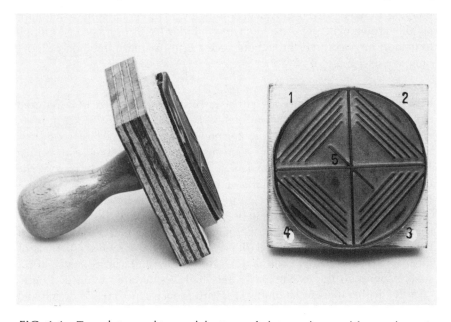

FIG. 1.1 Template used to mark bottom of plates to be used for, and matrix for inoculation according to, and interpretation of, the ecometric technique for the monitoring of culture media. Inocula of test organisms are streaked onto media under examination in the sequence one to five.

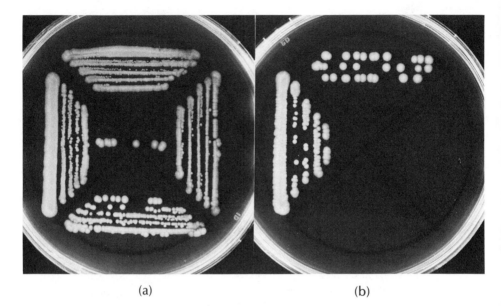

(a)   (b)

FIG. 1.2   Two typical results of ecometric evaluation of a culture medium:
(a) fully grown plate, i.e. Absolute Growth Index (AGI) = 5, because colony
formation has occurred throughout sector 5; (b) partial inhibition of inoculum; AGI = 2.

because these commodities are either intrinsically preserved by a reduced
a_w, pH or added antimicrobial substances (e.g. nitrite or sorbic acid), processed by heat, or else stored frozen or under refrigeration. These conditions
will induce sublethal lesions in organisms exposed (Mossel and van Netten
1984); hence resuscitation steps (Allen et al. 1952) should always precede
the application of selective isolation and enumeration procedures.

Relying on fortuitous repair during preparation of food macerates and
subsequent decimal dilutions is to be strongly discouraged, because this may
lead to insufficient recovery of the more severely impaired cells in a given
population. When macerates or dilutions are stored for longer periods of
time, however, repaired cells may start to grow and consequently affect
colony counts to the extent that falsely high results are obtained. Consequently, deliberate resuscitation steps, with proper experimental design and
empirical validation, should be used in all instances.

In presence-or-absence (P-A) tests (semi-quantitative assessment), maceration and dilution of samples and subsequent liquid medium repair ('nonselective pre-enrichment') can be adequate for recovering injured bacteria
present in the sample (Van Doorne and Claushuis 1979). With selective
colony counting procedures, liquid medium repair may sometimes lead to

complete revitalization of stressed cells (Mossel et al. 1980a); however, in many instances this may be inadequate. The solid medium procedure of Speck et al. (1975) is the most versatile one. It relies on recovery of injured cells by using a suitable solid medium followed by overlayering the recovery medium with a selective one; or as with strictly aerobic taxa, replica plating onto such a medium (Mossel et al. 1980b). The use of special, injury alleviating substances such as catalase or pyruvate in resuscitation media is sometimes essential to recover all viable colony forming units (van Netten et al. 1984). When such carefully devised resuscitation procedures are neglected, a substantial lack of reproducibility will occur.

There are indications that some selective media will not generally inhibit stressed populations and hence can be used without a resuscitation step. These media include: (1) Baird-Parker's glycine tellurite pyruvate egg yolk agar for the enumeration of *Staphylococcus aureus* (Idziak and Mossel 1980); (2) Mannitol egg yolk polymyxin agar for colony counts of *Bacillus cereus* (Rappaport and Goepfert 1978); and, (3) Skirrow's highly selective blood agar, relying on the use of a cocktail of antibiotics for the enumeration of *Campylobacter jejuni* (Waterman 1982; Hanninen 1982). However, omitting a resuscitation step when these media are employed entails a perennial risk. Different stresses such as heating versus freezing may differ in their effects, and moreover, the intensity of stress and hence of damage may vary widely, as illustrated by Fig. 1.3. This concern has recently been substantiated with respect to Baird-Parker's extensively tested medium. Mansfield et al. (1983) demonstrated that cells of *S. aureus* stored for an extended period of time in cured meats under anaerobic conditions might incur multifactorial damage leading to markedly reduced recovery on Baird-Parker's agar.

We have recently observed similar phenomena with *S. aureus* stored for many months in precooked frozen shrimps at about -25°C. As the data in Table 1.1 illustrate, such populations are only partially recovered on Baird-Parker agar at 37°C. An even lower recovery on this medium occurs when it is incubated at 42.5°C, despite the fact that incubation of Baird-Parker's agar at elevated temperatures has been found to completely recover populations of *S. aureus* stressed by heating or exposure to osmotic shock (van Doorne et al. 1982). On the other hand, solid medium repair allowed almost quantitative recovery of populations of *S. aureus* stressed by prolonged freezing, under any conditions of selective culturing.

Similarly, though it has recently been substantiated that selective media currently used for the enumeration of *Campylobacter jejuni* do not affect the recovery of *Campylobacter* populations exposed to heat injury (Palumbo 1984), this certainly does not apply to cold stress (Ray and Johnson 1984). Moreover the use of a nonprotective diluent could adversely affect colony counts of stressed cells of *C. jejuni* in the customarily used antibiotic containing media (Abram and Potter 1985).

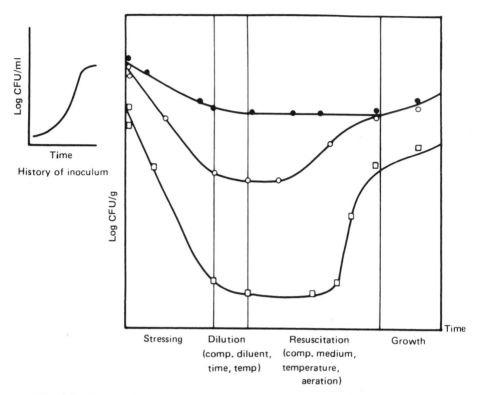

FIG. 1.3   Destruction-repair curve presenting the fate of a sublethally injured microbial population during incubation on nonselective medium ●——●, optimal selective medium ○——○, and suboptimal selective medium □——□; the latter two both recover noninjured populations quantitatively.

Ensuring Adequate Overall Consistency of Data

Monitoring of selective media and the use of proper resuscitation procedures are essential parts of every analytical procedure to be used in food microbiology. These measures alone, however, are by no means sufficient to ensure adequate reproducibility of P-A tests or colony counts.

As emphasized before, every effort should be made to guarantee the highest degree of reproducibility. This is imperative in view of the already relatively high coefficient of variation of colony counts (Mossel et al. 1980a), but especially of P-A procedures (Wood 1956; Pretorius 1961; Lear 1962). This applies even when these determinations are carried out by highly qualified staff, taking all possible precautions and adhering most accurately to

Table 1.1 Examination of Frozen Precooked Shrimps at 42.5°C Versus 37°C, Without and with Solid Medium Repair (SMR) on GTSYEP[a] Agar for 5 hr at 23 ± 2°C, Using Baird-Parker's Medium for Ultimate Assessment of Colony Forming Units (CFUs) of *Staph. aureus*

| | LOG_{10} CFU/G | | | | CFU Proportion | | CFU Proportion | |
| | 37°C | | 43°C | | | | | |
Sample	With SMR on GTSYEP	Without SMR	With SMR on GTSYEP	Without SMR	With SMR 37°C	With SMR 43°C	Without SMR 37°C	Without SMR 43°C
1	3.1	2.9	2.9	2.0	0.2			0.9
2	3.3	3.1	3.0	2.6	0.3			0.5
3	2.9	2.5	2.8	2.4	0.1			0.1
4	2.8	2.7	2.8	2.0	0.0			0.7
5	3.2	3.1	2.9	2.0	0.3			1.1
6	3.2	3.1	3.0	2.4	0.2			0.7
Average	—	—	—	—	0.2			0.7

[a]GTSYEP = buffered glucose tryptone soya peptone yeast extract agar with 100 mL egg yolk emulsion and 10g sodium pyruvate per 1 L of medium.

Table 1.2 Matrix to Be Followed When Developing Analytical Methods in Food Microbiology and in the Standardization of Procedures to Be Used in Trade and for Intra-Corporate Purposes

1. Sampling Plan
   a. randomization
   b. numbers to be drawn per predefined lot
2. Handling before examination
   a. transportation: time/temperature integral
   b. challenge
      - incubation
      - inoculation in case of survival studies or assessment of resistance against colonization.
3. Preparation for examination
   a. defrosting: time/temperature integral; squeezing to release fluid
   b. cleaning/disinfection of containers
4. Drawing of subsamples (aliquots)
   a. randomization
   b. size of subsample
   c. diminution and homogenization
5. Preparation of macerate and dilutions
   a. size of second subsample, i.e., aliquot to be examined
   b. preparation of macerate
      - composition of maceration fluid
      - procedure, including time/temperature regimen
      - mode of dispersion
      - preparation of serial dilutions
      - composition of diluent
      - procedure, including time/temperature regimen
6. Monitoring of culture media
   a. choice of test strains
   b. selection of inoculation procedure
   c. incubation, time, temperature and tolerances
   d. reading
   e. reference values to be used
7. Resuscitation procedure
   a. composition of resuscitation medium
   b. time/temperature program, including tolerances
   c. mode of processing of resuscitated system
8. Enumeration procedure
   a. composition of medium
   b. preparation of medium

(Continued)

Table 1.2 (*Continued*)

    c. decontamination of medium

    d. tempering of medium

    e. aseptic precautions during inoculation

    f. inoculation

       • procedure, qualitative

       • procedure, quantitative

       • holding or drying time/temperature

    g. incubation

       • procedure, qualitative

       • circulation, ventilation and temperature tolerances

       • duration, including tolerances

    h. reading

       • definition of target colonies

       • accuracy of colony counting

       • "emergency" handling of plates showing too few or too many colonies

       • reference values

    i. confirmation/identification

       • extent of picking per given type of colony

       • subculture for examination

       • preliminary taxonomic grouping

       • presumptive grouping

       • complementary testing: intramural/extramural

       • expression of results

    j. mathematical treatment of data and mode of recording of results

9. Essential annexes

    a. justification and documentation of techniques

    b. laboratory precautions to be observed ("GLP")

    c. reference centers available for consultation

    d. recommended reporting form(s)

    e. storage and retrieval of data

---

prescribed procedures. Several items requiring rigorous standardization are summarized in Table 1.2.

Unfortunately, all the precautions to be observed on the long way from drawing the sample to reporting the results elaborated in Table 1.2 are not consistently acknowledged in daily practice. Even the leading manuals in this field were, until recently, not always infallible in this respect.

The need for adequate sampling (Table 1.2, #1 and #4) and correct interpretation of results (Table 1.2, #8j) were, for the first time, emphasized in the monograph published in 1974 by the International Commission on Microbiological Specifications for Foods of the International Union of Microbiological Societies (ICMSF 1974). Indeed, the most difficult subject of how to account for severe stratification of colonization of foods has only been addressed occasionally (van Schothorst et al. 1966; Snijders et al. 1984; Habraken et al. 1986). Internationally, the most followed manuals are published by the American Public Health Association (Speck 1984) and the Association of Official Analytical Chemists (Andrews 1984). These publications pay adequate attention to purely analytical details listed in Table 1.2, #3 and #8. However, the imperative need for standardization and monitoring of selective enumeration media has only been recognized since about 1970 (Mossel et al. 1974; Corry 1982; Anon. 1983; Mossel et al. 1983a), while measures of control at the international level have not been suggested until recently (Baird et al. 1985). Indications for the need to abolish the direct use of selective media when determining microbial populations in foods that have incurred sublethal lesions were obtained over 40 years ago. Nonetheless, only recently were deliberate and accurately elaborated resuscitation steps introduced systematically and their impact on the use of reference values, i.e. allowing for the higher colony counts thereby obtained, accounted for (Mossel and van Netten 1984).

A wealth of scientific knowledge and laboratory experience is assembled in Table 1.2. The responsibility for ensuring that future optimal use of this is made lies with academic educators in food microbiology. Some educators reluctantly and very formally teach microbiological examination of foods, turning their students into no more than "methods freaks." However, the professorial staff should begin to emphasize the fascinating molecular and ecological facets of this branch of microbiology (Mossel and Dijkmann 1984; Sayler et al. 1985) and in this way provide enthusiasm for future generations of food microbiologists.

TENTATIVE TAXONOMIC GROUPING OF ISOLATES

Ecological Needs for Identification

Selective culture media in current use (Andrews 1984; Mossel et al. 1984, Speck 1984) are reasonably effective in allowing sought after taxa to develop, while inhibiting most interfering organisms. Consequently, for some purposes gross typical colony counts will suffice, particularly when adequate reference ranges have been generated and accurately standardized procedures have been established. For other purposes, however, identification of isolates, often termed 'confirmation' of counts, cannot be omitted.

In addition, sometimes an ecological reason for tentatively grouping isolates obtained in colony counts exists. It has become common practice to examine foods processed for safety, either before or after hermetic packaging, for marker organisms belonging to the *Enterobacteriaceae* (Mossel 1982; Leclerc et al. 1983). The entire group of these well-defined bacteria can be used for this purpose, because their presence above a certain level in processed foods indicates either inadequate heat treatment or post-process failure, e.g. reinfection of food and subsequent growth if this can occur (Mossel 1982). However, *Enterobacteriaceae* are not reliable markers for products that receive a sub-pasteurization level of heat treatment (Sheneman 1973). Last-minute addition of unprocessed condiments, such as grated aged cheese (Shelton 1961) or extensive handling after processing inevitably introduce low numbers of *Enterobactericeae* (Beckers et al. 1981). For these instances, we have suggested that the thermotrophic members of the group which are generally the pathogenic genera be used in addition to *Escherichia coli*, the classical marker (Mossel et al. 1986). Table 1.3 illustrates how well these organisms are recovered on the customarily used MacConkey-type selective media at 42.5°C. On the other hand, as demonstrated in Table 1.4, psychrotrophs are completely suppressed substantiating earlier observations of Mossel and Zwart (1960). When obtaining substantial counts from certain food products at this elevated temperature, further taxonomic grouping is necessary, allowing for differentiation of genera like *Klebsiella,* mostly of environmental origin, from the more relevant enteric types.

Another need for taxonomic grouping presented itself when studying the anaerobic microflora of dried weaning foods and their components (Mossel et al. 1973). These products are generally examined by inoculation of decimal dilutions of samples into sulphite iron polymyxin agar contained in oval cross-section tubes (which reduce oxygen penetration compared to circular cross-sectional tubes) so as to attain anaerobic conditions (Mossel 1959). When almost no black colonies are obtained from the first decimal dilution, products can be accepted. However, when substantial colony counts are observed, there is a need for tentative identification of the isolated organisms. It is particularly important to differentiate the butyric acid forming clostridia, *Desulfatomaculum nigrificans* and an occasional lactic acid bacterium from pathogens, including *Clostridium botulinum, Clostridium perfringens* and *Clostridium difficile.* The key, summarized in Table 1.5, has been found useful for this purpose.

Recommended Convenient Methods

Because the ingrained habit of "worship of numbers" (Wilson 1959) has long hindered food microbiology, few studies have been devoted to simple conventional systems for the approximate identification of isolates obtained from foods.

Table 1.3 Recovery ($\log_{10}$) of Thermotrophic Types of *Enterobacteriaceae* on MacConkey Agar (MCA) and Infusion Agar (IA) at 37°C and at 42.5 ± 0.5°C

	37°C		42.5°C	
Strain	IA	MCA	IA	MCA
Enterobacter	9.2	8.9	9.2	8.9
Escherichia				
coli 81	7.4	7.1	7.4	7.3
82	8.1	8.2	8.4	8.2
84	8.7	8.5	8.7	8.4
86	8.6	8.3	8.6	8.3
015	9.0	8.9	8.9	9.0
96	9.3	8.9	9.3	9.0
Klebsiella				
T 1	8.7	8.8	8.8	8.8
T 2	9.0	8.8	8.7	8.8
Kluyvera				
K	9.3	9.0	9.3	9.2
299	9.2	9.2	9.3	9.2
S36	9.2	9.2	9.3	8.9
Salmonella				
brandenburg	8.9	8.5	8.9	8.4
derby	9.0	9.2	9.0	9.2
eastbourne	8.8	8.6	8.8	8.7
enteritidis	9.3	9.2	9.3	9.3
hadar	9.1	8.5	9.1	8.4
heidelberg	8.9	8.8	8.9	8.6
indiana	7.2	7.3	7.2	7.2
london	8.9	9.2	9.1	9.1
montevideo	8.9	8.7	8.9	8.9
senftenberg	9.1	8.2	9.0	9.1
typhimurium	9.0	9.0	9.0	9.0
Shigella				
flexneri 2,H	7.9	7.9	8.0	7.7
flexneri 2,U	9.1	9.0	9.0	9.1
sonnei H	7.6	7.6	7.4	7.5
sonnei U	8.7	8.7	8.8	8.6

Data from Mossel et al. (1986)

Table 1.4 Recovery ($\log_{10}$) of Psychrotrophic Types of *Enterobacteri-aceae* on MacConkey Agar (MCA) and Infusion Agar (IA) at 30,37, and 42.5 ± 0.5°C

Strain	30°C IA	30°C MCA	37°C IA	37°C MCA	42.5°C IA	42.5°C MCA
Erwinia 96	8.7	7.2	8.7	7.9	< 2	< 2
240	—	—	8.8	8.9	< 2	< 2
Hafnia K	9.1	9.0	9.1	8.9	< 2	< 2
4	9.0	9.0	9.0	9.0	< 2	< 2
5	8.9	8.9	8.9	8.9	< 2	< 2
7	8.9	8.9	8.9	8.9	< 2	< 2
Yersinia enterocolitica serotype 0:3	9.0	8.9	9.0	8.9	< 2	< 2

Data from Mossel et al. (1986)

Table 1.5 Differential Characteristics of Some Clostridia[a]

	C. butyricum	*C. perfringens*	*C. botulinum*[b]	*C. difficile*
Gelatin	0	+	+	+
H$_2$S	0	+	+	0
Indole	0	0	0	0
Nitrate	D	+	0	0
Lactose	+	+	0	0
Sucrose	+	+	0	0
Mannitol	D	0	0	+
Spores	S/s	S/N	S/s	S/N
Motility	+	0	+	+

[a]0 = Negative result; S = Subterminal; N = Not swollen; s = Swollen.
[b]Isolates of *C. sporogenes* cannot, with certainty, be differentiated from *C. botulinum* without recourse to bioassays.

Bergan et al. (1982) and ourselves (Mossel et al. 1983b) have found that the determination of the microscopic morphology of organisms and a catalase test is useful as the first step in taxonomic grouping. Many valid conclusions can be drawn from these two simple tests. In practice, this is achieved by subculturing pure cultures of isolates in small tubes containing brain heart infusion broth to be incubated at 30°C. The growth obtained is subsequently examined by a Gram stain, while the sediment is tested for catalase activity by dispersing in a drop of freshly prepared 3% hydrogen peroxide, contained in wells of microtiter plates.

Further taxonomic grouping can be conveniently done with the aid of so-called 'polytropic' tubes. These are single tubes that allow for the determination of several taxonomic traits. The classical example of this type of tube is Kligler's glucose/lactose/iron agar (1918). Specific three-layer tubes have been developed for the examination of groups of organisms of special interest in food microbiology. Such tubes invariably contain (1) a bottom layer allowing fermentative attack on a carbon source to be assessed (Hugh and Leifson 1953); (2) a layer of water agar to prevent interference between the biochemical processes in the bottom and at the top; and, (3) a top layer ensuring anaerobic conditions in the bottom layer and allowing specific traits, including motility, oxidase reaction, pigment production and formation of indole, urea or H_2S to be determined.

In a few instances additional tests must be carried out, which cannot be combined with the traits determined in the polytropic master tube. These tests are done in microtiter plates or in square Petri dishes with 24 compartments. In Table 1.6, the various tests of this nature, which have been in use for over ten years, have been summarized. The use of polytropic tubes and microtiter plates allows considerable savings in work and cost, because relatively small volumes of media and reagents are required.

RETROSPECT

In food microbiology, monitoring line and end product samples for pathogens and marker ('indicator' and 'index') organisms is not the first priority. The most pressing assignment is *intervention* whereby implementation of suitable procedures will allow microbiologically safe food of high acceptability reaching the public's table. This change of priority applies without detriment to two essential functions of monitoring: (i) validation of safe processing and distribution practices (GMPs); (ii) prompt identification of the causes of outbreaks of food-transmitted disease or spoilage, allowing rapid remedies.

Table 1.6 Simplified Tentative Taxonomic Grouping of Bacteria Isolated from Foods After Having Been Examined for Gram Stain and Catalase Reaction

Type of bacterium	Polytropic Tube Composition	Traits determined	Supporting tests
Fermentative and nonfermentative Gram negative rod-shaped bacteria	Gram negative diagnostic tube, i.e. Bottom: violet red bile glucose agar; Top: SIM agar	Oxidase Anaerobic glucose dissimilation Motility Formation of H_2S, indole, and pigment	Open tube of glucose agar Multiwell plates with Simmons' citrate agar, urea agar When required, determination of lysine decarboxylase, DNase and attack on sorbitol
Escherichia coli	Bottom: MacConkey lactose agar Top: SIM agar Incubation at $44 \pm 0.1°C$	Formation of indole Anaerobic attack on lactose	Multiwell plates with Simmons' citrate agar
Yersinia enterocolitica	Bottom: sorbitol agar Top: lysine broth	Anaerobic dissimilation of sorbitol Lysine decarboxylase activity	Multiwell plates with Simmons' citrate agar
Vibrio parahaemolyticus	Bottom: 5% NaCL starch agar Top: MR-VP medium with 2% NaCl	Anaerobic dissimilation of starch VP-reaction	Reactions in Gram negative diagnostic tube (vide supra)

(*Continued*)

Table 1.6 (*Continued*)

| Type of bacterium | Polytropic Tube | | Supporting tests |
	Composition	Traits determined	
Gram positive bacteria	Bottom: glucose agar Top: tryptone agar	Anaerobic attack on glucose Catalase	Open tubes of glucose agar
Staphylococcus aureus	Bottom: mannitol agar Top: rabbit plasma	Anaerobic dissimilation of mannitol Coagulase	—
Lancefield group D streptococci	Bottom: kanamycin aesculin azide agar Top: 40% bile	Attack on aesculin Tolerance of azide, kanamycin and bile	—
Clostridium perfringens	Bottom: sulphite iron cycloserine agar Top: anaerobic motility medium Incubation at 46°C	Tolerance for cycloserine Thermotrophic Non-motile	Formation of indole
Other clostridia	Bottom: cysteine iron agar Top: sucrose agar Anaerobic incubation at 30°C	Formation of H_2S Attack on sucrose	Gelatin dissimilation Attack on lactose Attack on mannitol

In all instances where examinations are required they should rely on a minimum number of *criteria*, accurately selected from the point of view of the microbial ecology of every specific food. Existing *methods* should be carefully checked for validity, while new techniques should contain the analytical essentials shown in Table 1.2. Reference values ('standards') are always needed to gauge the results obtained. Such values should be derived exclusively from surveys on samples, drawn from factories adhering to validated GMPs. In the past, many of these principles of rational microbiological examination of foods have often been ignored, resulting in a marked decrease in credibility of food microbiology as an academic discipline.

This calls for an excellent type of academic education in food microbiology in the future. Like all University curricula, irrespective of the level—undergraduate or graduate—courses in food microbiology should be broad. Emphasis should be placed on scientific principles. Generally accepted, though nonetheless criticizable, approaches and techniques are to be abolished. A hazard which must be particularly taken into account is turning graduates into 'nit-picking' methods-freaks. This can best be avoided by continually emphasizing the wide confidence limits of all methods used in the microbiological examination of food, which make thinking in log cycles rather than in percentages compulsory. Microbial genetics, cytology, and ecology in addition to the sound analytical principles summarized in Table 1.2 are recommended as the core of theoretical and advanced practical classes. Awareness of literature cannot be overlooked, in the light of the rapidly developing character of the microbiological examination of foods and processing lines.

REFERENCES

ABRAM, D. D. and POTTER, N. N. 1985. Diluents and the enumeration of stressed *Campylobacter jejuni. J. Food Protect.* 48: 135–137.

ALCAIDE, E. and GARAY, E. 1984. R-plasmid transfer in *Salmonella* spp. isolated from wastewater and sewage-contaminated surface waters. *Appl. Environ. Microbiol.* 48: 435–438.

ALLEN, L. A., PASLEY, S. M., and PIERCE, M. A. F. 1952. Conditions affecting the growth of *Bacterium coli* on bile salts media. Enumeration of this organism in polluted waters. *J. Gen. Microbiol.* 7: 257–267.

ALTHERR, M. R. and KASWECK, K. L. 1982. In situ studies with membrane diffusion chambers of antibiotic resistance transfer in *Escherichia coli. Appl. Environ. Microbiol.* 44: 838–843.

ANDREWS, W. H. 1984. A perspective review of the developments of AOAC microbiological methods. *J. Assoc. Off. Anal. Chem.* 67: 661–663.

ANON. 1983. *Proceedings of the Second International Symposium on Quality Assurance of Microbiological Culture Media, 1982. Arch. Lebensm. Hyg.* 33: 137–175.

BAIRD, R. M., BARNES, E. M., CORRY, J. E. L., CURTIS, G. D. W., and MACKEY, B. M. (Ed.). 1985. *Quality Assurance and Quality Control of Microbiological Culture Media. Proceedings.* Third International Symposium, London, 9–13 January 1984. *Internat. J. Food Microbiol.* 2: 1–139.

BAUMAN, H. E. 1974. The HACCP concept and microbiological hazard categories. *Food Technol.* 28(9): 30–34, 74.

BECKERS, H. J., SCHOTHORST, M. VAN, SPREEKENS, K. J. A. VAN, and OOSTERHUIS, J. J. 1981. Microbiological quality of frozen pre-cooked and peeled shrimp from South-East Asia and from the North Sea. *Zentralbl. Bakt. Hyg. Abt. 1, Orig. B.* 172: 401–410.

BENSINK, J. C. and BOTHAM, F. P. 1983. Antibiotic resistant coliform bacilli, isolated from freshly slaughtered poultry and from chilled poultry at retail outlets. *Austral. Vet. J.* 60: 80–83.

BERGMAN, T., HOLLUM, A. B., and VANGDAL, M. 1982. Evaluation of four commercial test systems for identification of yeasts. *Europ. J. Clin. Microbiol.* 1: 217–222.

CORRY, J. E. L. (Ed.) 1982. Quality assessment of culture media by the Miles-Misra method. In *Quality Assurance and Quality Control of Microbiological Culture Media.* p. 21–37. G-I-T Verlag, Darmstadt.

DACK, G. M. 1956. Evaluation of microbiological standards for foods. *Food Technol.* 10: 507–509.

DIJKMANN, K. E. 1982. The optimal medium always the best choice? In *Quality Assurance and Quality Control of Microbiological Culture Media.* Corry, J. E. L. (Ed.). p. 175–180. G-I-T Verlag, Darmstadt.

GRASBECK, R. and ALSTROM, T. (Ed.). 1981. *Reference Values in Laboratory Medicine: The Current State of the Art.* Wiley, Chichester, England.

HABRAKEN, C. J. M., MOSSEL, D. A. A. and VAN DEN REEK, S. 1986. Management of *Salmonella* risks in the production of powdered milk products. *Netherl. Milk & Dairy J.* 40: in press.

HANNINEN, M. L. 1982. Effect of recovery medium on the isolation of *Campylobacter jejuni* before and after heat treatment. *Acta Vet. Scand.* 23: 416–424.

HUGH, R. and LEIFSON, E. 1953. The taxonomic significance of fermentative versus oxidative metabolism of carbohydrates by various Gram negative bacteria. *J. Bacteriol.* 66: 24–66.

ICMSF. 1974. International Commission on Microbiological Specifications for Foods. *Microorganisms in Foods. Vol. 2. Sampling for Microbiological Analysis: Principles and Specific Applications.* Univ. of Toronto Press, Toronto, Ontario.

IDZIAK, E. S. and MOSSEL, D. A. A. 1980. Enumeration of vital and thermally stressed *Staphylococcus aureus* in foods using Baird-Parker pig plasma agar (BPP). *J. Appl. Bacteriol.* 48: 101–113.

INGRAM, M. and ROBERTS, T. A. 1971. Application of the '12D-concept' to heat treatments involving curing salts. *J. Food Technol.* 6: 21–28.

KAYSER, A. and MOSSEL, D. A. A. 1984. Intervention sensu Wilson: The only valid approach to microbiological safety of food. *Internat. J. Food Microbiol.* 1: 1–4.

KLIGLER, I. J. 1918. Modifications of culture media used in the isolation and differentiation of typhoid, dysentery and allied bacilli. *J. Exper. Med.* 28: 319–322.

LEAR, D. W. 1962. Reproducibility of the most probable numbers technique for determining the sanitary quality of clams. *Appl. Microbiol.* 10: 60–64.

LECLERC, H., GAVINI, F., IZARD, D., and TRINEL, P. A. 1983. Les coliformes: mythe et realité. In *Les Bacilles à Gram Negatif, d'Intéret Medical et en Santé Publique: Taxonomie-Identification-Applications. Colloques Inst. Nat. Sante Recherch Med.* 114: 597–617.

MANSFIELD, J. M., FARKAS, G., WIENEKE, A. A., and GILBERT, R. J. 1983. Studies on the growth and survival of *Staphylococcus aureus* in corned beef. *J. Hygiene* 91: 467–478.

MASTERS, P. J. and PALMER, G. H. 1981. A note on the use of the spiral plates to study the in vitro effects of amoxycillin, spectinomycin and chloramphenicol on a porcine *Escherichia coli*. *J. Appl. Bacteriol.* 51: 253–255.

MEYER, K. F. 1931. The protective measures of the State of California against botulism. *J. Prevent. Med.* 5:261–293.

MOSSEL, D. A. A. 1959. Enumeration of sulphite-reducing clostridia occurring in foods. *J. Sci. Food Agric.* 10: 662–669.

MOSSEL, D. A. A. 1980. Assessment and control of microbiological health risks presented by foods. In *Food and Health*. Birch, G. G. and Parker, K. J. (Ed.). p. 129–166. Applied Science Publishers, London.

MOSSEL, D. A. A. 1982. Marker (Index and Indicator) organisms in food and drinking water. Semantics, ecology, taxonomy and enumeration. *Antonie van Leeuwenhoek* 48: 609–611.

MOSSEL, D. A. A. 1983. Essentials and perspectives of the microbial ecology of foods. In *Food Microbiology: Advances and Prospects*. Roberts, T. A. and Skinner, F. A. (Ed.). p. 1–45. Academic Press, London.

MOSSEL, D. A. A., BONANTS-VAN LAARHOVEN, T. M. G., LIGTENBERG-MERKUS, A. M. Th., and WERDLER, M. E. B. 1983a.

Quality assurance of selective culture media for bacteria, moulds and yeasts: An attempt at standardization at the International level. *J. Appl. Bacteriol.* 54: 313–327.

MOSSEL, D. A. A. and DIJKMANN, K. E. 1984. A centenary of academic and less learned food microbiology. Pitfalls of the past and promises for the future. *Antonie van Leeuwenhoek* 50: 641–663.

MOSSEL, D. A. A., EELDERINK, I., and SUTHERLAND, J. P. 1977. Development and use of single, 'polytropic' diagnostic tubes for the approximate taxonomic grouping of bacteria isolated from foods, water and medicinal preparations. *Zentralbl. Bakteriol. Parasitenk Abt. 1 Orig. A* 238: 66–79.

MOSSEL, D. A. A., HARREWIJN, G. A., and NESSELROOY-VAN ZADELHOFF, C. F. M. 1974. Standardization of the selective inhibitory effect of surface active compounds used in media for the detection of Enterobacteriaceae in foods and water. *Health Labor Sci.* 11: 260–267.

MOSSEL, D. A. A., HARREWIJN, G. A., and VAN SPRANG, F. J. 1973. Microbiological quality assurance for weaning formulae. In *The Microbiological Safety of Food.* Hobbs, B. C. and Christian, J. H. B. (Ed.). p. 77–87. Academic Press, London.

MOSSEL, D. A. A. and KAMPELMACHER, E. H. 1981. Prevention of salmonellosis. *Lancet* I: 208.

MOSSEL, D. A. A., RICHARD, N., GAYRAL, J. P., and BRISSUEL, C. 1983b. Etude comparative des tests préliminaires pour l'identification des bactéries isolées des matières alimentaires, des eaux et d'autres produits biologiques. *Science Aliments* 3: 91–115.

MOSSEL, D. A. A., VAN DER ZEE, H., CORRY, J. E. L., and VAN NETTEN, P. 1984. Microbiological quality control. In *Quality Control in the Food Industry.* Herschdoerfer, S. M. (Ed.). p. 79–168. Academic Press, London.

MOSSEL, D. A. A., VAN DER ZEE, H., HARDON, A. P., and VAN NETTEN, P. 1986. The enumeration of thermotrophic types amongst the Enterobacteriaceae, colonizing perishable foods. *J. Appl. Bacteriol.* (in press.).

MOSSEL, D. A. A. and VAN NETTEN, P. 1984. Harmful effects of selective media on stressed microorganisms—nature and remedies. In *The Revival of Injured Microorganisms.* Russell, A. D. and Andrew, M. H. E. (Ed.). p. 329–369. Academic Press, London.

MOSSEL, D. A. A., VELDMAN, A., and EELDERINK, I. 1980a. Comparison of the effects of liquid medium repair and the incorporation of catalase in McConkey type media on the recovery of Enterobacteriaceae sublethally stressed by freezing. *J. Appl. Bacteriol.* 49: 405–419.

MOSSEL, D. A. A., WIJERS, B., and BOUWER-HERTZBERGER, S. 1980b. The enumeration and identification of stressed *Escherichia coli* in foods using solid medium repair and Eljkman's thermotrophic criteria. *J. Appl. Bacteriol.* 49(3): xvii–xviii.

MOSSEL, D. A. A. and ZWART, H. 1960. The rapid tentative recognition of psychrotrophic types among Enterobacteriaceae isolated from foods. *J. Appl. Bacteriol.* 23: 185–188.

PALUMBO, S. A. 1984. Heat injury and repair in *Campylobacter jejuni. Appl. Environm. Microbiol.* 48: 477–480.

PRETORIUS, W. A. 1961. Investigations on the use of the roll tube method for counting *Escherichia coli* I in water. *J. Appl. Bacteriol.* 24: 212–217.

RAPPAPORT, H. and GOEPFERT, J. M. 1978. Thermal injury and recovery of *Bacillus cereus. J. Food Protect.* 41: 533–537.

RAY, B. and JOHNSON, C. 1984. Sensitivity of cold-stressed *Campylobacter jejuni* to solid and liquid selective environments. *Food Microbiol.* 1: 173–176.

REUSSE, U. 1982. The use of the stomacher and spiral plate methods in food microbiology. In *Quality Assurance and Quality Control of Microbiological Culture Media.* Corry, J. E. L. (Ed.). p. 59–61. G-I-T Verlag, Darmstadt.

SAYLER, G. S., SHIELDS, M. S., TEDFORD, E. T., BREEN, A., HOOPER, S. W., SIROTKIN, K. M., and DAVIS, J. W. 1985. Application of DNA-DNA colony hybridization to the detection of catabolic genotypes in environmental samples. *Appl. Environm. Microbiol.* 49: 1295–1303.

SHELTON, L. R. 1961. Frozen precooked foods—plant sanitation and microbiology. *J. Amer. Diet. Assoc.* 38: 132–134.

SHENEMAN, J. M. 1973. Survey of aerobic mesophilic bacteria in dehydrated onion products. *J. Food Sci.* 38: 206–209.

SNIJDERS, J. M. A., JANSEN, M. H. W., GERATS, G. E., and CORSTIAENSEN, G. P. 1984. A comparative study of sampling techniques for monitoring carcass contamination. *Internat. J. Food Microbiol.* 1: 229–236.

SPECK, M. L., RAY, B., and READ, R. B. 1975. Repair and enumeration of injured coliforms by a plating procedure. *Appl. Microbiol.* 29: 549–550.

SPECK, M. L. (Ed.). 1984. *Compendium of Methods for the Microbiological Examination of Foods.* 2nd ed. American Public Health Assoc., Washington, DC.

VAN DOORNE, H. and CLAUSHUIS, E. P. M. 1979. The quantitative determination of Enterobacteriaceae in pharmaceutical preparations. *Internat. J. Pharmaceutics* 4: 119–125.

VAN DOORNE, H., PAUWELS, H. P., and MOSSEL, D. A. A. 1982. Selective isolation and enumeration of low numbers of *Staphylococcus aureus* by a procedure that relies on elevated-temperature culturing. *Appl. Environ. Microbiol.* 44:1459–1462.

VAN NETTEN, P., VAN DER ZEE, H., and MOSSEL, D. A. A. 1984. A note on catalase enhanced recovery of acid injured cells of Gram negative bacteria and its consequences for the assessment of the lethality of l-lactic acid decontamination of raw meat surfaces. *J. Appl. Bacteriol.* 57: 169–173.

VAN SCHOTHORST, M., MOSSEL, D. A. A., KAMPELMACHER, E. H., and DRION, E. F. 1966. The estimation of the hygienic quality of feed components using an Enterobacteriaceae enrichment assay. *Zentralbl. Vet. Med.* 13: 273–285.

WALSH, T. J., VENANZI, W. E. and DIXON, D. M. 1985. Quantification of medically important *Candida* species and *Torulopsis glabrata* by a spiral inoculation system *J. Clin. Microbiol.* 22: 745–747.

WATERMAN, S. C. 1982. The heat-sensitivity of *Campylobacter jejuni* in milk. *J. Hygiene* 88: 529–533.

WILSON, G. S. 1935. *The Bacteriological Grading of Milk*. Med. Res. Council Spec. Rept. 206. p. 370. H.M. Stat. Office, London.

WILSON, G. S. 1955. Symposium on food microbiology and public health: General conclusions. *J. Appl. Bacteriol.* 18: 629–630.

WILSON, G. S. 1959. Faults and fallacies in microbiology. *J. Gen. Microbiol.* 21: 1–15.

WILSON, G. S. 1973. Introductory address. In *The Microbiological Safety of Food*. Hobbs, B. C. and Christian, J. H. B. (Ed.). p. xi–xii. Academic Press, London.

WOOD, P. C. 1956. The enumeration of *Escherichia coli* l in sea water. A comparison of counts determined by the 'most probable number' method in liquid medium with direct counts by the roll-bottle method. *J. Appl. Bacteriol.* 19: 26–30.

2

Regulatory Aspects of Microbiological Methodology

Carl S. Custer

USDA Food Safety Inspection Service
Washington, D.C.

The regulatory aspects of microbiological analytical methodology for food have both good news and bad news for microbiologists. The good news is that legislators have given microbiologists tremendous trust and leeway in selecting appropriate methods for analyzing foods. The bad news is that we are responsible for decisions affecting both the health and livelihood of our country's population; however, I think we can and should bear this responsibility well.

There are few regulatory aspects to microbiological food analysis because there are few regulatory microbiological requirements for food. That this paucity of requirements has a legal basis is useful information to scientists who are developing new microbiological methods, teaching the old ones, and to those who may be using present methods for quality control and compliance programs. Thus, this chapter is organized into three major areas: (1) the relationship of food safety laws and regulations to microbiology; (2) the application of analytical methodology to enforcing those laws and regulations; and (3) the adoption of future methods by regulatory agencies.

RELATIONSHIP OF FOOD SAFETY LAWS AND
REGULATIONS TO MICROBIOLOGICAL ASSAYS

The cardinal purpose of regulatory analytical methodology for food is to detect adulteration as defined by food safety laws or acts passed by the United States Congress. Table 2.1 lists definitions as they appear in the Federal Meat Inspection Act. This list is virtually identical to those contained in the Federal Poultry Inspection Act and the Food, Drug and Cosmetic Act. These lists are repeated again in the Code of Federal Regulations (CFR), the published rules by which regulatory agencies enforce the laws which Congress passes. For example, the USDA Food Safety and Inspection Service (FSIS) lists the definitions of adulteration in 9CFR 301.2(aa).

Adulteration of Foods

Federal regulatory agencies use microbiological analyses primarily for detecting two types of adulteration: (1) the presence of harmful substances, (m)(1); and (2) evidence that the food product was produced under insanitary conditions, (m)(4). In some cases, microbiological analyses can determine both: whether the product is composed of filthy or putrid substances (m)(3), or whether manufacturers complied with prescribed processing methods.

Interpreting what a harmful substance is might seem fairly simple, but Congress has placed two conditions in the definition of that type of adulteration; the first condition was in the original 1906 Act and is for added substances; the other is for naturally occurring substances and was added in the 1938 Act. The intent of these two conditions was to permit the sale of products such as spinach which naturally contains oxalic acid but *in amounts not ordinarily injurious to health*; at the same time it prohibits selling food with an added substance, such as formaldehyde *"which may render it injurious to health."* One example of how this provision works is in the FDA's approach to aflatoxin in corn. Originally, the FDA viewed this potent carcinogen as an added substance and thus banned it at the lowest detectable concentration, first 30 ppb then 20 ppb. Later research showed aflatoxin to be a natural contaminant of peanuts and corn not necessarily due to poor storage. Thus the FDA could not ban it in concentrations that may be injurious to health but only in concentrations that are ordinarily injurious to health. Therefore, they set tolerance levels ranging up to 200 ppb for animal feed shipped intrastate.

While legally interpreting what is an injurious substance may be complex, using microbiological results to prove that a product was produced under insanitary conditions is even more difficult. Both the FDA and the USDA

Table 2.1 Adulteration as Defined by 21 USCS Section 601(m)

The term "adulterated" shall apply to any carcass, part thereof, meat, or meat food product under one or more of the following circumstances:

(1) if it bears or contains any poisonous or deleterious substance which may render it injurious to health; but in case the substance is not an added substance, such article shall not be considered adulterated under this clause if the quantity of such substance in or on such article does not ordinarily render it injurious to health;

(2) (A) if it bears or contains (by reason of administration of any substance to the live animal or otherwise) any added poisonous or added deleterious substance (other than one which is (i) a pesticide chemical in or on a raw agricultural commodity; (ii) a food additive; or (iii) a color additive) which may, in the judgement of the Secretary, make such article unfit for human food;

(B) if it is, in whole or part, a raw agricultural commodity and such commodity bears or contains a pesticide chemical which is unsafe within the meaning of section 408 of the Federal Food, Drug, and Cosmetic Act (21 USCS ss 346a).

(C) if it bears or contains any food additive which is unsafe within the meaning of section 409 of the Federal Food, Drug, and Cosmetic Act (21 USCS ss 348).

(D) if it bears or contains any color additive which is unsafe within the meaning of section 706 of the Federal Food, Drug, and Cosmetic Act (21 USCS ss 376): Provided, That an article which is not adulterated under clause (B), (C), or (D) shall nevertheless be deemed adulterated if use of the pesticide chemical, food additive or color additive in or on such article is prohibited by regulations of the Secretary in establishments at which inspection is maintained under title I of this Act (21 USCS ss ss 601 et seq.);

(3) if it consists in whole or in part of any filthy, putrid, or decomposed substance or is for any other reason unsound, unhealthful, unwholesome, or otherwise unfit for human food;

(4) if it has been prepared, packed, or held under unsanitary conditions whereby it may have become contaminated with filth, or whereby it may have been rendered injurious to health;

(5) if it is, in whole or in part, the product of an animal which has died otherwise by slaughter.

have developed data bases on expected microbiological levels in a particular product produced under good manufacturing conditions. Bernard Surkiewicz, who worked for both of those agencies, gathered much of the initial data by surveying the industry producing a particular food product. His survey reports contained observations on the sanitary condition of individual plants and corrections made before sampling began. Surkiewicz' samples included raw materials, finished products, intermediate products, and, when available, frozen products from previous days' productions so the "before Surkiewicz" levels could be compared with the "after Surkiewicz" levels. The body of his data, along with that of others convincingly illustrates the effect of sanitation on the microbiological populations in various food products and has contributed greatly to the development of useful microbiological guidelines. However, even Surkiewicz' data does not always prove that a given microbiological level shows that a food product was produced under insanitary conditions.

A 1978 court case, *U.S. v. General Foods*, dealt with the issue of adulteration by filth resulting from production under insanitary conditions. The issue was whether the presence of *Geotrichum* mold in frozen green beans adulterated them as a filthy substance. The court made several interesting findings: (1) the mold fragments are filth; (2) if the product contains filth, then the Government need not prove that the product is injurious or unfit for consumption; (3) the court may overlook small unavoidable quantities (de minimis) of filth when no applicable defect action is in effect; (4) in applying a de minimis standard, the court must rely on the testimony of experts who are well acquainted with the product, the substance at issue and the state of the industry; (5) the purpose of the section defining as adulterated, product produced under insanitary conditions, is to prevent contamination, or nip it in the bud; actual contamination of finished product need not be shown. This particular court decision demonstrates the trust that the legal system has chosen to place in scientists for interpreting food safety issues (Cooper 1981).

Prescribed Process Control

Federal regulatory agencies have a policy of prescribing processing practices as their primary strategy for enforcing food safety laws. Some of these prescribed practices were designed to kill, inhibit, or avoid a particular pathogenic organism occurring in the raw ingredients of a food product. In practice these prescribed processes are indiscriminate and control other pathogens, even unknown and unsuspected ones. The success of this prescribed process policy is the prime reason for the virtual absence of mandatory Federal microbiological criteria for food.

The prescribed processes require a generally sanitary processing environment and may include minimum time-temperature treatments, minimum salt levels, or amounts of other inhibitors such as nitrite. The FDA and USDA regulations have many examples of these prescribed processes: for example: 21CFR 128.7 for control of *Clostridium botulinum* Type E in smoked fish; 9CFR 318.10 for control of *Trichinella spiralis* in processed pork; and 9CFR 318.17 for the control of *Salmonella* in roast beef.

Federal regulatory agencies have not required food processors to show compliance with the regulations by testing their products for pathogenic organisms, except for *Salmonella* in milk. Nor, with the exception of processes for the destruction of *Trichinella*, have the agencies permitted processors to substitute tests for prescribed treatments, mostly because of the indiscriminate nature of prescribed processes to pathogenic organisms.

Scientists and Regulators

Regulators establish processing rules and standards for food products while scientists provide methods for perceiving that those rules are followed. The rules decided on by the regulators are usually based on information provided by scientists. Yet, for all of the interaction and interdependence of scientists and regulators, there are differences that lead to misunderstanding, frustration, and even animosity between them.

First as a scientist and later as a regulator, I have experienced two major differences between their functions: the time frames and the end products. A scientist produces a consensus among colleagues that research data support a theory that may be readily abandoned or amended when new data so warrant. A regulator produces decisions resulting in hard and fast rules that are difficult to change because Congress has made it that way; then people build businesses, develop products, and make their livelihood dependent upon the relative consistency of those rules. In emergency cases, regulators must make fast decisions and take the risk of burdening the public with an incompletely thought out rule. To avoid this risk, regulators can publish "an interim final rule." This term is the closest thing to a regulatory scientific consensus; it means that the regulation has the full force of the law but it can be easily amended when new data (public comment) warrant.

The second major difference is the time frames under which scientists function. Scientists have the more consistent time frame: they have forever, their lifetime, or the end of the grant to investigate how the universe functions. Regulators necessarily take long periods of time to make decisions affecting the public so that those decisions will be as nearly perfect as possible. Further complicating and slowing this decision process are the facts that most regulatory issues have numerous sides and that the Executive Branch's regulatory philosophy may change every four years. However, public health emergencies completely change the regulatory time frame by requiring perfect decisions immediately.

Cooper's "Scientists and Lawyers in the Legal Process" (1981) eloquently summarizes some of the differences between our legal (adversarial) roles as regulators and our cooperative function as scientists. If as regulators we hesitate to make decisions it is partially because we are required to follow the motto of a former congressman from Tennessee, The Honorable Davy Crockett: "Be Sure You're Right; Then Go Ahead" with the additional proviso from the Administrative Procedures Act: publish your intentions in the Federal Register, receive public comments, then if they agree with you, go ahead. Davy Crockett would have been dismayed.

Having worked on both sides of the scientist-regulator fence, I have at times wondered, "why don't those yo yos outlaw that stuff before it kills somebody?" and later, "What do you mean he's not sure now? Last month he was 99% confident that it would be the best thing since sliced bread!" However, the reasons why regulators use certain analytical methods and choose particular strategies for insuring food safety are as valid as the reasons that research scientists have for amending a theory.

REGULATIONS AND MICROBIOLOGICAL METHODOLOGY

In The Code of Federal Regulations only one collection of microbiological methods is required to analyze food products to enforce a regulatory microbiological requirement; that is, the *Standard Methods for the Examination of Dairy Products* required in 7CFR 58.135 for raw milk. *Standard Methods*, first published in 1910 by the American Public Health Association and now in its fifteenth edition, is the most enduring collection of recognized microbiological analytical methods for food. It is predated only by the *Standard Methods for the Examination of Water and Wastewater*, (APHA 1905). One other collection of methods for examining foods mentioned in the CFR is the *Official Methods of Analysis of the Association of Official Analytical Chemists* (AOAC 1975), which the FDA requires for enforcement actions (21CFR 2.19). The AOAC methods are primarily chemical methods but many microbiological methods have been added in the past decade.

But neither the FDA nor the USDA limit their methods of analyses to those published in these two collections. The FDA also uses the *Bacteriological*

Analytical Manual or the "BAM," (U.S. FDA 1978) and the USDA has its *Microbiological Laboratory Guidebook* or "MLG" (USDA 1974) plus a looseleaf set of methods known as "Laboratory Communications." Both agencies, together with many academic/industry scientists, cooperated in the 1976 publication of the *Compendium of Methods for the Microbiological Examination of Foods* (Speck 1976), now in its second edition, published by the American Public Health Association under the aegis of the Intersociety/Agency Committee on Methods for the Microbiological Examination of Foods.

Since the regulations do not mention FDA and USDA methods, one may wonder then what methods are the regulatory agencies required to use to detect adulteration and to determine if manufacturers are in compliance with the processing regulations. The answer is that any method is acceptable as long as the regulators can convince a judge that the results are legitimate. In a 1933 court case (*U.S. v. Lesser et al.*) one of the defense's arguments was that the government used a nonstandard method to show adulteration of the defendant's product (the Government analyst had shown that the defendant's ginger extract was lethal to chickens as well as understrength). The judge's decision was eloquently stated, "On the contrary, it [adulteration] may be established in any other logical and convincing way." A similar decision was handed down in 1952 (*Woodard Laboratories Inc. et al. v. U.S.*) These court decisions demonstrate the judicial system's confidence in the regulatory agency's analysts.

Use of Methods by Federal Agencies

While Federal agencies may be permitted to use any method they please for regulatory analysis, they rarely go beyond the tried and true reference methods. In food poisoning cases the laboratories will generally supplement their usual methods with AOAC methods, and if time and sample size permit, any newer methods for evaluation and comparison.

Federal agencies use varied policies and strategies for detecting pathogens, toxins, and to determine whether a product was produced under filthy conditions or it contains decomposed or putrid substances.

Pathogens. The USDA's policy has been to recover and fully identify a culture of the pathogenic bacterium in question before it attempts to prosecute for adulteration. This policy may change if improvements in immunoassays continue but their previous history of uncollaboratable positives will probably keep immunoassays in their present place as only screening methods for several years hence.

USDA FSIS has maintained as policy that isolation of a single *Salmonella* in a ready-to-eat food product proves it is adulterated. This policy may seem in conflict with the theory that thousands of these bacteria are needed to cause sickness as well as the belief that these bacteria are natural unavoidable contaminants of raw meat. However, Blaser and Newman (1982) calculated that the actual dose in several outbreaks may have been less than 100 cells. USDA's policy has been maintained with the logic that properly processed products ought not contain any surviving salmonellae; the pathogen, thus, is an avoidable added contaminant. The courts have upheld this policy (see *U.S. v. 1,200 Cans Pasteurized Whole Eggs*).

Although *Trichinella spiralis* is not a bacterium, it is a pathogen that has been intimately associated with the regulatory policies of the USDA. Probably the first regulatory food safety method for food analysis was the trichinascopic method for detecting trichina cysts in pork. That method was abandoned by the USDA in the early part of this century in favor of both prescribed processing methods as well as educating consumers to cook pork thoroughly. At present, the USDA has gone full circle and recently proposed to exempt pork from prescribed processes when analysis has shown it negative for trichinosis. This change in policy is due to development of assays far more sensitive than the trichinoscope and a pork industry initiative to rid American pork of this pathogen. If successful, perhaps other pathogens could be targeted in the future.

Several years ago, USDA considered proposing a microbiological standard for staphylococci in fermented sausages; it would have condemned any sausage having 100,000 coagulase-positive staphylococci per gram. That standard was recommended in 1977 by a group of USDA scientists and regulators commissioned to study the problem of staphylococcal food poisoning outbreaks in those products. That recommended standard was well publicized but was never proposed for several reasons, including the fact that during the time necessarily taken by regulators to make a decision, tests better correlated to detectable toxin levels than coagulase-positive staphylococcal counts had been developed and more important, industry had implemented processing controls that apparently solved the problem. Although its effect was unplanned, this method for enumerating staphylococci had the desired regulatory purpose.

Toxins.   The two primary toxins assayed for in foods are botulinal toxin and staphylococcal enterotoxin (SET). Formerly, both detection methods used animal assays: mice for botulinal toxin, and monkeys and kittens for SET. The relative insensitivity of the animal assay for SET stimulated scientists to develop a satisfactory immunoassay for SET. The assays for SET are probably the most advanced technologically of any toxin assay; the immunochemical reaction has been amplified by using reverse passive hemagglutination or labeling the antibodies with radioisotopes, fluorescent compounds and more recently with enzymes.

As the sensitivity of the SET assay increases, the question arises, how much SET does it take to adulterate a food product? Dangerfield (1973) showed that only 0.00005 mg toxin per kg body weight could elicit a response in some individuals. The present policy holds any detectable toxin adulterates the product. For SET, this policy can be supported logically by the premise that the distribution of staphylococci and SET is so varied that finding any toxin is evidence that there is a larger amount somewhere on that lot of product and that this toxin is an avoidable contaminant.

Botulinal toxin assays are still based on inoculating mice but immunoassays have been developed. The mouse inoculation technique will probably remain the assay of choice for many years to come because the mice react equally to all botulinal toxins and the assay is sensitive. It is surprising that a dose lethal to a mouse can be recovered from the sera of a living human. Despite the assay's sensitivity, the presence of this toxin in any amount will probably remain evidence of adulteration, both because of its deadliness and the ease of avoiding its formation by reasonable processing practices.

Insanitary conditions and putrid or decomposed substances. Pathogens and toxins are interpreted as adulterants under the law. Using microbiological methods to prove adulteration under the "injurious to health" provision is far simpler than proving adulteration under the "filthy conditions or decomposed and putrid substances" provisions. To assess the general microbiological levels of food products, the Microbiology Division of USDA FSIS uses "the sanitation series," a set of standard microbiological tests, which includes aerobic plate counts at 20°C and 35°C, coliforms, staphylococci, salmonellae, gas-forming anaerobes, and any other tests that the product or situation might warrant. This sanitation series is the same set of tests used for the Surkiewicz surveys.

Products have been condemned voluntarily by the producer because of excessive levels of bacteria, after the USDA explained the gravity of the assay results. To the best of my knowledge, the USDA has not yet won a court decision on the basis of microbiological counts alone. About ten years ago the USDA brought legal action against someone for selling filthy and putrid meat in the District of Columbia. After the seized meat had been stored in a USDA freezer for about 18 months, the defendant's lawyer wanted laboratory analyses to determine the microbiological levels. Since the primary spoilage bacteria on meat are pseudomonads and they do not survive well in a laboratory freezer for 18 months, we anticipated low numbers of viable bacteria. Therefore, carefully documented Direct Microscopic Counts, in addition to the sanitation series and methods to help recover freeze-injured pseudomonads, were done on the meat samples. The court accepted microbiological data, but USDA won the case on testimony that the meat had an unacceptable odor and appeared unsound.

Food processors' use of methods.   Food processors use microbiological methods for their own quality control, to meet customers' specifications, and to gain an exemption from certain required processing controls. Only the latter use is relevant to this chapter.

USDA FSIS permits microbiological monitoring control to substitute for two processing controls, the midshift clean-up requirement and the prohibition against using fermented sausage rework in uncooked product. Neither of these processing controls is in the Code of Federal Regulations; they appear in the *Manual of Meat and Poultry Inspection*, an interpretation of the CFR for the use of inspection personnel.

Substituting a microbiological monitoring control program for the midshift clean-up requirement has proven successful. The USDA does not specify what microbiological methods and controls must be used; instead it asks the processor to propose a program of effective sanitation procedures, microbiological monitoring methods, and sampling protocols designed for his/her plant. If the USDA agrees that a given program is acceptable, then the plant has to provide data demonstrating its effectiveness in replacing midshift clean-up. In practice, the plant often discovers that some areas need more than a midshift clean-up and others can do without it. These monitoring programs are evaluated by the USDA FSIS Facilities, Equipment and Sanitation Division.

The other processing control for which microbiological monitoring can substitute, is the prohibition against adding fermented sausage rework back into new batches of sausage. Fermented sausage processors often generate a quantity of edible product that is not saleable as such, usually the ends and pieces left over from slicing or product from split casings. Without controls, the processor could unknowingly enrich new batches with enterotoxigenic staphylococci that have proved capable of surviving that fermentation process. Monitoring the rework before it is used can avoid enrichment with unusually high numbers of staphylococci. This successful voluntary program has contributed to processors' knowledge of the effect of their processing parameters on the staphylococcal levels in sausages.

ADOPTION OF MICROBIOLOGICAL METHODS BY REGULATORY AGENCIES

Regulatory agencies adopt analytical methodology for much the same reasons that any microbiology laboratory would: the method is reliable, it is sufficiently sensitive, it has the acceptance of the scientific community, and it is fairly inexpensive. Since regulatory analysis affects the health as well as the livelihood of the community, reliability of the method is perhaps the chief characteristic which a regulatory agency looks for.

Reliability

Collaborative testing procedures are the chief means by which regulatory methods are proven reliable. If the method does not yield similar results when performed by several competent laboratories, then the regulatory agency would neither risk the public health nor a false accusation of adulteration by using it. A successful collaborative test of a method is convincing evidence for the court that the method does yield valid and verifiable results. Collaborative testing is usually conducted under the aegis of the AOAC.

Before a method is validated by collaborative testing, the agency will have subjected it to in-house validation. Regulatory agencies performing this type of testing have a great advantage over most academic laboratories because of their access to thousands of routine food samples and the samples implicated in food poisoning outbreaks. Only after the agency is satisfied with the reliability of a method will it submit it to the AOAC. Within the USDA there are no hard and fast rules on how comparable results need to be before a method is deemed equivalent.

Future Regulatory Methodology: Some Speculations

These speculations are mine and do not necessarily reflect official FSIS planning or policy.

Scientists improving microbiological methodology are attempting to satisfy that primal human desire for instant gratification: we want more and better results and we want them faster. One of the slowest steps in present methodology is waiting while a culture grows so the analyst will have something to test. Future regulatory methods will probably eliminate or certainly reduce that growth step because there are no regulatory reasons to grow a culture if another method can otherwise reliably demonstrate adulteration. We no longer have to demonstrate that the *Salmonella* isolate causes enteritis any more than we have to demonstrate that a product will make kittens vomit to prove adulteration by staphylococcal enterotoxin.

Eliminating the common belief that we need to grow bacteria for food regulatory assays will stimulate present microbiological research on rapid methods. The DNA probes reported by Fitts (1985) or the immunoassays discussed by Swaminathan et al. (1985) hold great promise. The ideas Sharpe (1980) expressed in *Food Microbiology: A Framework For The Future* will help all of us to get out of the rut of the traditional "grow 'em up then look at 'em" methodology.

The U.S. Government's Office of Management and Budget recently emphasized its desire to replace Federal regulations with the demands of the market place. With respect to food safety, this concept has been rejected for thousands of years because food purchasers cannot always perceive adulteration in their prospective purchases. However, recent progress in rapid methods and the perceptive ability that they can offer to food purchasers may permit the market place to improve food safety.

Good rapid methods could aid in the continual improvement of food safety by giving buyers (processors as well as consumers) practical means of perceiving that their purchase is microbiologically safe. An example of how rapid methods have such an effect is the influence that the direct microscopic method and the California mastitis test have had on raw milk production. The dairy industry produces one of the most trusted and bacteriologically safe raw food ingredients; safety that has been stimulated by the technological advances in milk production as well as the producer's knowledge that potential purchasers of their product can analyze it for acceptability within minutes at the loading dock. Unfortunately, the industry does not yet have rapid assays for certain enteric pathogens.

Imagine what the effect of reliable loading dock tests for pathogens could have on producers as well as purchasers of raw agricultural products. Meat and poultry producers could test the efficacy of their management practices against the incidence of pathogenic bacteria in their flocks and herds, stimulated by the knowledge that they would get a better price for pathogen-free animals. The brucellosis testing programs already provide us an idea of how this kind of process could work. In another example, had loading dock tests for *Salmonella* in pork been readily available in 1976, the court decision for *Bona v. Turcotte* (1983) might have been different. Bona Limited, a Canadian fermented sausage manufacturer was sued because of a salmonellosis outbreak attributed to salmonellae surviving in their finished sausage. In turn, Bona sued Turcotte, the pork supplier, on the basis that Turcotte said that the pork was suitable for fermented sausage. Neither party was apparently aware of the high incidence of *Salmonella* in pork and their ability to survive mild fermentation processes (Goepfert and Chung 1970; Smith et al. 1975a,b). Nevertheless, according to English common law, Turcotte had guaranteed the ingredients to Bona and the court's decision favored Bona. Rapid test procedures might have prevented the outbreak in the first place and, had they been commonly available, Turcotte might not have sold *Salmonella* positive meat to Bona. Another example is perhaps easier to identify with personally. How many of us have eaten steak tartare or raw oysters fully aware that we are playing the odds against consuming an enteric pathogen? Wouldn't we eat more comfortably if we could improve those odds by having the product pretested? Reliable rapid tests could give producers both an additional incentive to rid their flocks and herds of foodborne pathogens and the money to fund eradication.

The general manner in which the food safety laws are written for public protection also offers versatility to regulators, industry and scientists for developing new methods to produce safe food. The courts have given microbiologists a great deal of trust in interpreting the law and in using and developing new methods for analysis. We must continue to earn that trust by both developing and applying microbiological methodology that is objective and scientifically sound.

REFERENCES

ANDERSON, J. M. and HARTMAN, P. A. 1985. Direct immunoassay for detection of Salmonellae in foods and feeds. *Appl. Environ. Microbiol.* 49: 1124–1127.

ANDREWS, W. H. 1985. A review of culture methods and their relation to rapid methods for the detection of *Salmonella* in foods. *Food Technol.* 39(3): 77–82.

AOAC. 1984. *Official Methods of Analysis.* 14th ed. Assoc. Official Analytical Chemists, Washington, DC.

APHA. 1980. *Standard Methods for the Examination of Dairy Products.* 15th ed. American Public Health Assoc., 1015 18th St., NW, Washington, DC.

APHA. 1980. *Standard Methods for the Examination of Water and Wastewater.* 15th ed. American Public Health Assoc., Washington, DC.

BLASER, M. J. and NEWMAN, L. S. 1982. A review of human Salmonellosis: I. Infective dose. *Rev. Infectious Diseases* 4: 1096–1106.

BONA FOODS LIMITED v. TURCOTTE AND TURMEL. 1983. Supreme Court of Ontario, September 1983.

COOPER, R. M. 1981. Scientists and lawyers in the legal process. *Food Drug Cosmetic Law J.* 36: 9–12.

DANGERFIELD, H. G. 1973. Effects of enterotoxins after ingestion by humans. ASM Annual Meeting, Miami, FL.

FITTS, R. 1985. Development of a DNA-DNA hybridization test for the presence of *Salmonella* in foods. *Food Technol.* 39(3): 95–102.

FLOWERS, R. S. 1985. Comparison of rapid *Salmonella* screening methods and the conventional culture method. *Food Technol.* 39(3): 103–108.

GOEPFERT, F. M. and CHUNG, K. C. 1970. Behavior of *Salmonella* during the manufacture and storage of a fermented sausage product. *J. Milk Food Technol.* 33: 185–191.

HAMILTON, P. B. 1984. Determining safe levels of mycotoxins. *J. Food Protection* 47: 570–575.

MATTINGLY, J. A., ROBINSON, B. J., BOEHM, A., and GEHLE, W. D. 1985. Use of monoclonal antibodies for the detection of *Salmonella* in foods. *Food Technol.* 39(3): 90–94.

SHARPE, A. N. 1980. *Food Microbiology: A Framework for the Future.* Charles C. Thomas, Springfield, IL.

SILLIKER, J. A. 1982. Selecting methodology to meet industry's microbiological goals for the 1980s. *Food Technol.* 36(12): 65–70.

SMITH, J. L., PALUMBO, S. A., KISSINGER, J. C., and HUHTANEN, C. N. 1975a. Survival of *Salmonella dublin* and *Salmonella typhimurium* in Lebanon bologna. *J. Milk Food Technol.* 38: 150–154.

SMITH, J. L., HUHTANEN, C. N., KISSINGER, J. C., and PALUMBO, S. A. 1975b. Survival of Salmonellae during pepperoni manufacture. *Appl. Microbiol.* 30: 759–763.

SPECK, M. L. (Ed.). 1976. *Compendium of Methods for the Microbiological Examination of Foods.* Am. Public Health Association, Washington, DC.

SWAMINATHAN, B., ALEIXO, J. A. G., and MINNICH, S. A. 1985. Enzyme immunoassays for *Salmonella*: One day testing is now a reality. *Food Technol.* 39(3): 83–89.

UNITED STATES CODE, Title 21, Ch. 12, section 601 et seq. The Federal Meat Inspection Act.

U.S. v. AN ARTICLE OF FOOD CONSISTING OF: 1,200 CANS. Article labeled in part(can) "30 lbs. Net Weight, PASTEURIZED WHOLE EGGS, distributed by FRIGID FOOD PRODUCTS, INC.-DETROIT, MICH." (coded 1937). 339 F. SUPP. 131 (N.D. Georgia 1972).

U.S. v. GENERAL FOODS CORPORATION, 446 F. SUPP. 740 (N.D. New York 1978).

U.S. v. MORTON-NORWICH PRODUCTS, INC. 461 F. SUPP. 760 (N.D. New York 1978).

U.S. v. NOVA SCOTIA FOOD PRODUCTS CORP., et al. 417 F. SUPP. 1364 (E.D. New York 1976).

U.S. v. 1232 CASES AMERICAN BEAUTY BRAND OYSTERS. 43 F. Supp. 749 (W.D. Missouri, 1942).

USDA. 1974. *Microbiology Laboratory Guidebook.* U.S. Dept. of Agric. Scientific Services, Food Safety and Inspection Service, Washington, DC.

U.S. FOOD AND DRUG ADM., DIV. OF MICROBIOLOGY. 1978. *Bacteriological Analytical Manual.* USFDA, Div. of Microbiology, Washington, DC.

WOODWARD LABORATORIES INC. et al. v. U.S. 198 F. 2d 995. (U.S.C.A. 9th Ct., 1952).

3

Methodology and Microbiological Criteria

David L. Collins-Thompson and O. Brian Allen
University of Guelph
Guelph, Ontario, Canada

Traditionally, texts on microbiological analysis have emphasized a system which consists of isolation, identification, and confirmation. For pathogens, we rely on all three components of the system; for others, we may use only one of these (e.g., Total Plate Count). This approach is perhaps a throwback from medical microbiology where the accent is on diagnosis. The correctness of the analysis could be confirmed or denied by the patient's condition. If the symptoms fitted the microbiological results, the methodology served its purpose. The size of the sample analyzed or the reproducibility of the method in terms of numbers to count was of little consequence. The intent was to find a method which had the selectivity to screen out pathogens from a mass of commensal organisms.

With the advent of food control in the area of microbiology, we transferred much of our knowledge from the medical field with reasonable success. Unfortunately, we also carried over certain assumptions which have isolated our thinking with respect to further developments. In the last decade or so, we have begun to realize that we need to widen our approach to methodology and control of foodborne organisms. This has come about as a result of two major occurrences: Consumer demand to improve both the quality and safety of our food supply and the centralization of food preparation in North American markets. Both of these changes have led to the idea of microbiological criteria as a possible control mechanism. Implementation of such criteria could perhaps insure the production of a safe and nutritious food supply. The idea of controlling imports by some discerning levels of bacteria is an appealing one. It is also difficult to argue against the thesis that there must be some levels of bacteria in foods that are unacceptable. It has been generally agreed that microbiological criteria serve three main purposes. The first is to control the level of pathogens in foods; the second is to control gross contamination, and finally to give an estimate of shelf life. It is in this context that the term 'criteria' is used in this discussion. The whole approach to the use of microbiological criteria as a control measure, however, is a complex issue (NRC 1985).

One of the drawbacks to our current thinking of microbiological criteria is the ingrained teaching of methodology and the early component system. Many of the current arguments against the use of criteria for foodstuffs stems from the perceived weakness in the methodology. Some of these arguments are perhaps justified in a few instances, but often it is the assumed accuracy about the sampling procedure which is at fault. We need to examine these early assumptions and errors built into methodology. We need to expand not only our concepts of what to include as part of the methodology, but also understand those factors that influence the methodology when it comes to applying microbiological criteria.

A few years ago, Cowell and Morisetti (1969) published a paper on statistical aspects and microbiological techniques. In the conclusion of this paper, it was suggested that unless sampling procedures are improved, the results of testing "may be rendered meaningless." They further explained that to determine if a food meets a criterion, two processes have to be undertaken. The first is the selection of a representative sample, and the second is use of a reliable test method. Thus it is necessary to link the sampling scheme to the test procedure.

When we look at methodology, we can see several components all linked to each other. The performance of a microbiological medium is related to its reliability, selectivity and reproducibility. This, in turn, is related to the amount and type of sample taken for the determination. Added to this is the important factor of the distribution of the organism of interest in the sample. We also have to consider the source of the sample, its condition, and the analyst's performance. Each of these components will influence the final result. Any errors in this system will affect the final result, so it is important to determine the nature and magnitude of them. If this is done, then such errors can be built into a criterion.

FACTORS IN METHODOLOGY AS RELATED TO CRITERIA

There are two major components in this section. The first relates to sampling and the second to media performance and reliability.

Sampling and Criteria

When one is faced with the need to know something about the microbiological quality or safety of a product, one cannot test all the product, either because of the excessive time and expense involved, or because testing is destructive. One is then forced to choose a sample of the product, test this, and on the basis of the results from the sample, draw conclusions about the product in general. If microbiological criteria are to apply to the product, these conclusions have to be based on sound statistical sampling procedures. It is therefore important to understand such procedures and the basis of assumptions used in sampling.

Microbiological measurements are subject to a great deal of unexplained variation. Total plate counts, for example, made from replicate samples of what is thought to be a uniform source will show variability in the count. For this reason, in order to obtain a good estimate of the level of contamination, one must choose several samples. To give some feeling for the magnitude of the variation, suppose one is sampling a tank of fluid milk in which there is, on average, two organisms per milliter. If the milk has been thoroughly mixed so that the organisms should occur at random throughout the milk, then there is a 5% chance of finding five or more organisms in 1 mL of sample. Because of the thorough mixing, the Poisson distribution is appropriate for computing these probabilities (Huntsberger and Billingsley 1981). Conversely, there is a 14% chance of finding no organisms. In food such as meats, where the bacteria will tend to be clumped, the variation will be much greater than that presented above. Hence, counts which are extreme (either very high or very low) will be more likely to occur.

Consider a second example. Suppose one wishes to detect the presence of *Salmonella* in a lot of canned egg powder and, in fact, 5% of the cans are contaminated. If there are no hints as to which cans are high risk candidates, the best strategy is to sample cans at random. However, in choosing five cans, there is a 77% chance that none of the five cans will be contaminated.

There is a 60% chance that none of a sample of ten cans will be contaminated. In order to be 95% certain of obtaining at least one contaminated can, 59 cans need to be sampled. This level of sampling assumes that the lot size is much larger than the sample size. If a significant portion of the whole lot is sampled, the required sample size declines.

The way a sample is selected can have a significant impact on both the validity of the sample and on the precision of the information obtained. Consider the example of an investigator who wishes to sample the product from a processing line. Unknown to him, problems usually occur at the start-up. If he consistently samples from the line after start-up, he will miss the problem no matter how many samples he takes!

In order to facilitate the discussion, certain terms should be defined. The quantity of product about which conclusions are made is referred to as the population. This could be the results of one day's production or it could be a batch of raw material which has arrived from a particular supplier. It could also be the product from a particular manufacturer on store shelves at a particular time. In a manufacturing process, it may be all of a product flowing past a valve during a 24-hour period. It is important that the population be clearly defined since this is an integral step in subsequently setting up a sampling plan.

The product that makes up the population can be divided into discrete "sampling units." Often the sampling unit is obviously defined, as in packaged foods. Sometimes, however, when the food is in bulk, the sampling unit may be arbitrary, for example, a 10 ml sample of fluid milk. The sampling unit is the unit on which a single measurement of microbiological quality is taken (i.e. a plate count or simply presence/absence of a pathogen).

In order to have the greatest chance of making accurate conclusions, and of being able to assess the precision of the conclusions, sampling units should be selected strictly at random. These are termed probability sampling schemes. There are a number of different probability sampling schemes available for microbiological analysis.

The simplest probability sampling scheme is simple random sampling. This is appropriate when nothing is known ahead of time about the likely distribution of organisms among the sampling units. Simple random sampling is a procedure for selecting the sample such that all possible distinct samples are equally likely to be the ones chosen. Suppose one has to choose a simple random sample of five units from among a population of 20 units. There are 15,504 distinct samples possible. Hence, one would like each of these 15,504 possible samples to have one chance in 15,504 of being the one chosen. Fortunately, there are relatively easy algorithms for achieving a simple random sample using random number tables (ICMSF 1974). This procedure is also easily implemented on a computer with a random number generator.

When the units are not naturally discrete, as for example with fluid milk in bulk tanks, randomization should still take place. Sampling may have to be modified depending on circumstances. If the milk is being pumped from the tank, it may be possible to take samples at randomly selected times. If the milk is not being pumped out, sampling units may be chosen from different locations within the tank. If so, the locations should be chosen randomly.

When something is known about the distribution of organisms in the population, this information should be used in the choice of sample. For example, suppose it is known that microbiological problems occur most frequently at either the beginning or the end of a production run. It would then be beneficial to stratify the run into, say three strata. These would be start-up, midportion and end of the run. The requirement that a fixed proportion of the units are selected from each stratum is then built into the sampling procedure. These proportions need not be equal. Within each stratum, a simple random sample of the specified size is then chosen. This procedure for choosing the sample is called stratified random sampling. It may result in a substantial increase in precision over simple random sampling.

In two-stage sampling or subsampling, the sample is selected in two stages. First a simple random sample of primary units is drawn. From each of the primary units, a simple random sampling of subunits is selected. This kind of sample is useful when the sampling units are naturally grouped together into primary units. A good example of this is canned goods where the primary sampling units could be cases and the subunits, cans. If all the cans in a case were produced about the same time, their microbiological quality may be very similar. This being the case, it would be most efficient from a statistical point of view to take only one can per case. Additional expense, however, is involved for every case that has to be opened. Thus, it is more cost efficient to sample all cans in the case.

The optimum sampling fraction, in order to minimize the costs for a fixed level of statistical precision, is somewhere between these extremes. To see how this works, suppose n represents the number of primary units sampled and m, the number of secondary from each primary unit. Further, suppose that the cost of sampling can be approximated by:

$$C = c_1 n + c_2 nm$$

where c_1 is the cost of obtaining each primary unit, and c_2 is the additional cost of sampling a secondary unit. Thus, in the above sample, c_2 would be the cost of the testing procedure (a total plate count for example) for a single can and c_1 would include the production cost of the case (assuming the remaining intact cans are not recoverable or were used in incubation studies) and selecting and transporting the case to the testing site. Then the optimum number of cans to test per case, in order to minimize the cost for a fixed level of statistical precision is:

$$ m_{opt} = \frac{S_2}{\sqrt{S_1^2 - S_2^2/m}} \cdot \sqrt{\frac{C_1}{C_2}} $$

where S_1^2 is the variance among primary units means, $\Sigma(\overline{Y}i - \overline{Y})^2/(n - 1)$ [Y is the measurement made on each can (e.g. total plate count)] and S_2^2 is the variance among subunits within the primary units, $\Sigma\Sigma(\overline{Y}ij - \overline{Y}i)^2/m(m - 1)$ [m is the total of subunits per primary unit]. If $m_{opt} > M$ or if $S_1^2 < S_2^2/M$, take m_{opt} to be M (that is, sample all subunits in the selected primary units). This is referred to as cluster sampling. Cluster sampling might be appropriate, for example when testing simply involves examining cans for dents, swelling or leakage. Since the cost of examining a can would usually be small relative to the cost of obtaining another case, C_1/C_2 will be large and m_{opt} will be M.

Another sampling procedure which can be used with criteria in mind is systematic sampling. It may often be convenient to take a systematic rather than a random sample of units. For example, in sampling units at a particular point in a production line, it might be more convenient to take every k^{th} item, rather than determining randomly the items to be selected. A systematic sample may be more or less precise than the corresponding simple random sample, depending on the nature of the pattern of responses as the units come along the line. If units adjacent on the line tend to be more similar than widely separated units, systematic sampling will tend to produce a more precise sample than simple random sampling will. If quality, however, tends to vary cyclically, a systematic sample may be very bad indeed. Consider for example, if the microbiological quality varies cyclically with a period of ten units (Fig. 3.1). Thus, if the systematic sample is taken at every 10th unit (or in general, every n^{th} unit where n is a multiple of 10), beginning with unit 6, a sample is obtained which badly underrepresents the average quality. On the other hand, beginning with unit 1 and taking every 10th unit would produce a sample which overrepresents the average quality. A more extensive discussion of these sampling procedures is presented by Cochran (1977).

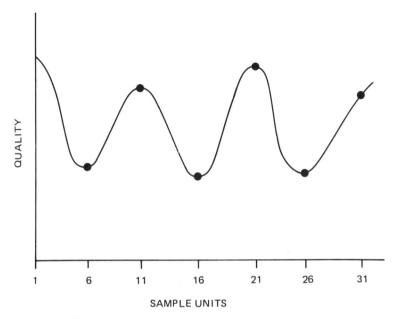

QUALITY

SAMPLE UNITS

1   6   11   16   21   26   31

FIG. 3.1 Cyclical variation in microbiological quality of a food product and systematic sampling procedure.

Sampling Plans

In some instances, the objective may simply be to estimate the level of microbiological contamination in a food. For this purpose, the various sampling techniques already presented are appropriate. In other instances, the objective is to make a decision as to whether a lot is acceptable or not. This may, for example, involve a raw material used in processing (chocolate, for example). Alternatively, it may be a shipment of a commodity seeking entry into the country. In either case, someone must make a decision to either accept or reject the lot based at least in part on its microbiological quality.

In this section, plans which allow acceptance or rejection of a lot based on an examination of a sample of the sampling units in the lot and for which the probability of making an incorrect decision can be calculated are discussed. These plans can be divided into two-class and three-class plans. The two-class plans assume that each sampling unit can be classified as either defective or acceptable. If, for example, total plate count is to be the measure of microbiological quality used, a number, m, (for example, $m = 10^5$) is chosen such that if the plate count is above m, the unit is judged to be defective, but if it is below *m*, the unit is acceptable. In practice, two-class plans are normally used for pathogenic organisms where $m = 0$.

A two-class attributes sampling plan then specifies that *n* units be chosen according to a simple random sampling procedure. Each unit sampled is classified as being defective or not. If there are more than *c* units defective the lot is rejected; otherwise, the lot is accepted. For example, ten units might be selected at random and the lot rejected if more than $c = 1$ are found to be defective. Provided that the units are selected at random and that there is no error involved in classifying the selected units, the probability of rejecting a good lot or of accepting a bad lot can be calculated. This probability will depend on *n*, *c*, and *p*, the true proportion of defective units in the lot. The probability of accepting the lot, plotted against *p*, is referred to as the operating characteristic curve. An example, for $n = 10$, $c = 1$, is given in Fig. 3.2. For the operating characteristic curves of other useful two-class attributes plans, see ICMSF (1974). From the operating characteristic curve, the appropriateness of a particular plan can be assessed. For example, from Fig. 3.2, with 5% of the units defective, there is a 91% chance of accepting the lot. With 10% defectives, the lot will be accepted 74% of the time. With 40% defectives, the lot would be accepted with probability 0.046. From this information, whether the plan possesses the desired properties can be assessed.

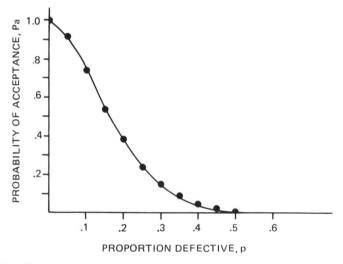

FIG. 3.2   Operating characteristic curve for $n = 10$ and $c = 1$, where *n* = number of samples taken and *c* = maximum allowable number of defectives.

If not, an alternative plan will need to be chosen. The ICMSF (1974) has plotted the operating characteristic curves for a variety of useful plans.

It is useful, when choosing a plan, to define producer and consumer risks. The producer risk is the probability that an acceptable lot will be falsely rejected. The consumer risk is the probability that an unacceptable lot will be falsely accepted. These risks can never be eliminated without sampling all units in the lot. However, they can be made as small as desired by appropriate choice of n and p. Suppose we wish to accept the lot with probability 0.95, if there are 10% ($p_1 = 0.10$) or fewer defectives (thus the producer's risk is $A_1 = 0.05$). Furthermore, we wish to reject the lot with probability 0.95 if there are 40% ($p_2 = 0.40$) or more defectives (consumer's risk is $A_2 = 0.05$). The region of 10% to 40% defectives is a sort of "indifference region" where it is not too serious whether the lot is accepted or rejected. The lot will be accepted anywhere from 95% of the time to 5% of the time as the proportion defective ranges from 0.10 to 0.40. A plan with the above characteristics can be chosen, approximately, using the normal approximation to the binomial distribution. The rule is to choose n to be the smallest integer greater than

$$n > \left[\frac{\sqrt{P_1^{(1-p_1)}}\, z_1 + \sqrt{p_2^{(1-p_2)}}\, z_2}{p_2 - p_1} \right]^2$$

and to choose c to be the largest integer less than

$$z_1 \sqrt{np_1(1 - p_1)} + np_1$$

where z_1 is the standard normal variate with area A_1 to the right (e.g., with $A_1 = 0.05$, $z = 1.645$). Similarly, z_2 is the standard normal variate with area A_2 to the right. For the example cited, the approximation yields $n = 19$ and $c = 4$. In fact, the exact producer and consumer risks are 0.035 and 0.070. If n is increased to 20 and c held at 4, the producer and consumer risks are almost exactly correct, at 0.043 and 0.051.

The two-class plans have been criticized because the distinction between an acceptable and a defective unit is often rather arbitrary. For example, if $m = 10^3$, the a unit with a count of 999 would be acceptable while a count of 10^3 would be defective. For this reason, Bray et al. (1973) developed three-class attribute plans. For these plans, the n units selected are judged as acceptable if the count is below m, marginal if the count is between m and M, and defective if the count exceeds M. The decision rule then says to choose a simple random sample of size n and to reject the lot if either more than c_1 units exceed M or if more than $c_1 + c_2$ units exceed m. Frequently, c_1 is taken to be zero. Operating characteristic curves must now be replaced by operating characteristic surfaces since the probability of acceptance now depends on the true proportion of defectives, p_d and on the true proportion of marginals, p_m, in the lot. The ICMFS (1974) have tabulated the operating characteristic surfaces for $n = 5$, 10 and 15, and for $c_2 = 1, 2$, and 3 $(c_1 = 0)$.

Attributes plans make no assumptions about the nature of the distribution of organisms in the food being sampled. These plans are appropriate for any distribution requiring only that the sampling units be selected at random and that each selected unit be categorized into its correct class (acceptable or defective, for a two-class plan). Consequently, when there is uncertainty about the correct distribution, the attributes plans represent a prudent choice. However, there are occasions when the appropriate distribution is known. In particular, Kilsby (1982) argued that the log normal distribution may often be appropriate. This being the case, the log count follows a normal distribution. Variables sampling plans take account of this fact and hence are able to make better use of the information provided by the sample. As with two-class attributes plans, the two-class variables plans, seek to control the proportion of defective units (that is, the proportion with counts above m). However, on each sampled unit, we now make use of the actual count rather than simply the number above m. In particular, the lot is rejected if, $\overline{X} + ks > m$ where $\overline{X}$ is the arithmetic average of the log counts, s is the standard deviation of the log counts, and k is a constant chosen so that the probability of rejecting a lot with proportion p defectives will be P. For example, we may wish to reject a lot with 20% defectives with at least 80% probability. In their original paper developing two-class variables plans, Jennett and Welch (1939), give an approximation which allows one to obtain k using standard normal tables. Brown (1984) has given a comprehensive review of two-class variables plans.

Just as two-class attributes plans can be extended to consideration of three classes, two-class variables plans may also be extended. Brown (1984) developed a three-class variables plan for which the lot is rejected if either:

$$\overline{X} + k_1 S > m$$

or if

$$\overline{X} + k_2 S > M$$

Procedures are given for determining appropriate values for k_1 and k_2 and for determining the operating characteristic surface, as a function of P_d, the proportion above M, and P_m, the proportion above m.

METHODS AND CRITERIA

If criteria are to play a role in the microbiological evaluation of foods, then it is necessary to assess the current status of the recommended methods. The first assessment is of the availability of the method. There are very few methods which can fulfill the needs or criticisms for a criterion. The application of criteria should only be used with organisms where there is an available method that can be used simply and efficiently. Such methods should also be acceptable in national and international laboratories. These conditions should also be tempered by a genuine need to protect the public from a particular hazard. Those organisms that are applicable are the pathogens. The application of *Salmonella* to a criterion is not limited by current methodology (NRC 1985). The detection of this organism in foods is perhaps the most studied and reported. There are other considerations, however, dealing with length of analysis and cost. These are dealt with later in this chapter.

The second organism for which the current methodology is adequate is *Staphylococcus aureus*. A review of this organism and applicable methodology was published by Tatini et al. (1984). The major question with *S. aureus* is whether the criterion should apply to the organism or the toxins it produces. There are reasonable arguments for both and it really comes down to the priority given to time and costs. In terms of sensitivity and accuracy, the toxin determinations are better.

The methodology for *Clostridium perfringens* is also adequate for detection and enumeration (NRC 1985). Its use in a criterion, however, is more limited than the other two organisms mentioned above. This is partly due to the conditions required to cause an outbreak of food poisoning.

Most other organisms associated with foodborne diseases lack the specificity required of a method. Examples of this are *Bacillus cereus*, *Shigella*, and enteropathogenic *Escherichia coli*. Identification of these particular organisms requires special expertise and is time-consuming. Although these organisms fit into the area of concern in public health, the lack of available methodology makes them poor candidates for use with criteria.

The methodology of indicator tests such as total plate count and the most probable number (MPN) are less reliable in terms of indicating specific adverse conditions in foods. Applying criteria to these tests requires very strict conditions. These conditions have been dealt with in the recent NRC report (1985). They can serve a useful purpose and can be used to define extreme states of food spoilage or safety. With these tests, we move out of the realm of making decisions based on presence, absence or direct relationships with hazardous conditions in food. The use of indicator tests introduces a judgment factor in the interpretation.

This judgment is based on a counting procedure which is prone to errors. The Poisson distribution can be applied to counting the number of bacteria in a volume of food sample. The assumptions required are that the bacteria are distributed at random throughout the material, the volume plated is constant, and that each bacterium or clump of bacteria give rise to one viable colony. These colonies must develop independently from each other, i.e., there must not be synergistic or antagonism effects between colonies. Deviations from theoretical distribution can also occur with defective media, variations in volumes plated (1 mL and 0.1 mL) and different incubation temperatures. If total counts are to be used in microbiological criteria, counting errors should be minimized. This means instructions for the method must be in detail and clearly laid out. Cowell and Morisetti (1969) looked at the relationship between number of colonies counted and the accuracy of the procedure with 95% confidence limits. With current practices of counting between 30 and 300, the precision varies 37% and 11%, respectively. If we use counts of 80 to 320, the precision varies only 22% and 11%, respectively. The difference may be important with restrictive criteria. In solid samples, one cannot assume the microbial population follows the Poisson distribution and other distributions have to be used. Kilsby and coworkers (1979, 1981, 1983) have advocated the statistical analysis of microbiological counts based on the log normal distribution. While empirical data may often justify this assumption, it is useful to examine theoretical models of bacterial growth which produce a log normal distribution of counts.

The log normal distribution is a continuous distribution defined on the interval $(0,\infty)$. Its theoretical properties are discussed by Johnson and Kotz (1970). For our purposes, it will suffice to note that if the count of bacteria follows a log normal distribution, then the log of the count follows a normal distribution. Since there is a vast and fairly complete statistical methodology developed for the normal distribution, it is natural that we transform to log counts in order to make use of this wealth of theory. One further point needs to be made. Since bacterial counts are discrete, but the log normal distribution is continuous, the log normal must be an approximation. However, if the counts are large, this approximation is of no great concern. The log normal distribution would not be appropriate for small counts or if there were a significant probability of a count of zero.

In the early stages of growth of a bacterial colony in an unlimiting environment, growth may be proportional to colony size. That is, if N_t is the colony size at time t, then:

$$\frac{dN_t}{dt} = CN_t$$

The solution to this differential equation is:

$$N_t = N_0 e^{ct}$$

where N_0 is the colony size at time 0. This says that the colony size is growing exponentially. Now suppose the food is contaminated at time 0 at a large number of sites, but with one organism at each site. This might be reasonable when the contamination is air- or waterborne. It is reasonable to suppose that the growth rates will vary among sites since there are many factors that will affect the growth rate of a colony. Among them is the genotype, the general viability of the founder organism, variations in temperature, moisture, and nutrients, and the number and kinds of various competitive microflora. Each of these factors has a small effect on growth rates so it is reasonable to suppose that the growth rate follows a normal distribution. This being the case, the log count at a fixed time t, follows a normal distribution. Although it was assumed initially that each colony began with a single founder organism as the duration of growth becomes longer, small variation in the initial colony size at time 0 will have a negligible effect on the final distribution.

Media Performance and Reliability

The reliability of most of the common procedures used to assess the state of foodstuffs have, at one time or another, been tested. We do so by use of the collaborative or comparative studies such as those by ICMSF (Brown and Baird-Parker 1982). Such studies are designed to give information about the method. They are set up to look not only at the reproducibility of the method under specified conditions, but also interrelations in methodology. It can compare analysts' performance, product-to-product variation with the method, and errors associated with the use of that method. These studies have revealed a number of interesting facts about the methods used and their possible application to criteria. The productivity or reliability varies with the food type (Silliker et al. 1979; Rayman et al. 1978). In an ICMSF study on the enumeration of *S. aureus*, the observation was made that the performance of the media was influenced by the food type. In a collaborative study, also part of the ICMSF method studies, a similar finding was noted with the MPN procedure and coliforms (Silliker et al. 1979). Difficulty in isolation of *Salmonella* in high moisture foods was noted by D'Aoust et al. (1983). It appears two factors may be responsible. The first is a synergistic effect with possible antimicrobial substances being produced by the competing flora; and the second, the components of the food itself. In the past, methods which applied to many food groups have been preferred to those for one or two foods. Evidence arising from collaborative studies now suggests this policy must change if we are to link such methods to criteria. The method must be specific for the food in question.

Another finding from such studies is that the errors in the selectivity of a medium are small compared to the errors in sampling. Furthermore, the errors surrounding such procedures as the MPN may be based on levels of contamination of the organism being tested. The errors in the MPN study clearly indicate a need for a better understanding of the errors involved. The authors point out that with this procedure, one should also state the "precision of the method used." Thus, if the MPN is to be used with a criterion, the errors in the method should be stated with the criterion. This enables the administrator of the criterion to make a responsible decision. This policy of stating errors of a method for official purposes is a standing recommendation by such organizations as the Association of Official Analytical Chemists (AOAC).

The stating of estimates of experimental error and among-analyst performance is an important function of collaborative/comparative studies. Comparative studies have reported that differences between methods are significantly smaller than differences between laboratories (Silliker et al., 1979; D'Aoust et al., 1983). Deviations from the norm are usually a result of the analysts' failure to identify contaminants correctly (Andrews et al. 1981). One reason for this is the laboratory environment. If this is controlled closely, then deviations between laboratories can be diminished. This means controlling media preparation, using experienced analysts and regulating the many activities in the monitoring laboratory. The analysts' performance can be used to develop estimates of variance. Using the statistical procedure given by Graybill (1976), Peeler et al. (1980) compared analysts in state milk-monitoring programs. By determining these estimates on a yearly basis among different laboratories and analysts, a record of their performance can be established. Comparison to recommended estimates of variance will reflect the value of the monitoring program. With new methodology, components of variance will vary and may require some time before stabilization to an acceptable value (Donnelly et al., 1960). These studies were also useful in demonstrating the need for alternate methods for the MPN procedure with *S. aureus*.

It is interesting to speculate on how collaborative studies represent the normal conditions one meets in food analysis. For one thing, the sample is preselected and its history is known. Often in the preparation, especially if it is artificially inoculated, a great deal of mixing occurs. This does not usually occur in naturally contaminated foods except liquids. Silliker et al. alludes to this mixing effect in an ICMSF study with the MPN (1979). The 95% confidence limits for a single determination for naturally contaminated samples showed a wider range in values than that of artificially inoculated samples. This was construed as a mixing effect associated with the preparation of the inoculated samples. The exhaustive mixing of the samples resulted in less variability between subsamples. This point of mixing was even more dramatically demonstrated by Brown and Baird-Parker (1982) using *Salmonella* inoculation into boneless meat. Prior to chopping of the meat, an inoculum of one *Salmonella* was added to 10g of meat. Using a 20 × 25 g sampling scheme, *Salmonella* was not detected in the meat. After bowl chopping, five of the 25 samples were positive for *Salmonella*. As a result of such experiments, these authors recommended careful selection of sampling sites in meats, larger sampling units, and thorough mixing of the units before analysis.

Apart from mixing, other factors which make up the sample history are also important. These factors will often introduce unknown parameters into the evaluation process. These cannot be estimated. Typical examples include abusive temperatures of storage during transportation or sale. Microbiological data from such samples would not represent the quality of the original lot, especially if part of the lot were stored or transported under ideal conditions. The age of samples for some foods will distort the true microbiological profile of the sample. The most familiar example is that of coliforms or *S. aureus* in cheese. Levels of these organisms decline considerably after five to six weeks of storage. Criteria based on detection of metabolites would be far more accurate than numerical criteria. The information obtained from chemical testing is direct and not based on estimates of numbers (e.g., measurement of toxin levels rather than numbers of coagulase positive *S. aureus*). This represents a clearer picture of the true condition of the food. The above aspects again demonstrate that the method per se is not at fault, only the sample selection.

The current concepts discussed in this article by no means eliminate the various concerns about microbiological criteria raised by Elliott and Michener (1961). A greater understanding of sampling procedures and statistical applications do diminish these concerns with regard to methodology. Other views expressed by the same authors, however, are not so easily dismissed. These concern economics, interpretation and application of criteria.

TIME, COSTS, AND THE JUDGMENT FACTOR

All methods suffer from a major drawback, the time factor. Foods that have to comply with criteria have to be held until the microbiological data have been processed and evaluated. This means higher storage costs, energy costs and perhaps loss of product quality. In the past, a great deal of time was invested in finding reliable methods that decrease the time for analysis. Successes have been modest because we still have to rely on bacterial growth as the indicator. We have chosen this approach for obvious economic reasons.

Sharpe (1978) in an article dealing with theoretical aspects of automation of microbiological methods places this choice into perspective. It is much simpler to allow bacteria to act as the detector for measurement rather than seek newer or most costly electronic methods of detection. When this is done, we trade off the time factor. We do this for other reasons too, for we achieve a sensitivity which may on occasions be "unequal in the physical world." It is also much cheaper to use a bottle of medium and a few petri plates than a machine costing several thousand dollars. In order to cut the time factor in methodology, we will have to change our whole concept towards our methods of measurement of bacteria. There is a need to develop methods that use other parameters of spoilage or safety, some of which may not even relate to bacterial growth.

Sharpe (1978) also raises an introspective view on the role of human judgment in methodology. The role of criteria often sharpens the judgment factor associated with methods. Using the example by Sharpe, this point is well illustrated. When a microbiologist sees a number of black shiny colonies with zones of clearing on Baird-Parker medium, he associates this with the possibility of enterotoxin being present in a food. The analyst makes this judgment even though the physical appearance of these colonies has nothing to do with the measurement of enterotoxin levels in the food. Criteria based on good historical evidence refines this judgment by addition of data relating numbers that are required for enterotoxin production in the food. The presence of a criterion associated with a method is an advantage since it generates a drive for a different approach to methodology and sharpens the judgement factor.

The addition of sampling plans to the analytical procedure raises the question of increase in costs. The report of the subcommittee evaluating microbiological criteria (NRC, 1985) makes the valid point that the correct way to look at costs is a cost/benefit analysis. Criteria, if linked to a method, will improve the decision-making process. In the case of food safety, less products containing pathogens should reach the market. This results in less recalls and bad publicity. With criteria and food quality, one could expect better process control to develop.

ACKNOWLEDGMENTS

The authors are indebted to Billie McGavin for her editorial and typing skills used in the preparation of this manuscript.

REFERENCES

ANDREWS, W. H., POELMA, P. L., and WILSON, C. R. 1981. Comparative efficiency of brilliant green, bismuth sulphite, salmonella-shigella, Hektoen enteric and xylose lysine desoxycholate agars for the recovery of Salmonella from foods: Collaborative study. *J. Assoc. Off. Anal. Chem.* 64: 899–928.

BRAY, D. F., LYON, D. A., and BURR, I. 1973. Three class attribute plans in acceptance sampling. *Technometrics* 15: 575.

BROWN, P. A. 1984. A three-class procedure for acceptance sampling by variables. M.Sc. thesis, Univ. of Guelph, Guelph, Ontario.

BROWN, M. H. and BAIRD-PARKER, A. C. 1982. The microbiological examination of meat. In *Meat Microbiology*. Brown, M.H. (Ed.). Applied Science Publications Ltd., London.

COCHRAN, W. E. 1977. *Sampling Techniques*. 3rd ed. John Wiley, New York.

COWELL, N. D. and MORISETTI, M. D. 1969. Microbiological techniques—some statistical aspects. *J. Sci. Fd. Agric.* 20: 573–579.

D'AOUST, J-Y., BECKERS, H. J., BOOTHROYD, M., MATES, A., McKEE, C. R., MORAN, A. B., SADO, P., SPAIN, C. E., SPERBER, W. H., VASSILIADIS, P., WAGNER, D. E., and WIBERG C. 1983. ICMSF methods studies. XIV. Comparison study on recovery of salmonella from refrigerated pre-enrichment and enrichment broth cultures. *J. Food Prot.* 46: 391–399.

DONNELLY, C. G., HARRIS, E. K., BLACK, L. A., and LEWIS, K. H. 1960. Statistical analysis of surface plate counts of milk samples split with state laboratories. *J. Milk Food Technol.* 23: 315–319.

ELLIOTT, H. P. and MICHENER, H. D. 1961. Microbiological standards and handling codes for chilled and frozen foods: A review. *Appl. Microbiol.* 9: 452–468.

GRAYBILL, F.A. 1976. *Theory and Application of the Linear Model.* Duxbury Press, North Scituate, MA.

HUNTSBERGER, D. and BILLINGSLEY, P. 1981. *Elements of Statistical Inference.* 5th ed. Allyn and Bacon Inc., Boston, MA.

ICMSF (International Commission on Microbiological Specifications for Foods). 1974. *Microorganisms in Foods. 2. Sampling for Microbiological Analysis: Principles and Specific Applications.* University of Toronto Press, Toronto.

JENNET, W. J. and WELCH, B. L. 1939. The control of portion defectives as judged by a single quality characteristic varying on a continuous scale. *J. Royal Stat. Soc.* Series B. 6: 80–88.

JOHNSON, N. L. and KOTZ, S. 1970. *Continuous Univarient Distribution.* Vol. 1, Ch. 14. Houghton Mifflin Co., Boston, MA.

KILSBY, D. C. 1982. Sampling schemes and limits. In *Meat Microbiology.* Brown, M.H. (Ed.). Applied Science Publications Ltd., London.

KILSBY, D. C. and PUGH, M. E. 1981. The relevance of the distribution of microorganisms within batches of foods to the control of microbiological hazards from foods. *J. Appl. Bacteriol.* 51: 345–354.

KILSBY, D. C., ASPENALL, L. J., and BAIRD-PARKER, A. C. 1979. A system for setting numerical microbiological specifications for foods. *J. Appl Bacteriol.* 46: 591–599.

NRC (National Research Council). 1985. An evaluation of the role of microbiological criteria in foods and food ingredients. Subcommittee on microbiological criteria. Committee on food protection. National Academy of Sciences, Washington, DC.

PEELER, J. T., MESSER, J. W., LESLIE, J. E., and HOUGHTBY, G. A. 1980. Variation in food microbiological tests used to evaluate analyst performance. *J. Food Prot.* 43: 729–732.

RAYMAN, M. K., DEVOYOD, J. J., PURVIS, U., KUSCH, D., LANIER, J., GILBERT, R. J., TILL, D. G., and JARVIS, G. A. 1978. ICMSF methods studies. X. An international comparative study of four media for the enumeration of *Staphylococcus aureus* in foods. *Can. J. Microbiol.* 24: 274–281.

SHARPE, A. N. 1978. Some theoretical aspects of microbiological analysis pertinent to mechanization. In *Mechanization Microbiology*. Sharpe, A. N. and Clarke, D. S. (Ed.). Charles A. Thomas Publishers, Springfield, IL.

SILLIKER, J. H., GABIS, D. A., and MAY, A. 1979. ICMSF methods studies. XI. Collaborative/comparative studies on determination of coliforms using the most probable number procedure. *J. Food Prot.* 42: 638–644.

TATINI, S. R., HOOVER, D. G., and LACHICA, R. V. F. 1984. Methods for the isolation and enumeration of *Staphylococcus aureus*. In *Compendium of Methods for the Microbiological Examination of Foods*. 2nd ed. Speck, M. E. (Ed.). American Public Health Assoc., Washington, DC.

4

Predictive Modeling of Food Deterioration and Safety

Jeffrey M. Farber

Health and Welfare Canada
Ottawa, Ontario, Canada

Traditionally, food microbiologists have relied on empirical data for information on ability of an organism to grow and/or produce toxin in a particular food environment. In these experiments, the important parameters governing growth such as pH, a_w, E_h, temperature, NaCl, etc. were defined, and maximum and minimum limits permitting growth were established (Table 4.1). From these data, shelf-life, microbiological stability and safety of foods have been evaluated. However, the value of studies that deal with only one variable at a time is limited because there are always at least three factors (pH, a_w, temperature) governing the growth of microbial populations, and in most cases there are interactive effects among them. These interactive or synergistic effects are well explained by the hurdle concept of Leistner and Rödel (1976) (Fig. 4.1), which attempts to describe how different extrinsic and intrinsic parameters affect an organism's ability to survive and initiate growth. In the first food product (Fig. 4.1, no. 1), five different hurdles of equal intensity combine to inhibit the organisms present. In a more likely situation (food product no. 2) four different hurdles of various intensities are sufficient

Table 4.1 Physical Methods for Control of Food-Poisoning Bacteria in Foods[a]

Bacteria	Growth temperature range (°C)	pH range permitting growth	Maximum brine permitting growth (%)	Minimum A_w permitting growth
Campylobacter jejuni (and *C. coli*)	31–45	6.0–9.5	2.0[b]	NK[c]
Clostridium botulinum:				
Types A	10–48	4.6	8.0	0.93–0.96
B	10–48	4.6	8.0	0.93–0.96
B (nonproteolytic)	>3.3	5.0	4.0	NK
E	3.3–45	5.0	4.0	0.96–0.97
F	10–48	4.6	8.0	NK
F (nonproteolytic)	>3.3	5.0	4.0	NK
C. perfringens	10–52	5.0–8.5	6.0	0.95–0.97
B. cereus	7–49	4.3–9.3	7.5	0.95
Salmonella spp.	5.2–45	4.0–9.6	8.0	0.95
S. aureus	6.7–46	4.0 ($+O_2$) 4.6 ($-O_2$)	16–18 ($+O_2$) 14–16 ($-O_2$)	0.83–0.86 ($+O_2$) 0.9 ($-O_2$)
S. aureus (enterotoxin production)	10–45	4.0 ($+O_2$) 5.3 ($-O_2$)	10 ($+O_2$) 9.5 ($-O_2$)	0.86 ($+O_2$) 0.94 ($-O_2$)
Vibrio parahaemolyticus	5–44	4.8–11.0	8.0[b]	0.94
V. vulnificus	5–42	NK	6.0[b]	NK
Yersinia enterocolitica	1–44	4.6–9.0	5.0[b]	0.96
Listeria monocytogenes	3–45	5.6–9.6	10.0[b]	NK

[a]Adapted from Genigeorgis (1981).
[b]Salt concentration.
[c]Not known.

for microbial stability. One can also have a food product with only two inherent hurdles (food no. 3), but these are sufficient for control of microbial growth (e.g., meat products can be stored unrefrigerated if the pH is ≤ 5.2 and the a_w is ≤ 0.95). In the last example, four hurdles of unequal intensity combine through direct as well as synergistic effects to secure microbial stability of the product. Although most foods are preserved by more than one hurdle, there is a lack of quantitative data available to allow us to predict the necessary levels of these hurdles. Some early investigators (Baird-Parker

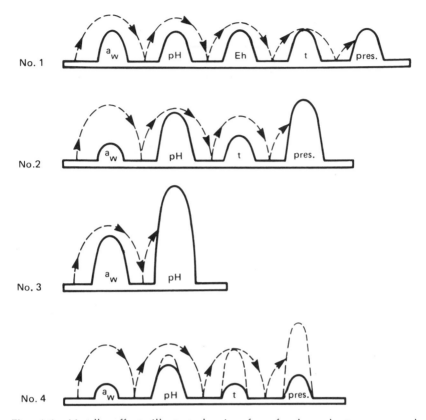

Fig. 4.1   Hurdle effect, illustrated using four food products as example. (*From Leistner 1978.*)

and Freame 1967; Ohye and Christian 1967; Matches and Liston 1972a,b; Roberts and Ingram 1973) saw the need to study the interactive effects of various parameters on microbial growth and toxin production. Roberts and Ingram (1973) described these interactions in the form of 3-dimensional ecograms. Figure 4.2 illustrates the interactive effects of pH, NaCl, and $NaNO_2$ on the growth of various strains of *Clostridium botulinum* in culture media. The limitation, however, in using graphical illustrations like ecograms is that only two independent variables can be included. Using mathematical models, however, many independent variables can be included, and several combinations of interactive effects can be studied simultaneously.

In the mathematical modeling procedure, certain regression equations are generated which may enable the investigator to predict the possibility or probability of microbial growth and/or toxin production in a certain food product. This information can be used advantageously in many situations:

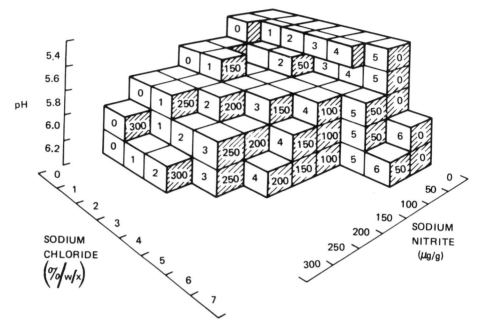

Fig. 4.2   Effect of pH, NaCl, and NaNO$_2$ on growth of *C. botulinum* at 35°C. Composite diagram of types A, B, E, and F. (*From Roberts and Ingram 1973.*)

1. to predict the relative microbial stability of a new food product, which may differ only slightly from an older established product;

2. to aid in the assessment of the direct and interactive effects on microbial growth of a novel combination of food preservatives (e.g. irradiation plus sorbate) in a food product;

3. to assess the safety of foods which are subjected to various degrees of temperature abuse as they pass through the wholesale, retail, and domestic outlets.

BASIC CONCEPTS IN MATHEMATICAL MODELING

"Mathematical modeling is a procedure leading to the description of a process or phenomena of interest by one or more mathematical equations" (Rand 1984). A brief overview of the basic concepts in mathematical modeling will be discussed. Successful application of modeling procedures requires knowledge of experimental design and regression analysis. No attempt will be

made here to delve into the statistics or to provide a comprehensive introduction. Interested readers should consult, for example, Draper and Smith
(1981), Afifi and Azen (1979), Daniel and Wood (1980), Neter and Wasserman (1974), or Himmelblau (1970).

The purposes of modeling are varied but in a particular application usually
include one or more of the following:

1. to describe the underlying process;
2. to predict a response from independent variables;
3. to study a particular variable after controlling for related variables.

Steps in the modeling procedure may be summarized as follows.

1. Planning. First and foremost in the planning stage is the clear and
specific statement of the problem. After this has been done, response variables
and independent variables which are believed to have an effect on the problem and are believed to be relevant should be identified.

2. Data collection. The relevant variables identified in (1) should be
measured at various levels. The levels should cover the ranges of interest
and sufficient measurements collected to permit adequate testing of the
model.

3. Model fitting. This consists of fitting different models which relate
the response variable and independent variables and then determining those
independent variables and the form of the model which best describes the
data. Procedures exist to provide guidance in the choice of models and
independent variables and for comparing competing models. An appropriate
source, e.g., Draper and Smith (1981) should be consulted for details.

4. Model validation. This involves evaluating the model using data not
used to fit the model. This can be accomplished by accumulating a new set
of data using different values for independent variables chosen within the
range covered by the model and by comparing the observed and predicted
values. Other procedures are outlined by Draper and Smith (1981) and
involve using part of a data set to generate the model and part to validate
it.

EXAMPLES OF PREDICTIVE MODELS IN FOOD MICROBIOLOGY SYSTEMS

Some companies in Canada, the United States, England, and Europe use
predictive modeling in their food operations, but their data are considered
proprietary. However, there are examples in the literature where investigators

have looked at specific food poisoning organisms and attempted to predict (1) the probability of toxin production in a model food system, (2) the probability of initiating growth in culture or a simulated food system, or (3) the extent of growth of a pathogen in a certain environment. The organisms that have been investigated include *Clostridium botulinum*, *Staphylococcus aureus*, *Clostridium perfringens*, *Bacillus cereus*, and *Salmonella* spp.

Clostridium botulinum

One of the significant factors controlling growth of *C. botulinum* in foods is the level of nitrite. Because of pressure to reduce the input of nitrite in foods, a clearer understanding of its role in the control of *C. botulinum* and its interaction with other control factors is needed. In an attempt to assess the relative importance of the various factors, a product risk evaluation system was devised whereby risk factors (derived from empirical data from many experiments) were assigned to each of the parameters thought to be important in the control of *C. botulinum* in cured meats (Jarvis and Patel 1979). The higher the numerical value assigned to the parameter, the greater the overall probability of toxin production (Table 4.2). A model pork slurry system (Rhodes and Jarvis 1976) was used for all experiments in studying the combined effect of parameters such as salt, nitrite, pH, storage temperature,

Table 4.2   Examples of Risk Factors Calculation[a]

(A)	Average present-day practice
	Salt (3.5%) + Nitrite (200) + P_{80}^b (6.7) + Storage (15°) + pH 6.0
	R = 1 × 1 × 1 × 1 × 1 = 1
(B)	Reduce salt and nitrite; increase temperature and pH
	Salt (2%) + Nitrite (50) + Storage (20°C) + pH (6.4)
	R = 4 × 10 × 5 × 4 = 800
(C)	Reduce nitrite and process; increase salt and temperature
	Salt (4.5%) + Nitrite (100) + Storage (20°C) + P_{80} (0.7)
	R = 0.5 × 3 × 5 × 3 = 22.5
(D)	As (C) + Polyphosphate
	C + Polyphosphate (0.5)
	R = 23 × 0.2 = 4.6

[a]From Jarvis and Patel (1979)
[b]Heat treatment (80°C; 6.7 min).

polyphosphates, and heat on the growth of *C. botulinum*. Although the relative extent of interactive effects on growth could be predicted, the risk factor assessment was generally imprecise. It was thus decided to see if a more precise mathematical modeling of the data could be performed.

A logistic regression model was then used to describe the relationships between the probability for botulinal growth and toxin production and the following parameters: salt, nitrite, polyphosphate, sorbate, heat, and storage temperature. Individual experiments were performed using a single set of parameters and a predictive regression equation was formulated for each experiment. The model used was of the form (Roberts et al. 1981c)

$$P_{ijk \cdots rst} = \frac{1}{(1 + e^{-\mu})} \quad \cdot \tag{1}$$

where $P_{ijk \cdots rst}$ = probability of toxin production under the combination of treatments defined by the subscripts $ijk \ldots rst$; and μ = expression for the individual terms derived by regression of a quantitative variable which varies over a defined range, e.g. β salt × (level of salt).

It is evident from this formula that any parameter which decreases the value of μ will reduce the probability of toxin formulation.

The predicted and observed values for toxin production after storage of meat slurries for three months in the presence of 3.5% brine (on water) is shown in Table 4.3. The observed and predicted values were similar. Comparisons of predicted values from several experiments demonstrated the effectiveness of parameters such as nitrite level, polyphosphates, and storage temperature in inhibiting toxin formation. The model also pointed out a marked inhibitory effect of polyphosphates, which had not been expected.

Roberts et al. (1981a, b, c; 1982) went one step further. Instead of using many predictive equations, mammoth experiments were conducted in order to obtain a single predictive or "overall" equation for the probability of toxin production by *C. botulinum*. It was hoped that this equation could aid in situations where product formulations required modifications or where product safety was in question. The model pork slurry system mentioned previously was used for inoculation of a mixture comprising five strains each of *C. botulinum* types A and B. The factors (and levels) listed in Table 4.4 were evaluated for their effects (singly and in combination) on the probability of toxin production by *C. botulinum*. Many significant two-factor interactions were observed (Roberts et al. 1981a) which support the observations of others that factors can combine or interact to secure microbial stability of food systems contaminated with *C. botulinum* (Baird-Parker and Freame 1967; Roberts and Ingram 1973). In most instances, the observed and predicted

Table 4.3 Observed (O) and Predicted (P) Values (%) for Toxin Production After Three-Month's Storage of Meat Slurries Containing 3.5% Salt-on-Water[a]

Input nitrite (μg/g)	Storage temp (°C)	Low heat[b] O	Low heat[b] P	High heat[c] O	High heat[c] P
75	15	60	53	7	5
	25	100	>99	90	96
175	15	10	24	0	1.5
	25	100	93	67	37
300	15	10	6	3	<1
	25	5	12	5	<1

[a]From Jarvis and Robinson (1983).
[b]$P_{80}°C = 0.65$ min.
[c]$P_{80}°C = 12.65$ min. See Rhodes and Jarvis (1976).

Table 4.4 List of Factors Used to Control Growth of *C. botulinum* Types A and B in Pasteurized, Cured Meats[a]

Factor	Units	Levels
NaCl	% on water (w/v)	2.5, 3.5, 4.5
$NaNO_2$	μg/g slurry	0, 100, 200, 300
$NaNO_3$	μg/g slurry	0, 500
Sodium isoascorbate	μg/g slurry	0, 1000, equimolar with $NaNO_2$
Polyphosphate	% w/v slurry	0, 0.3
Inoculum	Spores per bottle	0, 10^1, 10^3
Heat treatment	°C	0, 80°/7 min, 80°/7 min + 70° 1 hr
Storage temperature	°C	15, 17.5, 20, 35

[a]Adapted from Roberts et al. (1981a).

values obtained mimicked each other closely, although there were some large individual differences. From the data presented, given any combination of chemical additives, it was possible to predict (within the ranges tested) the probability of C. botulinum producing toxin in the pork slurry system. For example, if one looks at the data in Table 4.5, it would be possible to reduce the probability of toxin production in the pork slurry system in the presence of 2.5% salt from approximately 48–76% to 1–3% by raising the $NaNO_2$ level from 100 to 300 μg/g. Without changing the input level of nitrite it would be necessary to raise the NaCl level to at least 4.5% to achieve approximately the same level of protection. Although these probabilities cannot be applied directly to actual food products, the important consideration here is that "the assessment of the relative effect of changes in product formulation on toxin production by C. botulinum can be evaluated in terms of increased or decreased safety of the product" (Roberts et al. 1981c).

Roberts et al. (1982) estimated the probabilities of growth and toxin production by C. botulinum in a pork slurry system with the following variables: NaCl (2.5, 3.5, 4.5%), potassium sorbate (0, 0.26%), pH (5.7, 6.6) and incubation temperature (15, 17.5, 20, 35°C). The relative effect of potassium sorbate was the greatest at 3.5 or 4.5% salt, and at pH 5.7 (Table 4.6). Contrary to previously published results (Robach 1980), no interactions were

Table 4.5 Probability (%)[a] of Toxin Production by C. botulinum Types A and B in Pork Slurry Prepared From "Low" pH Meat,[b] Inoculum 10 Spores/Bottle[c]

NaCl (% on water)	NaNO (μg/g)[2]	Low heat[d]			
		15	17.5	20	35[e]
2.5	100	48	66	76	59
2.5	200	9	16	25	13
2.5	300	1	2	3	2
3.5	100	14	25	35	20
3.5	200	2	5	8	4
3.5	300	0	1	1	1
4.5	100	3	5	9	4
4.5	200	1	1	2	1
4.5	300	0	0	1	0

[a]The percentage probabilities are rounded to the nearest whole number.
[b]pH range 5.5–6.3
[c]Adapted from Roberts et al. (1981c).
[d]80°C for 7 min.
[e]Storage temperatures (°C).

Table 4.6 Probability (%)[a] of Toxin Production by C. *botulinum*
Types A and B, in Pork Slurry Containing 40 μg/g Sodium Nitrite, 550
μg/g Sodium Isoascorbate, Inoculum Ten Spores per Bottle[b]

NaCL (% on water)	pH	Potassium[c] sorbate (0.26 % w/v)	Low heat[d] 15	17.5	20	35[e]
2.5	5.7	−	40	67	83	60
2.5	5.7	+	15	34	55	28
2.5	6.6	−	69	90	97	98
2.5	6.6	+	36	70	88	93
3.5	5.7	−	10	27	49	39
3.5	5.7	+	3	9	20	14
3.5	6.6	−	29	67	88	97
3.5	6.6	+	9	34	65	90
4.5	5.7	−	5	17	38	47
4.5	5.7	+	1	5	14	18
4.5	6.6	−	17	53	82	98
4.5	6.6	+	5	22	54	92

[a]The percentage probabilities are rounded to the nearest whole number.
[b]Adapted from Roberts et al. (1982).
[c]Sorbate present + or absent − at stated level.
[d]80°C for 7 min.
[e]Storage temperatures (°C).

observed between salt and sorbate or storage temperature and sorbate. Generally, the authors felt that it would be unwise to lower sodium nitrite levels
for meats of high pH that could possibly be temperature abused, even when
0.26% (w/v) potassium sorbate was present in the formulation (Roberts et
al. 1982).

Problems encountered when doing an investigation of a model are illustrated by Robinson et al. (1982). When examining data on the sorbate
experiments (see above) and on the effect of pig breed, cut and batch of
meat on spoilage and toxin production by C. *botulinum* (Gibson et al. 1982),
it became evident that there were nonlinear effects of storage temperature
and salt concentration on toxin production, i.e., increasing the salt level from
3.5 to 4.5% in the sorbate study (see Table 4.6) did not reduce the probability
of toxin production significantly. When quadratic terms were included in
the regression equations, it was apparent that a better fit of the data to the
model existed. This led the investigators to re-examine data from previous

experiments (Roberts et al. 1981c) to see if a better fit of the regression model to the data could be obtained, which was the case. The nature of the nonlinearity proved to be similar in all cases and led to the inclusion into the regression equation of a quadratic term in storage temperature (T^2). Generally, the difference between the original and revised data was largest over the middle range of probabilities of toxin production.

Using a simpler approach to predictive analysis, Hauschild (1982) attempted to compile and analyze the wealth of data existing in the literature on challenge studies with *C. botulinum* in cured meat products.

The basic equation $P = MPN/s$ estimates the probability (P) of individual spores to grow out and produce toxin within a given period of temperature abuse. MPN is the most probable number of spores capable of toxin production per sample (e.g., can of pasteurized ham) and s the total number of spores per sample. MPN in turn may be calculated as $MPN = \ln(n/q)$ (Halvorson and Ziegler 1933), where n is the total number of samples and q the number of nontoxic samples.

Thus, if 50 samples were inoculated with 100 spores each, and if four samples became toxic, P would equal $\ln(50/46)/100 = 8.3 \times 10^{-4}$. The value log ($1/P$) was used to express the number of log units of spores needed for only one spore to germinate and produce toxin within a defined period of temperature abuse.

The calculations allowed the author to compare quantitatively the results of widely divergent challenge studies and led to a number of interesting conclusions. For example, the contribution of nitrite to the overall protection of cured meats was generally found to be small, e.g., the nitrite content of vacuum-packaged bacon contributed only one log unit to a total log $1/P$ value of six (Fig. 4.3). The study also showed that the protection of some high a_w products such as vacuum-packaged turkey rolls was about three log units less than that of bacon, yet paradoxically, the less protected products have generally received much less attention with respect to their potential botulism risk. The author concluded that selective reductions in nitrite input could be made safely, provided that other antibotulinal parameters such as salt, carbohydrate, and erythorbate contents were properly controlled (Hauschild 1982).

Staphylococcus aureus

Little work has been done in the past using mathematical modeling to predict staphylococcal growth and enterotoxin production in liquid culture or in foods. Genigeorgis et al. (1971a, b), using a factorial design experiment and multiple regression analysis, studied the effects of NaCl and pH on the log

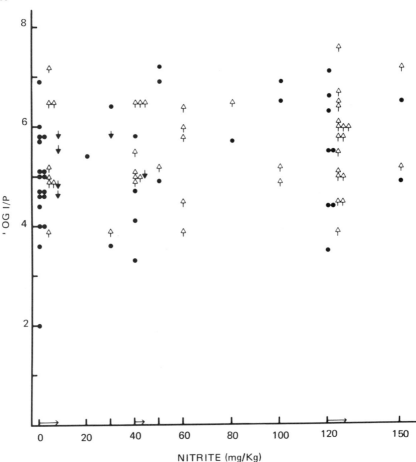

Fig. 4.3   Vacuum-packaged bacon. Number of C. *botulinum* spores required for one spore to grow out and produce toxin (1/P) during temperature abuse (average 27°C; 7 days) ↑ = data with the sign >; ↓ = data with the sign <; ● = finite values. (*From Hauschild 1982.*)

reduction of staphylococcal populations inoculated into Brain Heart Infusion (BHI) broth. From the following equation:

$$P = 1/\text{antilog}\ [\log\ (R_I/R_G)] \qquad (2)$$

where R_I = number of cells in inoculum and R_G = number of cells initiating growth, it was possible to determine the probability, P, of a single cell initiating growth in broth at a certain pH and NaCl level. For example, growth of *S. aureus* S-6 in BHI broth (pH 6.0) containing 5.0% NaCl was decreased by 1.69 log units compared to the control, and the probability of initiating growth was 2.04% (l/antilog 1.69). The authors found that the strain, pH, and NaCl concentration all significantly affected the magnitude of the log reduction in staphylococcal numbers.

The general regression equation used to predict the decimal reductions of the bacterial populations exposed to different environments was as follows:

$$Y_e = a + b_1X_1 + b_2X_2 + b_3X_1^2 + b_4X_2^2 + b_5X_1X_2 \qquad (3)$$

where Y_e = estimated log decrease of the bacterial population; a = intercept; X_1 = % NaCl (w/v); X_2 = pH level; and $b_1 \ldots b_5$ = regression coefficients.

When the data obtained from the models were compared to previous empirical work performed in liquid culture, close agreement was found between the two. However, when similar-type experiments were repeated in laboratory-prepared cured meats (Genigeorgis et al. 1971b), the results were inconsistent with the data derived from culture work with BHI broth. It appeared that S. aureus grew better on the cured meats, which meant that fewer cells initiated growth at a certain brine concentration and pH than could be predicted from equations derived from studies in broth.

Recognizing the imprecision of extrapolating from liquid culture to foods, Nderu and Genigeorgis (1975) devised a model meat system comprising 1.0-g portions of cooked ground beef discs which were adjusted to various pH levels (4.3, 6.1, 7.8) and brine concentrations (0, 4.8, 9.5, 14.6%). The discs were inoculated with different strains of S. aureus at various concentrations ranging from 10^0 to 10^6. The all-strains equation generated was as follows:

$$Dr = 23.27 + 0.61\,(\text{salt}\%) - 7.74\,(\text{pH}) - 0.06\,(\text{pH})\,(\text{salt}\%) \qquad (4)$$
$$- 0.001\,(\text{salt}\%)^2 + 0.616\,(\text{pH})^2 \pm 0.937$$

where Dr = decimal reduction of a staphylococcal population exposed to an environment of a certain pH and salt.

To test the reliability of the derived mathematical equations, various commercially processed meats (beef bologna, cooked beef, mortadella, cotto salami, and Italian-style dry salami) were inoculated with different S. aureus strains at various concentrations. Although no data were presented, the authors stated that, given the pH and brine concentration, one could reliably predict the extent of staphylococcal growth in commercially processed meats. The main conclusion drawn from the study was that unless large numbers of organisms other than staphylococci (usually lactic acid bacteria) are present, the potential for low numbers of S. aureus to initiate growth in processed meats is great.

Since little data existed on the various parameters affecting growth and toxin production of *S. aureus* in fermented sausages, and since staphylococcal food-poisoning outbreaks in fermented meat products such as Genoa and Italian-style dry salami had been only recently reported (CDC 1975, 1979), Metaxopoulos et al. (1981a) extended their studies to include fermented meats produced under commercial manufacturing conditions.

In those experiments, the ability of several *S. aureus* strains to grow and produce enterotoxin in commercially prepared Italian-style dry salami was investigated. Equations derived from stepwise multiple regression analysis were used to predict the ability of *S. aureus* to grow in the meat environment, as influenced by a number of parameters. The regression equation used was:

$$Y_i = a + b_1X_1 + b_2X_2 + b_3X_3 + b_4X_4 \tag{5}$$

where $Y_i = \log_{10}$ *S. aureus* counts g^{-1} salami at a given day of fermentation; b_1, b_2, b_3, b_4 = regression coefficients; X_1–X_4 = variables affecting the growth of *S. aureus*.

There was good agreement between the predicted and observed levels of *S. aureus* growing on the salami. Generally, the staphylococci inherent in the salami never exceeded 2×10^4 cells/g at any time during the fermentation. Even when artificially inoculated *S. aureus* reached levels greater than 1.0×10^7 cells/g of salami, no enterotoxin could be detected. This was probably due to interactive effects of pH, brine %, $NaNO_2$, a_w and lactic acid bacteria (Metaxopoulos et al. 1981a).

Outbreaks of staphylococcal food poisoning traced to Italian-style dry salami have occurred in instances where manufacturers have failed to add starter culture. Thus, the importance of keeping initial *S. aureus* levels down to a minimum in meats without starter culture is critical.

In a parallel series of experiments (Metaxopoulos et al. 1981b) the effect of starter culture and chemical acidulation on growth and toxin production by *S. aureus* strain S-6 in Italian-style dry salami was studied. *S. aureus* growth was affected most significantly by pH, followed by the numbers of staphylococci and lactic acid bacteria initially present. The initial pH, initial starter culture concentration, and the day of fermentation all significantly affected the levels of lactic acid bacteria at a particular day of fermentation. Many interactive effects on the levels of staphylococci and lactic acid bacteria were noted.

The addition of 0.4% glucono-delta-lactone (GDL) powder plus 10^5 cells of fresh starter culture was an effective combination in controlling *S. aureus* growth. A higher concentration of GDL appeared to have an inhibitory effect on the growth of the lactic acid bacteria.

Using regression equations similar to those described previously (see Eq. 5), the maximum population levels of *S. aureus* growing on salami of different initial pH and lactic acid bacteria levels were predicted, assuming an initial *S. aureus* count of 7×10^4 cells/g. This level was chosen because previous studies had shown that staphylococci counts at the time of stuffing were usually in the range of 1000 organisms/g. With the initial pH adjusted to 5.7, the predicted *S. aureus* levels on salami manufactured in two plants remained below 1×10^6 organisms/g, regardless of the initial levels of lactic acid bacteria (Table 4.7). Plant A was slightly more conducive to growth of the lactic acid bacteria and this was the probable reason for the decreased numbers of staphylococci observed in plant A relative to plant B (see Table 4.7). Overall, there was close agreement between the estimated and observed levels of *S. aureus*/g on any particular day of the fermentation.

The information obtained from the equations generated in these studies cannot be extrapolated to predict reliably the extent of *S. aureus* growth in products other than in similarly processed, Italian-style dry salami. However, the important consideration here is that the equations provide basic information which may be used as an aid by industry in approaching any production problems that may arise (Metaxopoulos et al. 1981b).

Broughall et al. (1983) described models whereby predictions of growth rate and duration of lag phase of *S. aureus* growing at different temperatures and a_w levels could be made. A nonlinear Arrhenius regression equation was used. Since the authors' main concern was microbial growth at or below ambient temperature during food processing or along the distribution chain, the kinetics dealt only with the low temperature (not high temperature)

Table 4.7 Effect of Changes in pH_0^a and LAB_0^b of Salami Formulation on the Maximum Growth of *S. aureus* During the First 7 Days of Processing in Two Plants[c,d]

	Log cells/g at following pH_0:			
	Plant A		Plant B	
LAB_0/g	6.1	5.7	6.1	5.7
10^4	6.35	5.03	6.86	5.32
10^5	5.88	4.68	6.32	4.83
10^6	5.48	4.33	5.74	4.33

[a]Initial pH.
[b]Initial lactic acid bacteria concentration.
[c]From Metaxopoulos et al. (1981b).
[d]Data based on regression equations reported in Metaxopoulos et al. (1981 b) and an initial *S. aureus* level of 7×10^4 cells/g.

inactivation portion of the Arrhenius plot. UHT milk was chosen as the model food system, with D-glucose being used to adjust the a_w. Briefly, generation and lag times were correlated to temperature and a_w using the nonlinear Arrhenius equation:

$$\frac{\dfrac{1}{K} \, P_{25} \, T_{298} \, \exp\left[\dfrac{H_A}{R} \cdot \left(\dfrac{1}{298} - \dfrac{1}{T} \right) \right]}{1 + \exp\left[\dfrac{H_L}{R} \cdot \left(\dfrac{1}{T_{1/2}L} - \dfrac{1}{T} \right) \right]} \qquad (6)$$

where R = universal gas constant; K = generation time; P_{25} = the growth rate at $25°$ C; T = temperature in degrees absolute; H = constant describing the enthalpy of low temperature inactivation of growth; T = temperature for 50% low temperature inactivation of the growth rate.

The Verhulst differential equation was then used to calculate the extent of microbial growth:

$$N = \frac{b}{1 + \dfrac{b - N_0}{N_0} \cdot \exp\left[\dfrac{-0.693 \, (t - L)}{K} \right]} \qquad (7)$$

where L = lag time; N = final concentration of bacterial cells at time t; N_0 = initial population; b = maximum cell population achievable; K = generation time at the maximum growth rate.

Both the predicted generation times of the model and experimental determinations observed were very similar, but the model fits were more exact for generation time data (Fig. 4.4) than for data derived from lag time. This may be due to the fact that the lag time does not represent a uniform physiological process (Broughall et al. 1983). The overall trend was for both the generation and lag time to increase for a given temperature as the a_w decreased. At $28°C$ the predicted generation times (h) of S. aureus at a_w values of 0.881, 0.90, 0.92, 0.94 and 0.96–0.98 were 5.0, 3.1, 1.7, 0.96, and 0.72, respectively, while at $16°C$, for the same a_w levels the generation times were 45.6, 24.0, 12.7, 6.5, and 3.4 hr, respectively. Generally, the staphylococci were able to survive at low a_w and temperature by undergoing lengthy lag phases of up to 35 days. This is in contrast to a Salmonella typhimurium strain which under extreme conditions of a_w and temperature had a maximum lag phase of only five days. The minimum growth temperature predicted (6.3–6.4°C) for S. aureus in the model system was very close to that observed

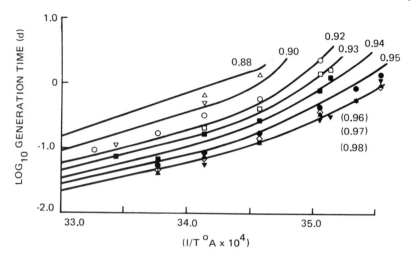

Fig. 4.4 Arrhenius plots of *Staphylococcus aureus* generation times. The lines show the predicted generation times of the model. The points represent experimental determinations at the following a_w values: ▼ 0.98; ▲ 0.97; ◇ 0.96; ● 0.95; ■ 0.94; □ 0.93; ○ 0.92; ▽ 0.90; △ 0.88. (*From Broughall et al. 1983.*)

experimentally (Angelotti et al. 1961). As with all models, certain shortcomings are evident. The main ones existing for this model are (1) only two limiting parameters (a_w and temperature) are accounted for; (2) one cannot use the model to describe situations in which food is stored above 30°C (because of possible high temperature inactivation); (3) the model is limited to foods with an a_w of 0.88 or greater; and (4) the model may predict greater risks than actually exist because *S. aureus* growth can occur at low temperatures without toxin production.

Expanding on the above work, Broughall and Brown (1984) introduced another variable into their mathematical formulations which resulted in three-dimensional models used for predicting microbial growth. An analysis of variance technique was used to give an objective measure of generation time and lag times derived from growth-curve data thus improving on the techniques used previously (Broughall et al. 1983).

The models presented demonstrated the effects of a_w and pH on the growth of *S. aureus* and *S. typhimurium* in UHT milk held at temperatures from 10 to 30°C. Higher growth temperatures allowed the bacteria to overcome the a_w/pH hurdles that were sufficient to control microbial growth at lower temperatures.

The most useful application of these three-dimensional models may be in the prediction of microbial growth in foods which have been subjected to several time/temperature cycles. Additionally, the models could be used to assess the time required for a certain pathogen to reach critical levels in food containing known inherent hurdles (Broughall and Brown 1984).

Clostridium perfringens

Yip and Genigeorgis (1981) studied the direct and interactive effects of pH (5, 7, 9), NaCl (0.5, 4.0, and 7.5%), and NaNO$_2$ (0, 20, 40 ppm) on the survival of four different *C. perfringens* strains in BHI broth. Using a factorial-designed experiment and a most probable number technique, the decimal reductions of the organism exposed to a particular environment were calculated from the ratio:

$$\log \left(\frac{\text{initial inoculum}}{\text{cells initiating growth}} \right)$$

i.e., with a log ratio of three, 1 in 1000 cells would have survived in the particular environment studied. These decimal reduction (DR) values were used in (a) statistical analysis to determine which of the single or interactive factors tested significantly reduced the DR value, (b) formulation of mathematical regression equations used to predict to what extent cells could survive in a certain environment, and (c) to determine the probability of one cell initiating growth in a particular environment (P = 1/antilog DR). Highly significant interactions were observed for pH, NaCl%, a_w, strain $\times$ pH, NaCl and a_w; pH $\times$ NaCl and a_w; strain $\times$ pH $\times$ NaCl; and strain $\times$ pH $\times$ a_w, on the DR of the *C. perfringens* populations tested. Generally, growth was very poor in the presence of 7.5% NaCl, even under otherwise optimal conditions. The greatest reduction in DR was found at pH 5.0 (6–7 DR compared to 1.3 DR at pH 9.0). Surprisingly, there were no significant effects of up to 48 ppm NaNO$_2$ (first or second order interactions) on the DR value.

Using multiple regression analysis, a single regression equation was obtained for the four *C. perfringens* strains.

$$DR = a + b_1 X_1 + b_2 X_2 + b_3(X_3) - b_4(X_4) \tag{8}$$

where X_1 = pH; X_2 = NaCl; X_3 = $(\text{pH})^2$; X_4 = $(\text{NaCl})^2$.

Some examples of the average DR and P values for four *C. perfringens* strains growing in different environments are shown in Table 4.8. If one wanted to obtain the right combination to use in a formulation to reduce the level of *C. perfringens* by greater than four DR, this could be readily

Table 4.8 Regression Equation for Four *C. perfringens* Strains[a]

$$DR = a + b_1X_1 + b_2X_2 + b_3X_3 + \cdots \pm SE$$
$$DR = 22.49 - 5.65 \; (\text{pH}) + 1.4 \; (\text{NaCl}) + 0.37 \; (\text{pH})^2 - 0.1 \; (\text{NaCl})^2 \pm$$
1.2
R = Multiple Correlation Coefficient = 0.875
P = Probability of 1 Cell to Initiate Growth = 1/Antilog DR

Examples	pH	NaCl%	DR	Antilog	P %
	5	0.5	4.29	1.95×10^4	0.005
	7	4.0	5.38	2.4×10^5	0.0004
	6	0.5	2.58	3.84×10^2	0.26
	7	0	1.07	1.17×10^1	8.5
	9	0	1.61	4.07×10^1	2.5
	7	6	5.95	8.91×10^5	0.0001

[a]From Yip and Genigeorgis (1980).

accomplished by looking at the combination of pH and salt outside the curve for four DR (Fig. 4.5). It should be pointed out that these data do not allow prediction of *C. perfringens* growth in foods.

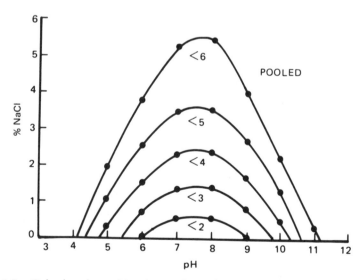

Fig. 4.5 Calculated combinations of NaCl and pH which will result in 2, 3, 4, 5, and 6 decimal reductions of *C. perfringens* populations. (*From Yip and Genigeorgis 1980.*)

Bacillus cereus

Similar experiments to those with *C. perfringens* in BHI broth were done with
B. cereus, using five strains, four NaCl levels (0, 2.5, 5.0, and 7.5%), and four
pH values (4.6, 6.1, 7.5, and 8.8) (Raevuori and Genigeorgis 1975). Multiple
regression analysis of the data generated equations which related the DR of
B. cereus to the levels of NaCl and pH (Fig. 4.6). Attempts were then made
to predict the DR value of *B. cereus* growing in cooked meat and rice. It was
evident that the organism grew to a much greater extent in the foods rather
than in culture, and thus the predicted DR values were in many instances
grossly overestimated. For example, the predicted and observed DR values
at pH 5.0 for *B. cereus* strain 01552 in rice and BHI broth was 1.02 and 5.03,
respectively. This demonstrates that regression equations derived from culture studies cannot be used to predict growth behavior of the organisms in
food systems. Similar observations were made previously with *S. aureus* (see
above).

Salmonella

Since *Salmonella* is one of the leading causes of foodborne illness worldwide,
it is surprising that very little published data exist on the interactive effects
of various parameters on growth and survival of this organism. In one of

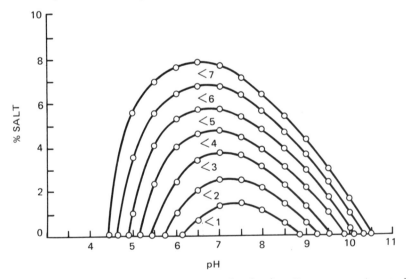

Fig. 4.6   Pooled calculated log decreases for the five *B. cereus* strains studied. (*From Raevuori and Genigeorgis 1975.*)

the few studies, Genigeorgis et al. (1977) attempted to evaluate the ability of various *Salmonella* serotypes to initiate growth in BHI broth and on discs of meat at various pH values and NaCl levels.

A highly significant overall effect ($P < 0.0001$) of pH, NaCl and pH × NaCl was observed on the growth of *Salmonella* in both the broth and meat systems. All strains tested were similarly affected by given growth environments, except in the trials where extreme pH levels (no NaCl) were used. For example, at pH 4.05 and 9.18 *S. infantis* required an inoculum of greater than 11 and 5 cells/mL, respectively, to initiate growth, while under the same conditions populations of $> 4.5 × 10^5$ and $> 5 × 10^4$ cells/mL of *S. typhimurium*, respectively, were required. Such a diversity of strains (as exists in the genus *Salmonella*) presents problems in predictive modeling.

It would be prudent to use at least four or five representative strains of each species and develop an average overall regression equation from the observed behavior of the strains in the model test system. On the other hand, under certain circumstances (e.g. food which is known to support growth of *Salmonella* and which is destined for consumer groups with increased susceptibility) it may be wise to choose the equation from data generated by the organism which grew under the most stringent conditions tested.

At a_w levels of 0.94 (meat) or 0.95 (broth) an inoculum of greater than 10^7 *Salmonella* cells/mL was required to initiate growth. These data are consistent with the present literature which states that 0.95 is the lowest a_w value supporting growth of *Salmonella* (Leistner and Rödel 1976). Under conditions of extreme pH and increasing levels of brine, heavier inocula were needed to initiate growth. Also, as the pH decreased or increased from its optimum value, lower brine concentrations were required to inhibit growth.

From the regression equations, the authors were able to predict the percentage of salmonellae able to initiate growth in a culture or meat system of a certain pH value and/or brine concentration (Fig. 4.7).

The predictive type of experiments described above can be used as an aid in the development of minimum contamination or safety standards for high-risk foods (Genigeorgis et al. 1977). Of course, this could be accomplished much more readily for foods with standards of identity. In some cases, this might actually lessen the stringent safety standards imposed on foods. For example, 10^1 *Salmonella* organisms/g might be tolerated in a food product of pH 5.0 and 5.0% brine composition if this combination would predictably cause a three log reduction in bacterial numbers (see Fig. 4.7) by the time it reaches the consumer.

Using a different approach Broughall et al. (1983) developed mathematical models to describe the interactive effects of a_w and temperature on the growth kinetics of *S. typhimurium*. The overall observed and predicted values obtained were very similar (Fig. 4.8) although one atypical area of prediction

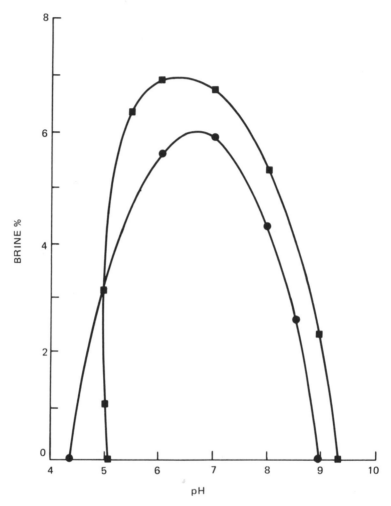

Fig. 4.7   Comparison of calculated combinations of pH and brine which will cause three log reductions to *Salmonella* populations inoculated in broths (●) and cooked meats (■). (*From Genigeorgis et al. 1977.*)

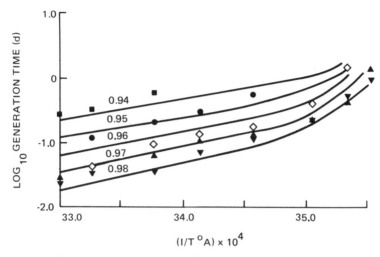

Fig. 4.8 Arrhenius plots of *Salmonella typhimurium* generation times. The lines show the predicted generation times of the model. The points represent experimental determinations at the following a_w values: ▼ 0.98; ▲ 0.97; ◇ 0.96; ● 0.95; ■ 0.94. (*From Broughall et al 1983.*)

occurred for lag times at low temperature i.e., at 8°C the predicted lag phase was longer at a_w 0.98 than at 0.97.

In agreement with current literature (Matches and Liston 1972b), the predicted minimum growth temperature for *S. typhimurium* was 6.0°C with a lag period of five to six days. As was shown for *S. aureus* (Broughall et al. 1983) the interactive effects of temperature and a_w were important in controlling the growth of *Salmonella,* with growth occurring at high temperatures at a_w values that restricted growth at lower temperatures. Subsequent models incorporated another variable into the mathematical equations which allowed the construction of three-dimensional models; these could be used to predict the combined effect of a_w, pH, plus temperature on the growth of *S. typhimurium* (Broughall and Brown 1984).

Because lag and exponential periods can be predicted separately by the models of Broughall and co-workers, it may be possible to use this information in Hazard Analysis Critical Control Point (HACCP) techniques applied to process and distribution chains with several time/temperature cycles (Broughall et al. 1983). This could lead to better applications of HACCP techniques, where traditionally the effects of various interaction parameters on the growth of microorganisms is neglected.

FOOD SPOILAGE

Besides the traditional biochemical approaches to predicting the shelf-life of foods (Ingram and Dainty 1971), attempts have been made to use mathematical methods to predict shelf stability.

Milk

Muir and Phillips (1984) predicted the shelf-life of refrigerated raw milk using generation time data and weighted-mean distribution curves for growth of psychotrophic bacteria in raw milk.

Data on bacterial generation times accumulated from over 150 individual milk samples stored at 4, 6, and 8°C, were used to construct distribution curves (generation times vs. % frequency of occurrence) (Fig. 4.9). Although there was a large variation in reported generation times at any one temperature, it was possible to assign a probability value to a particular rate of growth.

For example, if milk samples with an initial count of 2.5×10^5 CFU/mL were stored for 24 hr at 4, 6, and 8°C, the probability of the count exceeding the rejection level (5×10^6 CFU/mL) would be 3, 4, and 15%, respectively. The derivation of the rejection level was based on the author's work and other published data which demonstrated that changes in milk quality were detectable only when bacterial numbers exceeded 5×10^6 CFU/mL. The probability values were derived by initially calculating the apparent generation time, i.e.

$$\frac{0.301 \times \text{storage time [24 hr]}}{\log_{10} \text{(final count) } 6.7 - \log_{10} \text{(initial count)} 5.4} = 5.55 \text{ hr}$$

and then calculating the area under the distribution curve for this rate of growth (see Fig. 4.9). Additionally, a probability table was drawn up for three different storage periods (24, 48, and 72 hr), five initial bacterial levels and three temperatures (4, 6, and 8°C). Minor differences in storage temperature and initial microbial loads in milk were found to be very significant in terms of "safe" storage life.

As a rough approximation, the authors suggested that if there were a greater than 10% probability of raw milk reaching a rejection level (prior to manufacture) the milk should be rejected. The major disadvantage of the above method is that the initial bacterial count must be known.

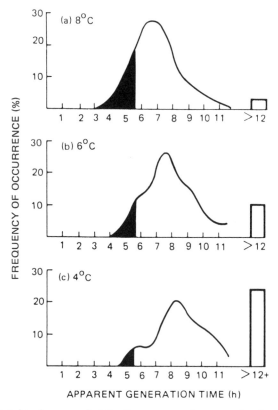

Fig. 4.9 Weighted-mean distribution curves for growth of psychrotrophic bacteria in raw milk. (*From Muir and Phillips 1984.*)

Meat

Rödel et al. (1976) demonstrated that limited growth or spoilage predictions can be made without any mathematical data evaluation. On the basis of published data and his own experimentation involving incubation of representative commercial meat products, he related microbial growth or no growth versus pH and water activity of nonsterile meats when the following minimal parameters were met; (a) $a_w \leq 0.95$ *and* pH ≤ 5.2, or (b) $a_w < 0.91$, or (c) pH < 5.0.

These limits were accepted in 1976 as EEC guidelines (Rödel and Leistner 1982), with the exception of a stricter pH limit of < 4.5 instead of < 5.0, apparently to ensure complete inhibition of *C. botulinum* under otherwise optimal conditions of growth.

Poultry. Daud et al. (1978) predicted the remaining shelf-life of poultry tissues by incorporating the general spoilage curve of Olley and Ratkowsky (1973) into an instrument called the temperature function integrator. This electronic-integrator device, which was originally developed by Nixon (1977) to assess storage conditions in fish-holds, can (a) give a read-out of equivalent days of spoilage at 0°C, and (b) predict the remaining shelf-life of the product at 0°C.

When the authors compared the relative growth rates (rate at temperature t/rate at 0°C) of spoilage bacteria in poultry predicted by the integrator with experimental values, there was close agreement between the two at storage temperatures up to 16°C. Above this temperature, significant deviations between the two values occurred.

Using available data from the literature on poultry spoilage, Pooni and Mead (1984) compared the general spoilage curve of Olley and Ratkowsky (1973) with a new model developed by Ratkowsky et al. (1982), to assess their potential in determining the shelf-life of nonfrozen poultry-meat products. Although the model proposed by Ratkowsky et al. (1982) appeared the most appropriate, there were still certain inadequacies in the method, the major one again being large deviations from the observed data at storage temperatures above 15°C.

A new model, however, described recently by Ratkowsky et al. (1983) appears to adequately describe the relationship between bacterial growth rate and temperature over a wide temperature range. A temperature function integrator incorporating this model into its circuitry would appear to have great potential for monitoring the residual shelf-life of chilled flesh foods which are temperature abused.

There remain problems, however, with this predictive method mainly because other functions which are important in determining the spoilage rate of flesh foods such as initial microbial loads and substrate differences within a food product are neglected.

Fish

Charm et al. (1972) developed a graphic method that correlated spoilage of fish at temperatures of 0–8°C and for periods up to the end of shelf-life, to the number of days of ice storage (0.6°C) that allowed the same degree of spoilage (Fig. 4.10). The graphs were obtained as follows:

1. Samples held at 1, 4, 6, and 8°C for various periods were evaluated by a trained panel for odor and given scores that expressed the equivalent number of days at 1°C.

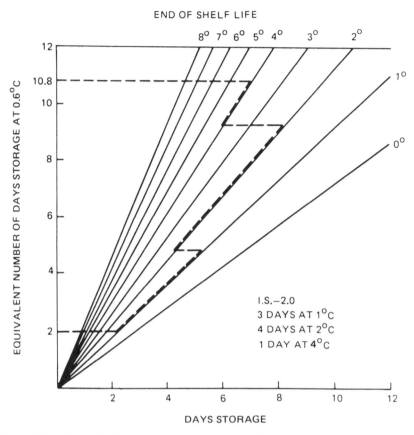

END OF SHELF LIFE

Fig. 4.10 Graphical method for estimating the final quality of cod fillets after storage under a given set of temperature conditions. Horizontal dotted lines represent change in storage temperature, and diagonal dotted lines represent number of days at the indicated temperatures. (*From Charm et al. 1972.*)

2. The rate constants K for spoilage at given temperatures were calculated as the average ratio of estimated storage at 1°C over the actual days of storage.

3. Rate constant values plotted against temperature indicated that fish spoilage occurred at a constant rate at any given temperature in the range of 1–8°C.

4. The resulting K values were plotted against K at 0.6°C (Fig. 4.10) to correlate the number of days at any temperature up to 8°C to the number of days on ice that would lead to the same degree of spoilage.

Final quality scores may also be calculated as

$$CS = IS + K_n T_n \qquad (9)$$

where CS = calculated score (days at 1°C); IS = initial score; K_n = rate constant for temperature n; T_n = number of days at temperature n.

If fish is stored at a number of different temperatures, then the scores can be calculated as:

$$CS = IS + \sum K_n T_n \qquad (10)$$

To assess the accuracy of the mathematical model, fish were stored at five different storage conditions (e.g., storage condition A—2 days at 1°C, 2 days at 4°C, and 3 days at 6°C) and predicted scores were compared with panel scores. Under all storage conditions, the predicted scores derived from the above formula were very similar to the actual panel scores.

An example of determining CS graphically is given in Fig. 4.10 (dotted lines), which also shows that the final score is independent of the order in which the temperature variations occur. Based on these data, Ronsivalli and Charm (1975) developed a "shelf-life prediction slide rule" which, by a series of simple operations, allows a rapid estimate of the remaining shelf-life of cod. The authors claim that the slide rule could be an effective predictor of storage shelf-life for most other varieties of lean fish as well, such as eviscerated whole haddock and haddock fillets.

In addition to the above graphical-type prediction methods, other investigators (James and Olley 1971; Olley and Ratkowsky 1973) have proposed models relating fish spoilage rate to temperature. Incorporation of these models into a temperature function integrator (see section on poultry) could provide a means for predicting the shelf-life of refrigerated fish, although newer models recently developed by Ratkowsky et al. (1982, 1983) appear more promising.

SUMMARY AND CONCLUSION

Recently, Roberts and Jarvis (1983) questioned the traditional approach of food microbiologists who perform experiments to determine the limits of microbial growth, usually varying only one parameter at a time, while holding all other parameters constant within an optimum range. The authors wondered whether we need a review of attitudes in food microbiology, and whether the area of predictive microbiology could be developed, thus supposedly eliminating the need for costly, duplicated, and often uncomparable experiments that try to define minima for growth.

Once accepted, predictive microbiology could be used to predict what would happen to foods as they pass through the distribution, retailing and domestic chain, and accumulated data banks might eventually eliminate the need for much of the routine food microbiological analyses that are carried on at present.

Roberts and Jarvis (1983) suggested that standardized systems be developed for computer compatible data acquisition, formatting, and storage in all areas of microbiology, and that possibly an international data bank be organized. The authors feel that with a coordinated research program of 5–10 years duration, enough data could be obtained to adequately predict the response of many food products to "normal" and abusive storage conditions, thus eliminating a large percentage of the "traditional" microbiology.

That this concept of data collection is feasible has already been demonstrated by IN FOODS, an international organization which has as its mandate the acquisition and exchange of standardized data on the nutrient composition of foods and beverages (Rand and Young 1984).

It has already been demonstrated that carefully controlled experiments in different labs can be used as data bases to predict microbial growth and/or toxin production in foods (Table 4.9). Although experiments using predictive modeling as a tool have many advantages over separate empirical experiments, there are certain limitations:

1. One should not extrapolate and make predictions beyond the limits of the experiment.

2. Experiments done in culture should not be used to predict growth and/or toxin production in food systems (Genigeorgis et al. 1971b; Raevuori and Genigeorgis 1975).

3. Definitive statements about an organism's ability to grow and/or produce toxin in a certain food environment cannot be made. Only a comment on the relative effects of treatment combinations can be made with certainty, since small changes in food production and/or formulation with a resultant increased or decreased probability of growth and/or toxin production can occur (Roberts et al. 1981c).

A panel of 30 experts in the area of food microbiology, using the Delphi technique of intuitive forecasting, predicted that the assessment of shelf-life by computer prediction (based upon the use of data banks of information on growth of spoilage organisms) had an 80% probability of being widely

Table 4.9 Probability of Toxin Production (%) by *Clostridium botulinum* Types A and B in Pasteurized Cured Meat Slurries[a]

Salt (% w/v)	NaNO$_2$ (μg/g)	Probability of toxin production after 6 months at 20°C: low heat process (L)[b]	
		MRI[c]	LFRA[d]
2.5	100	62	76
	200	16	34
	300	2	7
4.5	100	5	13
	200	1	2
	300	0	0

[a]From Roberts and Jarvis (1983). pH of pork slurry 5.5–6.3. Inoculum 10 spores per bottle (replicate).
[b]80°C for 7 min.
[c]Meat Research Institute data from Roberts et al. (1981c). Results rounded to the nearest whole number, i.e. '0' = < 0.49%.
[d]Leatherhead Food Research Association data from Jarvis and Robinson (1983). '0' = 'very much less than 1%'.

used by the year 1993. However, at least 25% of the panel were unconvinced that the predicted method could become acceptable even by the year 2001 (Jarvis 1983). It is really up to us as food microbiologists to decide whether or not we want to force the required changes in attitude that are necessary.

ACKNOWLEDGMENT

The author thanks S. Malcolm for his guidance in the statistical aspects of this paper. The valuable comments and advice of Dr. A. Hauschild were also greatly appreciated.

REFERENCES

AFIFI, A. A. and AZEN, P. S. 1979. *Statistical Analysis: A Computer Oriented Approach.* Academic Press, New York.
ANGELOTTI, R., FOSTER, M. J., and LEWIS, K. H. 1961. Time-temperature effects on salmonellae and staphylococci in foods. 1. Behaviour in

refrigerated foods. 2. Behaviour at warm holding temperatures. *Am. J. Public Health.* 51: 76–88.

BAIRD-PARKER, A. C. and FREAME, B. 1967. Combined effect of water activity, pH and temperature on the growth of *Clostridium botulinum* from spore and vegetative cell inocula. *J. Appl. Bacteriol.* 30: 420–429.

BROUGHALL, J. M., ANSLOW, P. A., and KILSBY, D. C. 1983. Hazard analysis applied to microbial growth in foods: Development of mathematical models describing the effect of water activity. *J. Appl. Bacteriol.* 55: 101–110.

BROUGHALL, J. M. and BROWN, C. 1984. Hazard analysis applied to microbial growth in foods: development and application of three-dimensional models to predict bacterial growth. *Food Microbiol.* 1: 13–22.

CENTER FOR DISEASE CONTROL. 1975. Staphylococcal food poisoning associated with dry salami. *Morbidity Mortality Weekly Report* 24: 374, 379.

CENTER FOR DISEASE CONTROL. 1979. Staphylococcal food poisoning associated with Genoa and hard salami. *Morbidity Mortality Weekly Report* 28: 179–180.

CHARM, S. E., LEARSON, R. J., RONSIVALLI, L. J., and SCHWARTZ, M. 1972. Organoleptic technique predicts refrigeration shelf-life of fish. *Food Technol.* 26: 65–68.

DANIEL, C. and WOOD, F. S. 1980. *Fitting Equations to Data.* Wiley, New York.

DAUD, H. B., McMEEKIN, T. A. and OLLEY, J. 1978. Temperature function integration and the development and metabolism of poultry spoilage bacteria. *Appl. Environ. Microbiol.* 36: 650–654.

DRAPER, N. and SMITH, H. 1981. *Applied Regression Analysis.* 2nd ed. John Wiley and Sons, Inc., New York.

GENIGEORGIS, C. A. 1981. Factors affecting the probability of growth of pathogenic microorganisms in foods. *J. Am. Vet. Med. Assoc.* 179: 1410–1417.

GENIGEORGIS, C., MARTIN, S., FRANTI, C. E., and RIEMANN, H. 1971a. Initiation of staphylococcal growth in laboratory media. *Appl. Microbiol.* 21: 934–939.

GENIGEORGIS, C., NYCHAS, A., and LOULLIS, C. 1977. Interaction of *Salmonella* with food environments. In *Proceedings*, 7th Int. Symp., World Assoc. Vet. Food Hygienists. Vol. I, pp. 269–274.

GENIGEORGIS, C., SAVOUKIDIS, M., and MARTIN, S. 1971b. Initiation of staphylococcal growth in processed meat environments. *Appl. Microbiol.* 21: 940–942.

GIBSON, A. M., ROBERTS, T. A., and ROBINSON, A. 1982. Factors controlling the growth of *Clostridium botulinum* types A and B in pasteurized cured meats. IV. The effect of pig breed, cut and batch of pork. *J. Food Technol.* 17: 471–482.

HALVORSON, H. O. and ZIEGLER, N. R. 1933. Application of statistics to problems in bacteriology. *J. Bacteriol.* 25: 101–121.

HAUSCHILD, A. H. W. 1982. Assessment of botulism hazards from cured meat products. *Food Technol.* 36(12): 95–104.

HIMMELBLAU, D. M. 1970. *Process Analysis by Statistical Methods.* John Wiley and Sons, Inc., New York.

INGRAM, M. and DAINTY, H. 1971. Changes caused by microbes in spoilage of meats. *J. Appl. Bacteriol.* 34: 21–39.

JAMES, D. G. and OLLEY, J. 1971. Spoilage of shark. *Aust. Fish.* 30: 11–14.

JARVIS, B. 1983. Food microbiology into the twenty-first century - a delphi forecast. In *Food Microbiology: Advances and Prospects.* T. A. Roberts and F. A. Skinner (Ed.). Academic Press, New York.

JARVIS, B. and PATEL, M. 1979. The occurrence and control of *Clostridium botulinum* in foods. *Leatherhead Fd. R.A. Res. Rep.* No. 686.

JARVIS, B. and ROBINSON, A. 1983. Predictive modeling of *Clostridium botulinum* toxin production in model cured meat systems. *Leatherhead Fd. R.A. Res. Rep.* No. 414.

LEISTNER, L. 1978. Microbiology of ready-to-serve foods. *Fleischwirtschaft* 58: 2008–2111.

LEISTNER, L. and RÖDEL, W. 1976. The stability of intermediate moisture foods with respect to micro-organisms. In *Intermediate Moisture Foods.* R. Davies, G. G. Birch, and J. K. Parker (Ed.). Applied Science Publishers Ltd., London.

MATCHES, J. R. and LISTON, J. 1972a. Effects of incubation temperature on the salt tolerance of *Salmonella. J. Milk Food Technol.* 35: 39–44.

MATCHES, J. R. and LISTON, J. 1972b. Effect of pH on low temperature growth of *Salmonella. J. Milk Food Technol.* 35: 49–52.

METAXOPOULOS, J., GENIGEORGIS, C., FANELLI, M. J., FRANTI, C., and COSMA, E. 1981a. Production of Italian dry salami I. Initiation of staphylococcal growth in salami under commercial manufacturing conditions. *J. Food Prot.* 44: 347–352.

METAXOPOULOS, J., GENIGEORGIS, C., FANELLI, M.J., FRANTI, C., and COSMA, E. 1981b. Production of Italian dry salami: Effect of starter culture and chemical acidulation on staphylococcal growth in salami under commercial manufacturing conditions. *Appl. Environ. Microbiol.* 42: 863–871.

MUIR, D. D. and PHILLIPS, J. D. 1984. Prediction of the shelf-life of raw milk during refrigerated storage. *Milchwissenschaft* 39: 7–11.

NDERU, F. M. K. and GENIGEORGIS, C. A. 1975. Prediction of sta-phyloccocal growth in cured meats. *Proc. 20th World Vet. Congr.* 1: 812–813.

NETER, J. and WASSERMAN, W. 1974. *Applied Linear Statistical Models*. Richard D. Irwin, Inc., Homewood, Illinois.

NIXON, P. A. 1977. Temperature function integrator. U.S. Patent 41,061,033.

OHYE, D. F. and CHRISTIAN, J. H. B. 1967. Combined effects of tem-perature, pH and water activity on growth and toxin production by *Clos-tridium botulinum* types A, B and E. In *Botulism*. M. Ingram and T.A. Roberts (Ed.). Chapman and Hall, London.

OLLEY, J. and RATKOWSKY, D. A. 1973. Temperature function inte-gration and its importance in the storage and distribution of flesh foods above the freezing point. *Food Technol. Aust.* 25: 66–73.

POONI, G. S. and MEAD, G. C. 1984. Prospective use of temperature function integration for predicting the shelf-life of non-frozen poultry-meat products. *Food Microbiol.* 1: 67–78.

RAEVUORI, M. and GENIGEORGIS, C. 1975. Effect of pH and sodium chloride on growth of *Bacillus cereus* in laboratory media and certain foods. *Appl. Microbiol.* 29: 68–73.

RAND, W. M. 1984. Development and analysis of empirical mathematical kinetic models pertinent to food processing and storage. In *Computer-Aided Techniques in Food Technology*. I. Saguy (Ed.). Marcel Dekker, Inc., New York.

RAND, W. M. and YOUNG, V. R. 1984. Report of a planning conference concerning an international network of food data systems (IN FOODS). *Am. J. Clin. Nutr.* 39: 144–151.

RATKOWSKY, D. A., LOWRY, R. K., McMEEKIN, T. A., STOKES, A. N., and CHANDLER, R. E. 1983. Model for bacterial culture growth rate throughout the entire biokinetic temperature range. *J. Bacteriol.* 154: 1222–1226.

RATKOWSKY, D. A., OLLEY, J., McMEEKIN, T. A., and BALL, A. 1982. Relationship between temperature and growth rate of bacterial cultures. *J. Bacteriol.* 149: 1–5.

RHODES, A. C. and JARVIS, B. 1976. A pork slurry system for studying inhibition of *Clostridium botulinum* by curing salts. *J. Food Technol.* 11: 13–23.

ROBACH, M. C. 1980. Interaction of salts, potassium sorbate and tem-perature on the outgrowth of *Clostridium sporogenes* PA 3679 spores in a pre-reduced medium. *J. Food Sci.* 45: 742–743.

ROBERTS, T. A., GIBSON, A. M., and ROBINSON, A. 1981a. Factors controlling the growth of *Clostridium botulinum* types A and B in pasteurized, cured meats. I. Growth in pork slurries prepared from 'low' pH meat (pH range 5.5–6.3). *J. Food Technol.* 16: 239–266.

ROBERTS, T. A., GIBSON, A. M., and ROBINSON, A. 1981b. Factors controlling the growth of *Clostridium botulinum* types A and B in pasteurized, cured meats. II. Growth in pork slurries prepared from 'high' pH meat (range 6.3–6.8). *J. Food Technol.* 16: 267–281.

ROBERTS, T. A., GIBSON, A. M., and ROBINSON, A. 1981c. Prediction of toxin production by *Clostridium botulinum* in pasteurized pork slurry. *J. Food Technol.* 16: 337–355.

ROBERTS, T. A., GIBSON, A. M., and ROBINSON, A. 1982. Factors controlling the growth of *Clostridium botulinum* types A and B in pasteurized, cured meats. III. The effect of potassium sorbate. *J. Food Technol.* 17: 307–326.

ROBERTS, T. A. and INGRAM, M. 1973. Inhibition of growth of *Cl. botulinum* at different pH values by sodium chloride and sodium nitrite. *J. Food Technol.* 8: 467–475.

ROBERTS, T. A. and JARVIS, B. 1983. Predictive modelling of food safety with particular reference to *Clostridium botulinum* in model cured meat systems. In *Food Microbiology: Advances and Prospects.* T.A. Roberts and F.A. Skinner (Ed.). Academic Press, New York.

ROBINSON, A., GIBSON, A. M., and ROBERTS, T. A. 1982. Factors controlling the growth of *Clostridium botulinum* types A and B in pasteurized, cured meats. V. Prediction of toxin production: Non-linear effects of storage temperature and salt concentration. *J. Food Technol.* 17: 727–744.

RÖDEL, W. and LEISTNER, L. 1982. Critical appraisal of shelf-life prediction of meat products on the basis of a_w and pH value. *Fleischwirtschaft* 62: 288–291.

RÖDEL, W., PONERT, H., and LEISTNER, L. 1976. Einstufung von Fleischerzeugnissen in leicht verderbliche, verderbliche und lagerfähige Produkte. Fleischwirtschaft 56: 417–418.

RONSIVALLI, L. J. and CHARM, S. E. 1975. Spoilage and shelf-life prediction of refrigerated fish. *Marine Fisheries Rev.* 37: 32–34.

YIP, B. and GENIGEORGIS, C. 1981. Interactions of *Clostridium perfringens* and certain curing factors in laboratory media. In *Proceedings.* World Congress of Foodborne Infections and Intoxications, Berlin 1980. Paul Parey Publishers.

5

Membrane Filtration Systems

Phyllis Entis

QA Laboratories Limited
Toronto, Ontario, Canada

INTRODUCTION

Membrane filters are available in a wide diversity of materials, pore structures, and pore sizes. Plastics used to manufacture them include cellulose derivatives (acetates, nitrates, and esters), polycarbonates, polysulfones, and polyvinyl chlorides, among others (Brock, 1983). Filters can be laminated or cast on nylon supports during manufacture to increase their strength. The microstructure of most membrane filters is "sponge-like" in appearance; some filters have straight cylindrical pores. Membrane filters are usually white, often imprinted with a counting grid, but black filters are also available.

This variety is in sharp contrast to the situation in 1922, when a U.S. Patent was issued to Zsigmondy for a method to produce a membrane filter (cited by Geldreich 1975). First nitrocellulose and then cellulose acetate membrane filters became available to researchers. In 1951, Goetz and Tsuneishi (1951) and Clark et al. (1951) reported independently on the use of membrane filters for microbiological analysis of water. The former group described in detail the properties of membrane filters (which they referred to as "molecular filter membranes"), and reported on microbiological detection and enumeration techniques they had devised using these filters. During the 1950's and early 1960's, McCarthy and his colleagues focused on water-related applications for membrane filters, principally relating to coliform enumeration procedures (McCarthy and Delaney 1958; McCarthy et al. 1961). Clark et al. (1957), Geldreich (1975), and Morgan et al. (1965) studied the performance of membrane filters, and sounded a few cautionary notes. Their concerns included sample size, statistically valid counting ranges, differential recognition of coliforms in the presence of noncoliforms, and problems with the coliform enumeration medium then in use (M-Endo broth). Also, researchers have detected and reported on manufacturer variations in bacterial recovery on membrane filters (Presswood and Brown 1973; Sogaard 1976).

Food microbiologists were also trying to make use of membrane filters. Nutting et al. (1959) attempted to adapt the coliform enumeration method used for water to the analysis of ice cream. They postulated, correctly, that membrane filtration would eliminate the problem of false positive coliform reactions resulting from the presence of sucrose in the product. In conventional cultural methods, sucrose contained in ice cream is introduced into the culture medium in high concentrations; consequently, sucrose-positive noncoliforms produce colonies resembling those produced by coliforms. Nutting et al. (1959) encountered several problems in applying this approach: fat globules impeded filtration; it was necessary to allow particles (e.g., fruit and nuts) to settle prior to analysis and the presence of stabilizers in the ice cream affected filtering performance. Chocolate ice cream presented additional problems due to the presence of large numbers of chocolate particles. Use of a surfactant (Triton X-100) increased the filterability of ice creams, with the exception of chocolate. An unsuccessful attempt was made to centrifuge chocolate ice cream in order to remove the particles. While Nutting et al. recovered coliforms quantitatively by the procedures outlined in their paper, the difficulties inherent in their approach appear to have discouraged their contemporaries from pursuing this method.

Kirkham and Hartman (1962) described a membrane filter method for detection and enumeration of *Salmonella* in egg albumen. They encountered many of the same difficulties as Nutting et al. and once again, despite an apparent success in recovering *Salmonella*, the method did not gain acceptance.

In general, three problems appear to have impeded the broad application of membrane filtration to food microbiology. Many foods are inherently difficult to filter through a 0.45μ membrane filter; food particles which collect on the filter during filtration can make accurate counting of colonies and interpretation of reactions difficult; and standard membrane filters have a very limited reliable counting range. With respect to this last factor, standard procedures (American Public Health Association, 1980) specify that for total coliform counts, only filters containing 20–80 colonies should be counted. In the case of fecal coliforms, the counting range is limited to 20–60 colonies. Even without the other problems, this limited counting range would make membrane filtration an impractical approach for many foods.

DIRECT MEMBRANE-SPREAD METHOD

In 1975, Anderson and Baird-Parker side-stepped the problem of food filtration by introducing another approach to using membrane filters for food analysis. They developed a method referred to as the "membrane-spread" technique. Their method entailed laying a membrane filter onto the surface of an agar plate and spread-plating the inoculum over the filter. Although this procedure forfeits many of the benefits usually associated with membrane filter methods, it does allow the inoculum to be moved from place to place without disturbance. In the application described by Anderson and Baird-Parker and modified by Holbrook et al. (1980), the filter is inoculated while resting on a nonselective agar and is left on that medium for several hours after inoculation to allow repair of injured cells. Then it is lifted off the medium, transferred to a selective agar medium for *E. coli*, namely Tryptone Bile agar, and incubated overnight at elevated temperature. Finally, the filter is removed from the selective medium and placed on filter paper which has been soaked in indole reagent. Typical *E. coli* biotype I colonies turn pink from the indole reaction and can be enumerated directly. This method has been subjected to an international comparative study under the auspices of the International Commission on Microbiological Specifications for Foods and is recognized as a valid method by that body (Rayman et al. 1979).

DIRECT EPIFLUORESCENT MICROSCOPY TECHNIQUE

One means of avoiding the problem of a limited counting range was reported by Pettipher et al. (1980), who described a direct microscopy technique using membrane filtration. In Direct Epifluorescent Microscopy (DEFT) a sample is filtered through a membrane filter, stained with a fluorescent dye, and examined microscopically. The number of fluorescing bacterial cells on the filter is determined and multiplied by the appropriate dilution factor to establish the count per gram or milliliter in the original sample. The principal advantage of this method is its speed. Since filters are not incubated for growth, counts can be obtained in under 30 min (Pettipher and Rodrigues, 1981), allowing rapid clearance, for example, of incoming raw milk shipments. DEFT-type methods have been developed for milks and creams (Pettipher and Rodrigues 1981), coastal surface films (Sewell et al. 1981), and determining yeast and bacteria levels in wineries (Cootes and Johnson 1980) and breweries (Day and Meyling 1983). The drawbacks to DEFT are two fold. Operator fatigue can be a significant factor in any microscopy, but is especially so in fluorescent microscopy, and particles can interfere with counting the bacterial cells. These problems probably were the source of poor repeatability and reproducibility of DEFT in a collaborative study conducted in six laboratories (Pettipher et al. 1983).

A semi-automated counting system for DEFT filters has been described (Pettipher and Rodrigues 1982a). While the authors noted that at low levels automated DEFT counts were higher than the corresponding manual counts, they postulated that this might be due to problems in discriminating between bacteria and small particles of stain or debris by the automated system. At higher counting levels, reasonable correlation was obtained between the manual and automated counts. Application of DEFT is limited to products with few, if any, particles and with counts in the range 6000–10,000,000 bacteria/g or mL (Pettipher et al. 1983). Differential or selective counts, such as coliforms, *E. coli*, etc., are not possible with this sytem.

HYDROPHOBIC GRID MEMBRANE FILTER

An elegant solution to the problem of limited counting range was found by Sharpe and Michaud (1974) with their invention of the hydrophobic grid membrane filter. They determined that certain nontoxic water repellant materials, such as some waxes, were capable of limiting physically the size and degree of spreading of bacterial colonies. The hydrophobic grid enabled the counting of up to 10^4 colonies on one filter (Sharpe and Michaud 1975a). A patent was issued on the hydrophobic grid membrane filter in 1975 (Sharpe and Michaud 1975b), and Sharpe and his colleagues explored some potential applications of HGMF, mainly in the realm of water microbiology (Sharpe and Michaud 1975a; Hendry and Sharpe 1975). While the HGMF enabled microbiologists to count a substantially larger number of colonies on a single membrane filter, "conventional wisdom" insisted that membrane filtration could not be applied successfully to food microbiology analyses. Sharpe and his various colleagues (Sharpe et al. 1978, 1979; Peterkin and Sharpe 1980;

Peterkin et al. 1982.) established otherwise. They surveyed a large variety of food homogenates prepared using conventional blenders and "Stomacher" and determined the filtration rates of these homogenates under controlled conditions. They found that many food homogenates could be filtered quite readily at levels consistent with current conventional limits of detection. Other foods could be filtered by using a surfactant, or an enzymatic digestion. Also, they determined that "Stomached" homogenates filtered more easily than those prepared by conventional blending. These reports rekindled the interest of food microbiologists in membrane filtration as an analytical tool.

A practical means of eliminating the problem of food particles was reported by Entis et al. (1982a). They investigated the use of a stainless steel woven wire cloth pre-filter as a means of eliminating particles from a homogenate immediately prior to filtration. Their initial work was carried out with a 10μm nominal pore size screen. Later, they validated a 5μm screen. They carred out aerobic plate counts on naturally contaminated food homogenates immediately before filtration through the screen and repeated the same counts on the filtrate. No significant differences were found between the homogenate and filtrate counts. The validity of this type of filtration was corroborated by Pettipher and Rodrigues (1982b), who used nylon (5μm) or stainless steel (4μm) mesh prefilters.

Since then, food microbiology applications of the hydrophobic grid membrane filter have been reported for aerobic plate count, yeast and mold, total coliforms, fecal coliforms, *E. coli*, *S. aureus*, *V. parahaemolyticus*, fecal streptococci, *Salmonella* and *Yersinia enterocolitica* (Entis et al. 1982b; Brodsky et al. 1982a, b; Entis and Boleszczuk 1983, 1984). In most of these applications, one or more of the properties of the HGMF have allowed a more rapid test result to be obtained. Several of these analyses have received "official" status (Association of Official Analytical Chemists 1984; Anon. 1985).

Salmonella

Developing a rapid, sensitive *Salmonella* detection method has long been a priority for food microbiologists. Published methods include fluorescent antibody (Silliker et al. 1966), enrichment serology (Banwart and Kreitzer 1969; Sperber and Deibel 1969), radiometry (Stewart et al. 1980), enzyme-linked immunosorbent assay (Robison et al. 1983), and DNA probe (Fitts et al., 1983). Entis et al. (1982b) described a semi-automated HGMF method for *Salmonella* that took advantage of the concentrating and colony-isolating properties of the HGMF. This method was further refined since the original publication and consists of the following steps (Entis, 1985):

1. Overnight pre-enrichment at 35°C.
2. Selective enrichment in tetrathionate brilliant green broth (TBG) at 35°C for 6 hr.
3. Filtration of 1 mL of TBG culture and incubation of the HGMF on selective agar for 24 hr.
4. Examination of the HGMF and subculture of suspicious colonies to biochemical screening media for overnight incubation.
5. Examination of biochemical reactions and performance of serology and any additional biochemical confirmation.

With this method, food samples that produce no suspicious colonies on the HGMF can be cleared within 48 hr from the time analysis is begun, with biochemical and serological screening results available within 72 hr of initiation. This time saving over conventional tests is due largely to the shortened selective enrichment step. The use of filtration instead of streak plating allows a significantly larger volume of TBG to be analyzed. This enables detection of lower levels of *Salmonella* in the medium and, therefore, a significantly shortened incubation period. Furthermore, the hydrophobic grid prevents other flora which might be present in the TBG from overgrowing the *Salmonella* colonies.

This rapid HGMF method can detect *Salmonella* at levels at least as low as one viable cell per 25g sample and is capable of detecting biochemically atypical strains. It has been validated in an AOAC collaborative study and found to be equivalent in sensitivity to the conventional cultural method (Entis 1985). Table 5.1 lists the serotypes used in the study, while the results have been summarized in Table 5.2. This method was adopted by the Association of Official Analytical Chemists (AOAC) as an Official First Action method in October, 1984 (Anon, 1985).

Escherichia coli

The HGMF method for enumerating this species has been adapted from Anderson and Baird-Parker's membrane spread procedure (*vide supra*). A resuscitation step is used routinely, followed by incubation on Tryptone Bile agar (TBA) at 44.5°C. At the end of a 24-hr incubation period, the HGMF is removed fromTBA and placed on filter paper which has been soaked with

Table 5.1 Salmonella Serotypes Used to Inoculate Collaborative Study Samples[a]

Sample no.	Serotype				
	Chocolate	Pepper	Cheese powder	Egg powder	Nonfat dry milk
1	S. infantis	S. st. paul	Control[b]	S. give[c]	S. montevideo
2	S. eastbourne	S. infantis	S. thompson	S. infantis	S. kentucky[d]
3	Control	Control	S. typhimurium	S. typhimurium	Control
4	S. infantis	S. typhimurium	S. enteritidis	S. hvittingfoss	S. typhimurium
5	S. chester	S. blockley	S. infantis	Control	S. infantis
6	S. typhimurium	Control	S. infantis	S. typhimurium	Control
7	S. haardt	S. cubana	Control	S. bareilly	S. infantis
8	S. typhimurium	S. typhimurium	S. arizonae	S. infantis	S. tennessee
9	Control	S. agona	S. typhimurium	Control	S. nevington
10	S. indiana	S. infantis	S. senftenberg	S. heidelberg	S. typhimurium

[a]Raw poultry samples were naturally contaminated.
[b]Uninoculated control sample.
[c]H_2S-negative strain.
[d]Lactose-positive strain.

Table 5.2 Comparison of *Salmonella* Detection by AOAC/BAM and HGMF Methods

| Product | No. of samples[a] | No. positive samples | | |
		AOAC/BAM	HGMF	Combined[b]
Chocolate	68	68	67	68
Raw poultry meat	150	131	133	138
Ground black pepper	84	56	57	61
Cheese powder	136	80	81	89
Whole egg powder	104	45	51	59
Nonfat dry milk	129	72	68	87

[a]Negative control samples excluded from statistical analysis.
[b]Reflects combined results of AOAC/BAM and HGMF methods (i.e., no. of samples positive by at least one method).

Table 5.3 Comparison of *Escherichia coli* Counts Obtained by AOAC 3-Tube MPN and HGMF Methods

| Food | Geometric mean MPN/g | |
	AOAC	HGMF
Fish	15	35
Poultry	24	96[a]
Walnuts	1.6	6.2[a]
Pepper	3.1	11[b]
Cheese	27	30

[a]Significantly higher than AOAC method (ANOVA; $P \le 0.05$).
[b]Significantly higher than AOAC method (ANOVA; $P \le 0.01$).

a modified indole reagent. *E. coli* biotype I colonies stain bright pink within 10–15 min at room temperature, and indole negative colonies are yellow to beige in color. The *E. coli* confirmation rate of indole positive colonies with this method is 97–99% (Entis 1984a). In an AOAC collaborative study (Entis 1984b), the HGMF method compared favorably with the conventional three-tube MPN procedure, as demonstrated by the data summarized in Table 5.3. The HGMF *E. coli* method is an AOAC Official Method (AOAC, 1984).

Total Coliforms

Coliforms are enumerated by incubating the HGMF on mFC agar without rosolic acid for 24 hr at 35°C. Lactose positive colonies are various shades of blue on the filter, and lactose negative colonies are yellow to beige. Confirmation rates of positive colonies on this medium approach 100% (Entis 1984a). AOAC collaborative studies of this HGMF procedure were carried out in 1982 (Entis 1983) and 1983 (Entis 1984b). The results of the latter study are summarized in Table 5.4. It is evident from these data that the HGMF procedure is at least equivalent in sensitivity to the conventional three-tube MPN method used as the reference procedure in this study. The HGMF coliform method is an Official Method of AOAC (AOAC, 1984).

Fecal Coliforms

This method is very similar to the total coliform procedure, except that a resuscitation step is employed prior to placing the filter onto mFC agar, and incubation is carried out at 44.5°C rather than 35°C. The confirmation rate for this test has been reported as 98% (Entis 1984a). The HGMF fecal coliform method has AOAC Official Method status (AOAC, 1984).

Aerobic Plate Count

This was one of the first reported food applications of HGMF (Brodsky et al. 1982a). Initially, the method consisted of preparing a food homogenate, diluting (if necessary), filtering through a pre-filter and HGMF and incubating

Table 5.4 Comparison of Coliform Counts Obtained by AOAC 3-Tube MPN and HGMF Methods

Food	Geometric mean MPN/g	
	AOAC	HGMF
Fish	39	45
Poultry	170	200
Walnuts	34	41
Pepper	3.8	63[a]
Cheese	76	55

[a]Significantly higher than AOAC method (ANOVA; $P \leq 0.01$).

the HGMF on Standard Plate Count (SPC) agar at 35°C for 48±3 hr. Colonies on the filter were visualized by removing the HGMF from the agar and floating it on a safranin solution. Colonies were stained red, providing good contrast against the nearly white filter. More recently, we have eliminated the staining step by incorporating a nontoxic dye, fast green FCF, into the culture medium at a concentration of 0.25 g/L and have replaced SPC agar with Tryptic Soy agar. The HGMF method using Tryptic Soy Fast Green (TSFG) agar performed equivalently to conventional pour plate methodology in our lab (see Table 5.5). A collaborative study sponsored by the AOAC is in progress.

Yeast and Mold Count

This HGMF method was also first described in 1982 (Brodsky et al. 1982a). Yeast and mold counts on HGMF were carried out in much the same way as the aerobic plate count, except that filters were incubated on antibiotic-supplemented Potato Dextrose agar (PDA) for 48 ± 3 hr at 25°C. Once again, safranin was used to stain the colonies. In 1984, Lin and Fung reported on the effect of various stains and dyes on the growth of yeast. One of these dyes, trypan blue, was among those found to have no toxic effect, and also was taken up by both yeasts and molds, resulting in blue colonies. Lin et al. (1984) compared counts obtained on HGMF incubated on PDA with and without trypan blue. Their work was carried out on naturally contaminated samples, and showed no significant differences between the two media. Comparisons have also been carried out between the conventional PDA pour plate method and the HGMF method using PDA with trypan blue (P. Hall, personal communication). Data from those comparisons are summarized in Table 5.6. An AOAC collaborative study is being planned for the HGMF yeast and mold method, and will likely take place in 1985.

LOOKING AHEAD

It is evident from the work reported to date that the hydrophobic grid membrane filter is a very versatile microbiological tool. In addition to the analyses mentioned above, methods are in the process of being developed in our laboratory for *Clostridium perfringens* and *Bacillus cereus*. Other possible applications could include *Lactobacillus*, *Campylobacter*, *Shigella*, or any other organism of interest to the food microbiologist.

The greatest potential extension of HGMF methodology, however, is in

Table 5.5 Comparison of Total Aerobic Count Obtained by Pour Plate and HGMF Methods

Product	Mean count/g or mL	
	Pour plate	HGMF
Raw milk	1.3×10^4	3.8×10^4
Fresh, raw ground beef	1.2×10^5	2.2×10^5
Fresh raw ground pork	6.9×10^5	2.6×10^6
Frozen, raw ground chicken	1.1×10^5	7.9×10^4
Instantized skim milk powder	1.0×10^3	9.2×10^2
Corn meal	6.8×10^2	1.0×10^3
Peanut butter	6.8×10^1	5.1×10^1
Fig paste	8.0×10^1	3.6×10^2
Ground black pepper	2.6×10^5	4.8×10^5
Nondairy coffee whitener	8.5×10^1	7.4×10^1
Paprika	9.7×10^5	8.8×10^5
Dark rye flour	1.3×10^5	2.3×10^5
Fresh mushrooms	1.3×10^6	8.3×10^5
Fresh bean sprouts	5.8×10^7	4.7×10^7
Long grain brown rice	3.9×10^3	2.8×10^3
Sunflower seeds	5.7×10^3	4.7×10^3
Pecan pieces	2.4×10^2	1.4×10^2
Fresh shrimp	5.0×10^5	5.1×10^5
Fresh oysters	1.1×10^3	2.7×10^3
Frozen beef pies	7.8×10^2	1.6×10^3
Part skim (2%) milk	7.6×10^3	1.0×10^4
Liquid whole egg	4.8×10^2	1.6×10^2
Whole egg powder	6.7×10^1	1.2×10^2
All purpose flour	4.2×10^2	4.1×10^2
Semi-sweet chocolate	1.2×10^5	1.0×10^5

the area of rapid confirmation. Peterkin and Sharpe (1984) developed an enzyme-linked immunosorbent assay to detect and enumerate enterotoxigenic *S. aureus* colonies on a membrane filter. Even more interesting is the potential use of DNA-DNA colony hybridization as a confirmation tool (Hill et al. 1983). If the volume of research being carried out in this area continues to accelerate at its present pace, current cultural and serological confirmation techniques could be largely replaced by genetic and/or immunological confirmation within a decade.

Table 5.6 Comparison of Yeast and Mold Counts Obtained by Pour Plate and HGMF Methods

	Geometric mean count/g	
Food	Pour plate[a]	HGMF[b]
Roquefort cheese	5.5×10^4	7.8×10^4
Corn meal	2.2×10^4	2.3×10^4
Ground black pepper	0.6×10^1	1.8×10^1
Mayonnaise	2.6×10^2	2.5×10^2
Ground coriander	1.7×10^4	2.1×10^4
Ground cinnamon	1.6×10^2	1.7×10^2
Ground nutmeg	3.4×10^1	3.8×10^1
Crushed red pepper	2.7×10^2	3.0×10^2
Active dried bakers yeast	3.7×10^9	3.7×10^9
Frozen orange juice	1.2×10^2	1.8×10^2

[a]Incubated 5 days at 25°C.
[b]Incubated 48 ± 3 hr at 25°C.

REFERENCES

ANDERSON, J. M. and BAIRD-PARKER, A. C. 1975. A rapid and direct plate method for enumerating *Escherichia coli* biotype I in food. *J. Appl. Bacteriol.* 39: 111–117.

ANON. 1985. *Salmonella* in foods. Hydrophobic grid membrane filter method. First action. In *Official Methods of Analysis*, 14th ed., First supplement. sec. 46.A06–46.A11. Association of Official Analytical Chemists, Arlington, VA.

AOAC. 1984. *Official Methods of Analysis*, 14th ed., sec.46.030–46.034. Association of Official Analytical Chemists, Arlington, VA.

APHA. 1980. *Standard Methods for the Examination of Water and Wastewater*, 15th ed. American Public Health Association, Washington, DC.

BANWART, G. J. and KREITZER, M. J. 1969. Rapid determination of *Salmonella* in samples of egg noodles, cake mixes, and candies. *Appl. Microbiol.* 18: 838–842.

BROCK, T. D. 1983. *Membrane Filtration: A User's Guide and Reference Manual.* Science Tech, Inc., Madison, WI.

BRODSKY, M. H., ENTIS, P., ENTIS, M. P., SHARPE, A. N., and JARVIS, G. A. 1982a. Determination of aerobic plate and yeast and mold counts in foods using an automated hydrophobic grid-membrane filter technique. *J. Food Prot.* 45: 301–304.

BRODSKY, M. H., ENTIS, P., SHARPE, A. N., and JARVIS, G. A. 1982b. Enumeration of indicator organisms in foods using the automated hydrophobic grid-membrane filter technique. *J. Food Prot.* 45: 292–296.

CLARK, H. F., GELDREICH, E. E., JETER, H. L., and KABLER, P. W. 1951. The membrane filter in sanitary bacteriology. *Pub. Health Rpts.* 66: 951–977.

CLARK, H. F., KABLER, P. W., and GELDREICH, E. E. 1957. Advantages and limitations of the membrane filter procedure. *Water and Sewage Works* 103: 385–387.

COOTES, R. L. and JOHNSON, R. 1980. A fluorescent staining technique for determination of viable and non-viable yeasts and bacteria in wineries. *Food Technol. Australia* 32: 522–524.

DAY, A. and MEYLING, J. C. 1983. Practical experience with rapid methods of detecting yeasts in breweries. *J. Inst. Brew.* 89: 204–206.

ENTIS, P. 1983. Enumeration of coliforms in nonfat dry milk and canned custard by hydrophobic grid membrane filter method: collaborative study. *J. Assoc. Off. Anal. Chem.* 66: 897–904.

ENTIS, P. 1984a. Enumeration of total coliforms, fecal coliforms, and *Escherichia coli* in foods by hydrophobic grid membrane filter: supplementary report. *J. Assoc. Off. Anal. Chem.* 67: 811–812.

ENTIS, P. 1984b. Enumeration of total coliforms, fecal coliforms, and *Escherichia coli* in foods by hydrophobic grid membrane filter: collaborative study. *J. Assoc. Off. Anal. Chem.* 67: 812–823.

ENTIS, P. 1985. Rapid hydrophobic grid membrane filter method for *Salmonella* detection in selected foods. Collaborative study. *J. Assoc. Off. Anal. Chem.* 68: 555–564.

ENTIS, P. and BOLESZCZUK, P. 1983. Overnight enumeration of *Vibrio parahaemolyticus* in seafood by hydrophobic grid membrane filtration. *J. Food Prot.* 46: 783–786.

ENTIS, P. and BOLESZCZUK, P. 1984. Rapid detection of *Yersinia enterocolitica* in dairy products by hydrophobic grid membrane filter. Presented at the 44th Annual Meeting of the Institute of Food Technologists, Anaheim, CA.

ENTIS, P., BRODSKY, M. H., and SHARPE, A. N. 1982a. Effect of prefiltration and enzyme treatment on membrane filtration of foods. *J. Food Prot.* 45: 8–11.

ENTIS, P., BRODSKY, M. H., SHARPE, A. N., and JARVIS, G. A. 1982b. Rapid detection of *Salmonella* spp. in food by use of the ISO-GRID hydrophobic grid membrane filter. *Appl. Environ. Microbiol.* 43: 261–268.

FITTS, R., DIAMOND, M., HAMILTON, C., and NERI, M. 1983. DNA-DNA hybridization assay for detection of *Salmonella* spp. in foods. *Appl. Environ. Microbiol.* 46: 1146–1151.

GELDREICH, E. E. 1975. Performance variability of membrane filter procedures. Presented at the Conference of Public Health Laboratory Directors, Chicago, IL.

GOETZ, A. and TSUNEISHI, N. 1951. Application of molecular filter membranes to the bacteriological analysis of water. *J. Amer. Water Works Assoc.* 43: 943–969.

HENDRY, G. S. and SHARPE, A. N. 1975. Superior performance of hydrophobic grid membrane filters for membrane total coliform determinations of recreational lake waters. Presented at the 43rd Annual Meeting of the Canadian Public Health Association, Toronto, Ontario, Canada.

HILL, W. E., PAYNE, W. L., and AULISIO, C. C. G. 1983. Detection and enumeration of virulent *Yersinia enterocolitica* in food by DNA colony hybridization. *Appl. Environ. Microbiol.* 46: 636–641.

HOLBROOK, R., ANDERSON, J. M., and BAIRD-PARKER, A. C. 1980. Modified direct plate method for counting *Escherichia coli* in foods. *Food Technol. Austral.* 32: 78–83.

KIRKHAM, W. K. and HARTMAN, P. A. 1962. Membrane filter methods for the detection and enumeration of *Salmonella* in egg albumen. *Poultry Sci* 41: 1082–1088.

LIN, C. C. S. and FUNG, D. Y. C. 1984. Effect of dyes on the growth of food yeasts. Presented at the 44th Annual Meeting of the Institute of Food Technologists, Anaheim, CA.

LIN, C. C. S., FUNG, D. Y. C., and ENTIS, P. 1984. Growth of yeast and mold on trypan blue agar in conjunction with the ISO-GRID system. *Can. J. Microbiol.* 30: 1405–1407.

McCARTHY, J. A. and DELANEY, J. E. 1958. Membrane filter media studies. *Water and Sewage Works* 104: 292–296.

McCARTHY, J. A., DELANEY, J. E., and GRASSO, R. J. 1961. Measuring coliforms in water. *Water and Sewage Works* 107: 238–243.

MORGAN, G. B., GUBBINS, P., and MORGAN, V. 1965. A critical appraisal of the membrane filter technique. *Health Lab. Sciences* 2: 227–237.

NUTTING, L. A., LOMOT, P. C., and BARBER, F. W. 1959. Estimation of coliform bacteria in ice cream by use of the membrane filter. *Appl. Microbiol.* 7: 196–199.

PETERKIN, P. I. and SHARPE, A. N. 1980. Membrane filtration of dairy products for microbiological analysis. *Appl. Environ. Microbiol.* 39: 1138–1143.

PETERKIN, P. I. and SHARPE, A. N. 1984. Rapid enumeration of *Staphylococcus aureus* in foods by direct demonstration of enterotoxigenic colonies on membrane filters by enzyme immunoassay. *Appl. Environ. Microbiol.* 47: 1047–1053.

PETERKIN, P. I., SHARPE, A. N., and WARBURTON, D. W. 1982. Inexpensive treatment of frozen dairy products for membrane filtration. *Appl. Environ. Microbiol.* 43: 486–487.

PETTIPHER, G. L., FULFORD, R. J., and MABBITT, L. A. 1983. Collaborative trial of the direct epifluorescent filter technique (DEFT), a rapid method for counting bacteria in milk. *J. Appl. Bacteriol.* 54: 177–182.

PETTIPHER, G. L., MANSELL, R., MCKINNON, C. H., and COUSINS, C. M. 1980. Rapid membrane filtration-epifluorescent microscopy technique for direct enumeration of bacteria in raw milk. *Appl. Environ. Microbiol.* 39: 423–429.

PETTIPHER, G. L. and RODRIGUES, U. M. 1981. Rapid enumeration of bacteria in heat-treated milk and milk products using a membrane filtration-epifluorescent microscopy technique. *J. Appl. Bacteriol.* 50: 157–166.

PETTIPHER, G. L. and RODRIGUES, U. M. 1982a. Semi-automated counting of bacteria and somatic cells in milk using epifluorescence microscopy and television image analysis. *J. Appl. Bacteriol.* 53: 323–329.

PETTIPHER, G. L., and RODRIGUES, U. M. 1982b. Rapid enumeration of microorganisms in foods by the direct epifluorescent filter technique. *Appl. Environ. Microbiol.* 44: 809–813.

PRESSWOOD, W. G. and BROWN, L. R. 1973. Comparison of Gelman and Millipore membrane filters for enumerating fecal coliform bacteria. *Appl. Microbiol.* 26: 332–336.

RAYMAN, M. K., JARVIS, G. A., DAVIDSON, C. M., LONG, S., ALLEN, J. M., TONG, T., DODSWORTH, P., McLAUGHLIN, S., GREENBERG, S., SHAW, B. G., BECKERS, H. J., QVIST, S., NOTTINGHAM, P. M., and STEWART, B. J. 1979. ICMSF methods studies. XIII. An international comparative study of the MPN procedure and the Anderson-Baird-Parker direct plating method for the enumeration of *Escherichia coli* biotype I in raw meats. *Can. J. Microbiol.* 25: 1321–1327.

ROBISON, B. J., PRETZMAN, C. I., and MATTINGLY, J. A. 1983. Enzyme immunoassay in which a myeloma protein is used for detection of salmonellae. *Appl. Environ. Microbiol.* 45: 1816–1821.

SEWELL, L. M., BITTON, G., and BAYS, J. S. 1981. Evaluation of membrane adsorption-epifluorescent microscopy for the enumeration of bacteria in coastal surface films. *Microb. Ecol.* 7: 365–369.

SHARPE, A. N., DIOTTE, M. P., DUDAS, I., and MICHAUD, G. L. 1978. Automated food microbiology: potential for the hydrophobic grid-membrane filter. *Appl. Environ. Microbiol.* 36: 76–80.

SHARPE, A. N. and MICHAUD, G. L. 1974. Hydrophobic grid-membrane filters: new approach to microbiological enumeration. *Appl. Microbiol.* 28: 223–225.

SHARPE, A. N. and MICHAUD, G. L. 1975a. Enumeration of high numbers of bacteria using hydrophobic grid-membrane filters. *Appl. Microbiol.* 30: 519–524.

SHARPE, A. N. and MICHAUD, G. L. 1975b. Apparatus for enumerating microorganisms. U.S. Patent 3,929,583. Dec. 30

SHARPE, A. N., PETERKIN, P. I., and DUDAS, I. 1979. Membrane filtration of food suspensions. *Appl. Environ. Microbiol.* 37: 21–35.

SILLIKER, J. H., SCHMALL, A., and CHIU, J. Y. 1966. The fluorescent antibody technique as a means of detecting salmonellae in foods. *J. Food Sci.* 31: 240–244.

SOGAARD, H. 1976. A comparison of Seitz and Millipore membrane filters for the enumeration of fecal coliforms. *Acta Vet. Scand.* 17: 25–31.

SPERBER, W. H. and DEIBEL, R. H. 1969. Accelerated procedure for *Salmonella* detection in dried foods and feeds involving only broth cultures and serological reactions. *Appl. Microbiol.* 17: 533–539.

STEWART, B. J., EYLES, M. J., and MURRELL, W. G. 1980. Rapid radiometric method for detection of *Salmonella* in foods. *Appl. Environ. Microbiol.* 40: 223–230.

ZSIGMONDY, R. 1922. *Cited by* Geldreich, E.E. (1975). U.S.Patent 1,421,341. June 27.

NOTE ADDED IN PROOF: The HGMF aerobic plate count method was adapted as an Official Method of AOAC in October, 1985.

6

Plating Systems

Samuel Schalkowsky

Spiral System Instruments, Inc.
Bethesda, Maryland

INTRODUCTION

The use of nutrient gel plates for the observation of the presence and features of microorganisms dates back to the early days of microbiology. The important role which such plating methods have played, and continue to play, can be attributed to the fact that (1) they provide a *direct* means for enumerating viable bacteria; (2) they allow for a distinction between the original bacterium deposited onto the plate—as represented by the presence of a colony—and subsequent progeny in the colony; (3) they allow for indirect observation of bacterial growth rate by virtue of change in colony size; and (4) they provide a visual means for observing distinguishing features of different types of bacterial colonies.

The following describes advances in the utilization of plating systems deriving from the spiral plating method.

SPIRAL PLATING FOR BACTERIAL ENUMERATION

The spiral plater was developed at the Bureau of Foods of the U.S. Food and Drug Administration in the early 1970's (Gilchrist et al. 1973). This development addressed the inefficiency of bacterial enumeration based on serial dilutions of the sample. Typically, three (or more) such dilutions are used to prepare pour plates or spread plates. But after incubation, only plates for one dilution would be retained for a colony count since the others will either be too crowded or contain too few colonies for a reliable count. There is thus considerable waste—in analyst time, materials, and laboratory space—associated with such standard enumeration methods. The spiral plating method provides the desired result by using only one 10 cm petri dish to cover about three decades of bacterial concentrations.

Pre-poured agar plates are used for the spiral plating method. The liquid sample is deposited on the agar surface in a controlled manner such that variable amounts of sample volume in different regions of the plate, although quite small, are known with accuracy and are highly repeatable from plate to plate.

A spiral plater is shown in Fig. 6.1 while Fig. 6.2 shows the plater mechanism. To operate the spiral plater, the liquid sample is drawn in by vacuum through a stylus into a hollow plunger syringe. Opening or closing a valve above the plunger controls the filling procedure. Normally, the stylus tubing and syringe would first be completely filled with sterile water. The stylus is then lowered into a 5 mL cup containing the sample and the valve opened and quickly closed so as to limit the amount of sample drawn into the stylus tubing. This procedure, aside from being frugal with the use of sample, is particularly desirable when dealing with materials containing particulate matter—a frequent occurrence when testing food products. Thus, the sample is allowed to stand for a few minutes to allow the heavier particulates to settle and produce a small region of supernatant. Placing the stylus just below the surface and drawing in the few drops needed for plating, usually avoids the inclusion of particulates.

The pre-poured agar plate is placed on the turntable, the stylus lowered so its tip rests freely on the surface, and the start switch pressed to initiate two simultaneous actions: (1) the turntable rotates and the carriage holding the stylus assembly moves radially away from the center so that a spiral path is generated by the stylus on the surface of the agar, and (2) the cam follower mechanism, which controls the rate at which the sample is expelled from the syringe, varies the amount deposited on the agar surface. The shape of the cam is such that a large volume is expelled first (near the center of

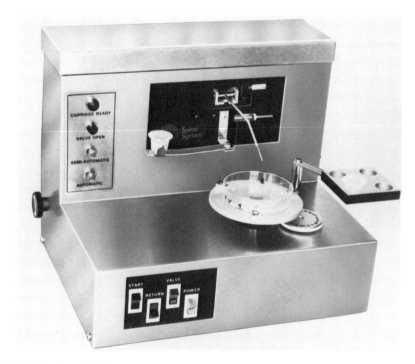

FIG. 6.1 Spiral plater.

the plate), decreasing logarithmically along the spiral path as it progresses toward the outside of the plate.

After incubation, colonies appear along the track made by the deposited sample with spacing between colonies increasing toward the outer region of the plate. Figure 6.3 shows a set of spiral plates prepared from serial dilutions of a mixed culture. The plate marked with the number 2 represents a concentration of about 200,000 CFU/mL, which is near the practical upper bound for accurate counting (a higher concentration would be countable if the colonies were smaller). Since the entire plate is counted for low bacterial numbers, the lower bound is a function of the minimum number of colonies needed to stay within the desired limits of statistical variability.

Enumeration is done by placing the plate over the pie-shaped grid illustrated in Fig 6.4, and counting the colonies in the sectors of the pie, starting with the outermost one and continuing until at least 20 colonies have been counted. The sector containing the twentieth colony is fully counted. Then the same sectors in the opposite side are also counted to average out nonuniformities in the plating and counting procedure. (The second count

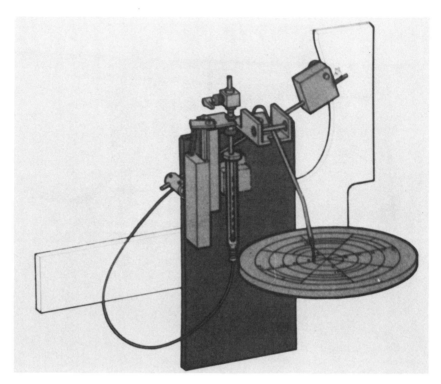

FIG. 6.2   Spiral plating mechanism.

represents, in effect, a replicate.) The total count is divided by the known volume of liquid deposited in the counted sectors, to provide the CFU/mL of the plated sample.

The spiral plating method has been evaluated for a wide range of applications (Donnelly et al. 1976; Gilchrist et al. 1977; Peeler et al. 1977; Jarvis et al. 1977; Hedges et al. 1978; Zipkes et al. 1981). It is an approved AOAC method (Association of Official Analytical Chemists 1984) and is a recommended APHA alternate to the standard plate count method (American Public Health Association 1978). It is also included in the FDA *Bacteriological Analytical Manual* (Food and Drug Administration 1984).

The spiral plater was first introduced commercially in late 1976. Since then spiral plating has gained worldwide recognition as an effective and economical method for performing direct bacterial enumeration. It also allows for more extensive testing in situations which otherwise would be too costly or impractical, e.g., enumeration on differential media or for extended challenge tests.

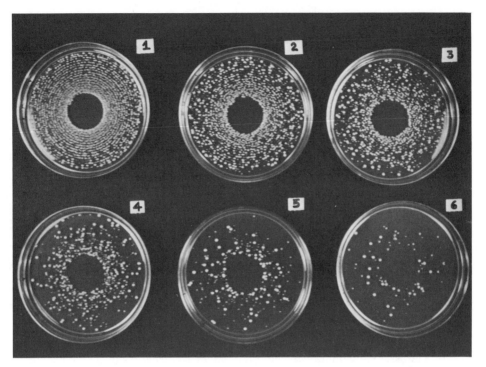

FIG. 6.3 Spiral plates prepared from serial dilutions of a mixed culture.

COMPUTER-ASSISTED PLATE COUNTS

The manual counting of colonies on agar plates—whether pour plates or spiral plates—is a tedious activity and therefore subject to fatigue errors when more than a few plates are counted on a routine basis. Automatic colony counters seek to overcome this problem but, while not subject to tedium errors, have their own limitations. Thus, they are generally unable to distinguish between colonies on the one hand, and air bubbles, particulate matter or agar imperfections, on the other (Brodsky et al. 1979; Devenish et al. 1984). Furthermore, the optical scanners used in automatic colony counters can count as one colony two or more colonies which are overlapping. Attempts to correct for these missed counts by applying an experimentally determined factor are of questionable value since the error is a function not only of the number counted but also of their size; however, the correction is generally made only on the basis of numbers (Brodsky et al. 1979).

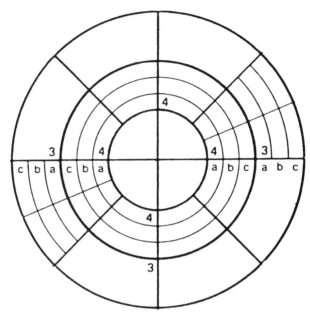

FIG. 6.4   Grid for counting 10-cm spiral plates.

The essentially unlimited computational capacity currently available with low cost, high speed microprocessors offers an opportunity to surmount automatic colony counter deficiencies and to seek not only to match manual counting performance but, preferably, to improve on it both in terms of reliability as well as accuracy. CASBA™, an acronym for Computer Assisted Spiral Bio-Assay, represents such a development (patent pending).

CASBA utilizes the laser scanner of Fig. 6.5 to transfer 2,000 sets of data from a 4 sec, spiral scan of the plate into the dedicated CASBA microprocessor shown in Fig. 6.6. The CASBA Enumeration Program, which operates on the above data, will complete a comprehensive analysis of the plate in less than 10 sec.

CASBA Enumeration Program

Plate analysis follows the spiral path produced by the plater, starting from the outside and progressing towards the center. The unit for analysis is a quarter of a spiral track, to be referred to as a segment. Typically, 50 such segments will be available for analysis on a standard 10 cm plate.

The first question addressed by the program in evaluating segment data is the validity of the colony count reported by the scanner for the segment.

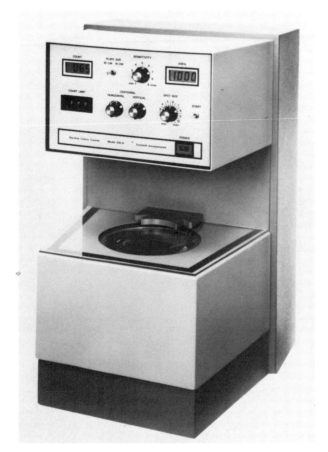

FIG. 6.5   Laser-beam scanner.

This is done by means of a model which predicts the number of missed counts on the basis of colony density and average colony size in the segment. The reported colony count is corrected accordingly. However, if the correction exceeds a reliable limit (when the number missed is about equal to the number counted), the segment is rejected from participation in subsequent analyses.

The second level of analysis utilizes a group of eight segments, denoted as a subsample. If most of the segments in the first, outer subsample of the plate were rejected because of excessive count correction, the entire plate is judged to be not countable and reported as such. Otherwise, analysis of the subsample proceeds to evaluate segment acceptability on the basis of (1) mean colony size and (2) their statistical distribution.

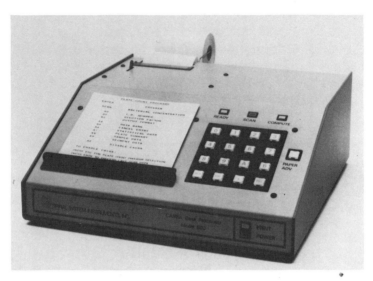

FIG. 6.6   CASBA data processor.

Segment qualification for mean colony size is intended to exclude segments which contain size anomalies, such as spreaders. It is accomplished by rejecting segments whose average colony size is significantly different from the average size of all the colonies in the subsample.

Segments of the subsample which survived the count correction and size qualifications procedures are subjected to an additional test intended to detect a wide range of anomalies, such as air bubbles or numerous particles. The basis for discriminating between colonies and such extraneous matter is the fact that colonies tend to follow a Poisson frequency distribution along spiral track lengths containing equal sample volumes, while extraneous matter is likely to produce deviations from such a Poisson distribution. The coefficient of variation is used as a measure of distribution, with that predicted for a Poisson distribution serving as a criterion of acceptability of segments within a subsample. Specifically, the coefficient of variation is computed with and without the individual segments being evaluated and the result used to reject the segments if it causes a deviation from the Poisson value. The final ratio of actual to Poisson coefficients of variation is used as a measure of "distributional quality" and retained for subsequent trade-off analysis.

An estimate of the sample CFU/mL is made from (1) the corrected colony count in the qualified segments of the subsample and (2) the known volume of sample deposited in these segments. The analysis then proceeds to the next subsample on the plate.

The final decision to be made by the program is how to best utilize the consecutive subsample estimates of bacterial concentration. The strategy implemented in the current bacterial enumeration program—considering sampling errors, counting accuracy, and bacterial crowding effects—selects among subsample results on the basis of their distribution quality and stops the analysis when a preset minimum number (about 300) of colonies has been used in qualified segments.

The CASBA enumeration program applies to spiral plates as well as to pour plates or spread plates; the difference is that, for spiral plates, the program expects variable colony densities corresponding to the logarthmically changing sample volumes as deposited by the plater, while for pour or spread plates it assumes sample distribution to be uniform. Illustrative performance data for spiral plates and pour plates follows.

CASBA Enumeration of Spiral Plates

The plates of Fig. 6.3 represent one set of serial dilutions of a mixed culture used to evaluate CASBA performance. Results are summarized in Table 6.1 in which hand counts and CASBA counts are the means of three replicate plates at each dilution.

A linear regression analysis of the above data yields a correlation coefficient of 0.995 for the hand count referred to the true count; 0.993 for the CASBA count referred to the true count; and 0.999 for the CASBA count referred to the hand count. Coefficients of variation computed for the three

Table 6.1 Comparison of Manual and CASBA Estimation of the CFU/mL of a Spirally Plated Mixed Culture

Dilution no.	True value[a]	Manual count[b]	CASBA count
2	184,000	154,000	139,000
3	61,300	66,100	62,300
4	20,400	19,100	22,300
5	6,810	7,050	8,010
6	2,270	2,270	2,240
7	757	667	629

[a]Values obtained by multiplying the manual count of dilution no. 6 (the anchor point)—where sampling and counting errors are expected to be small—by the appropriate dilution factor.
[b]Count determined with the manual grid system.

replicates in each dilution ranged from about 3–17% for hand counting and from 1–18% for the CASBA counts. For mixed cultures, but in the absence of major anomalies, CASBA performance is thus comparable to hand counting of spiral plates.

CASBA ability to cope with the presence of size anomalies, e.g. spreaders or molds, is illustrated by data from four replicate plates of a skim milk sample. Two of the spiral plates contained molds. Four replicate pour plates were also prepared from the same skim milk sample. Hand count results of the four pour plates were 14,600, 15,600, 14,000 and 14,000 CFU/mL (coefficient of variation = 5.2%). The CASBA counts of the two spiral plates without size anomalies gave 13,600 and 12,500 CFU/mL while with the molds the result was 15,500 and 12,800 CFU/mL (coefficient of variation for all four plates of 9.9%). The mean CFU/mL of 13,600 for the four CASBA counts of the spiral plates compares well with a mean CFU/mL of 14,600 obtained from the four replicate pour plates, illustrating the ability of CASBA to effectively exclude regions of the plate containing spreaders.

CASBA Enumeration of Pour Plates

Test data provided below is derived from routine raw milk samples of a large East Coast dairy. The plates were prepared and manually counted by personnel of the dairy laboratory in accordance with *Standard Methods* guide lines (APHA 1978). CASBA counts were made either at the dairy—by dairy personnel—or at the author's facility, or both.

Table 6.2 summarizes manual and CASBA assays of plates obtained from sequential twofold dilutions of two raw milk samples. (Only plates having a total count in the range of about 30–400 are included.)

CASBA estimates the total plate count from a selected portion of the plate. This also applies to manual counting for pour plates having more than 300 colonies, for which *Standard Methods* also prescribes the counting of only a portion of the plate. However, in the latter case, *Standard Methods* considers the result to be an "estimate" (APHA 1978).

A linear regression analysis of all the data in Table 6.2 yields a correlation coefficient of 0.996 for manual counts referred to the true values; 0.993 for CASBA counts referred to true values; and 0.997 for CASBA counts referred to manual counting. Thus, in the presence of anomalies normally encountered in raw milk plates, CASBA produces satisfactory results, comparable to those obtained by the analyst who counted the same plates.

For the range of total plate counts considered in additional studies, the dilution and crowding errors are relatively small (Wilson 1935). The coefficients of variation illustrated in Fig. 6.7 therefore represent, essentially, the

Table 6.2 Manual and CASBA Estimation of the Plate Count (CFU/mL) of Raw Milk Duplicate Pour Plates

Sample no.	Dilution no.	True value[a]	Replicate A		Replicate B	
			Manual count	CASBA count	Manual count	CASBA count
88	1	412	387	398	422	424
88	2	206[c]	212	212	189	212
88	3	103	(54	65)[d]	123	112
88	4	52	53	44[b]	42	42[b]
88	5	26	34	31[b]	39	38[b]
806	3	386	380	402	379	401
806	4	193[c]	201	184	194	192
806	5	96	113	124	116	134
806	6	48	73	91	71	85
806	7	24	25	22[b]	40	37[b]

[a]See footnote a, Table 6.1.
[b]Number of colonies on plate too small for segment qualification: CASBA reports total based on scanner count only.
[c]Anchor point used to obtain true values from multiplication by appropriate dilution factor.
[d]Excluded from linear regression analysis—apparent dilution error.

overall assay accuracy, reflecting the combined effect of sampling and counting errors. The solid curve in Fig. 6.7 represents the theoretical (Poisson) sampling error (given by the inverse of the square root of the mean count): it is the best accuracy obtainable with zero counting errors. As shown in Fig. 6.7, the overall assay accuracy of the CASBA counts is about the same as that of the analyst who manually counted these plates.

SPIRAL PLATING FOR ANTIMICROBIAL INTERACTION TESTING

The spiral plater has been used to evaluate interactions between bacteria and mutagenic substances by observing the change in numbers of colonies at different concentrations of the mutagenic substance deposited by the plater (Couse and King 1982; deFlora 1981). Its use to study the effect of one bacterial population on the viability of another was reported by Shelaih et

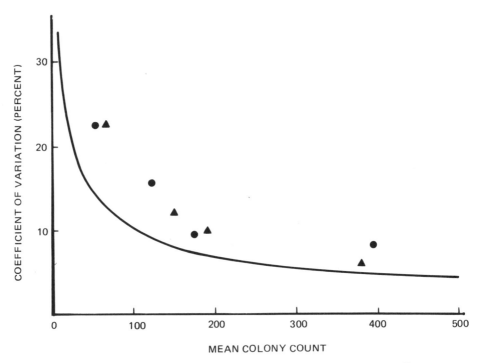

FIG. 6.7   Percent error in manual and CASBA counts of raw milk pour plates: ● manual; ▲ CASBA. Solid curve is theoretical (Poisson) sampling error.

al. (1985) and Gamay et al. (1984). The spiral gradient antimicrobial inter-action test is an alternative to broth dilution, agar dilution, or spot diffusion tests used to evaluate the inhibiting effect of antimicrobial agents on the growth of bacterial populations. It is simple to perform and allows for the testing of many different strains against an antimicrobial agent using one petri dish. The spiral gradient test provides greater sensitivity in the quan-titative determination of an MIC (Minimum Inhibitory Concentration) end-point and allows for the qualitative discrimination between biocidal and biostatic interactions.

For this application, a stock solution of the antimicrobial agent is deposited by the spiral plater to produce a radial gradient of concentrations in the agar, increasing from the outside to the center. (Fifteen centimeter petri dishes are preferable for this purpose to provide a larger range of test con-centrations.) After a few hours, a uniform vertical concentration is estab-lished. However, because the difference in antimicrobic concentrations between adjacent spirals is small, there is relatively little radial diffusion over the test interval. The desired radial gradient is retained with minor change, except near the center and outer edge where diffusion takes place into the regions where the antimicrobial was not deposited. Because of the latter effect the maximum available gradient of about 1:600—determined by the volumetric deposition rates of the plater—is reduced to a useable range of about 1:300 over a radial distance of about 42 mm (Schalkowsky et al. 1985). The volume of stock solution deposited at any location on the plate (microliters per square millimeter of surface area) is known. This quantity divided by the agar height (in mm) is a dimensionless number (since a microliter is approximately one cubic millimeter) which, when multiplied by the concentration of anti-microbic in the stock solution, yields the concentration in the agar at the selected location.

The bacterial suspension is deposited onto the surface of the agar by means of a sterile swab to produce a radial streak starting at the outer edge and ending at a radial distance of about 20 mm from the center. After incubation there will be growth in the outer region where the concentration of the antimicrobic is not high enough to inhibit it. This is illustrated in Fig. 6.8, in which the plate was photographed over a circular grid with 5 mm separations between circles.

Typical broth or agar dilution tests use twofold dilutions, which represents a sensitivity of ±100%. Reproducibility between laboratories with standard strains is exemplified by the fourfold range between the high and low values (plus or minus one twofold dilution) given by the NCCLS for the agar dilution method (National Committee for Clinical Laboratory Standards, 1983). The spiral gradient endpoint test offers greater sensitivity primarily because antimicrobic concentrations are known directly and continuously, rather than incrementally. To benefit from this greater sensitivity, it is necessary to define the transition between growth and no-growth in more detail. In the process of doing so, it is also possible to discriminate between biocidal and biostatic interactions.

Biocidal-Biostatic Endpoint Features

It is useful to distinguish between the outer, solid growth region of the streak and the subsequent tail which forms the transitional region to no growth. The biostatic interaction is characterized by greater continuity of change from growth to no-growth, i.e. there are no sharp distinctions at either end of the tail. In a biocidal interaction there are two types of discontinuity: (1) better differentiation of tail boundaries, and (2) greater variation of colony

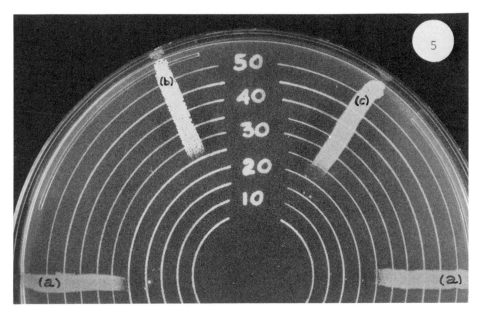

FIG. 6.8 Spiral gradient antimicrobial susceptibility plate. Gentamicin against (a) *E. coli* ATCC 25922, (b) *S. aureus* ATCC 29213, (c) *P. aeruginosa* ATCC 27853.

sizes in the tail, including the likely presence of a few larger colonies at the higher antimicrobic concentrations (see Fig. 6.8).

The character of a biostatic tail derives from the very nature of biostatic interaction, i.e., the effect is to reduce growth rate (and/or lag time) with increasing antimicrobic concentration. This is illustrated in Fig. 6.9, in which each curve was derived from the measurement of the average colony size of an *E. coli* culture on a plate containing the indicated concentration of chloramphenicol. Up to a diameter of about 1 mm, colony size changes linearly with incubation time and the slope is inversely proportional to generation time (Pirt, 1975). At a fixed incubation time there will thus be gradually decreasing colony sizes with increasing antimicrobic concentrations. The endpoint of a biostatic interaction is therefore a very elusive quantity, highly sensitive to incubation time.

A biocidal interaction, as expressed in colony formation on an agar plate, typically exhibits little effect until a threshold region of antimicrobic concentration is reached. This threshold region is represented by the end of the solid growth area and beginning of the tail. Within the tail itself, colony size

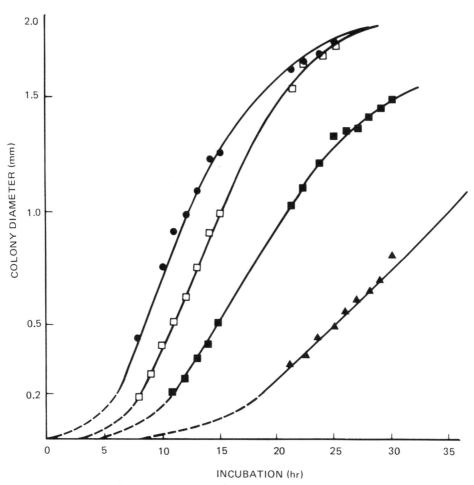

FIG. 6.9   Colony size as a measure of growth rate. Chloramphenicol in agar at fixed concentrations; *E. coli* ATCC 25922 spirally plated to provide separated colonies: ● Control (0 μg/mL); □ 0.75 μg/mL; ■ 1.50 μg/mL; ▲ 2.5 μg/mL.

will tend to be variable since it is determined, at least in part, by the biocidal interference with colony growth. Another factor, which is largely responsible for the appearance of large colonies at higher concentrations, is attributable to statistical selectivity.

Figure 6.10 shows a plate prepared with a special cam on the spiral plater so as to expand the tail of the biocidal interaction of gentamicin with *E. coli*.

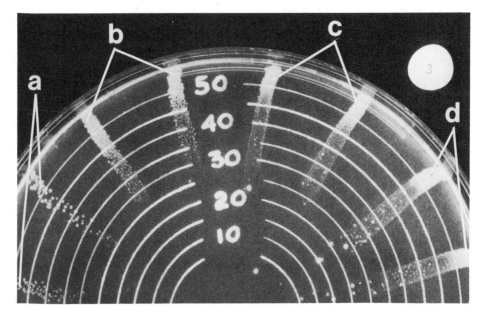

FIG. 6.10   Expanded tail of biocidal interaction. Gentamicin against *E. coli* ATCC 25922 swabbed at concentrations of (a) 10^5/mL;(b) 10^6/mL;(c) 10^7/mL;(d) 10^8/mL.

Specifically, in the radial advance region of 5–50 mm shown, gentamicin concentration varied only by a factor of about 1:3.5. The frequency of appearance and the size of the individual, larger colonies increase at the higher concentrations of the deposited bacterial suspension. As shown by Dean and Hinshelwood (1955), this is consistent with the expectation that resistance-related properties of individual bacteria in a population would have a frequency distribution about a mean value. But low frequency events, e.g., a cell having a high resistance and short lag time, would only materialize in a large population. These seemingly "abnormal," larger colonies should not be considered in defining the end-point for quantitative purposes as they represent the extreme end of the resistance frequency distribution.

Exclusion of the above colonies from MIC quantitation should not obscure the fact that their presence clearly provides additional information. On a relative basis, for example, the size of the tail and the extent of outlying, larger colonies may be indicative of relative distribution variances, i.e., the likelihood of developing a resistant subpopulation. Also, in a broth dilution test, one such resistant cell could cause a positive growth reading at a high dilution and therefore contribute to greater variability of MIC determinations.

In a biocidal spiral gradient plate, e.g. as illustrated in Fig. 6.8, the tail can seem to be nonexistent. However, subculturing the agar region immediately adjacent to the endpoint may show the presence of viable colonies; they are simply too small to have become visible during the overnight incubation period.

MIC Determination

The MIC in broth or agar dilution tests is defined as the first dilution which exhibits no growth, i.e., it is defined as a no-growth endpoint. In the spiral gradient test two endpoints can be defined: (1) the transition from solid growth to the start of the tail—to be referred to as the Nominal Inhibitory Concentration (NIC) and (2) the end of the tail, referred to as the Final Inhibitory Concentration (FIC). While these spiral gradient endpoints may have independent utility, e.g., the NIC could define a biocidal threshold concentration, it is necessary to relate spiral gradient growth endpoints to the MIC no-growth endpoint.

When using a swab to streak the bacterial suspension, it was found that a bacterial concentration of about 10^8 per mL will produce approximately the same surface density (about 200 cells per square mm) as that defined for agar dilution tests by NCCLS (1983) (Schalkowsky et al. 1985). A bacterial concentration of 10^8 also facilitates visual observation of the endpoint. To obtain the MIC, the FIC value obtained for a 10^8 streak is multiplied by two in order to approximate the equivalent next, twofold dilution corresponding to no-growth in broth or agar-dilution tests.

Spiral gradient MICs were obtained for the standard strains recommended by NCCLS for agar dilution testing. A comparison of these MICs with the MIC ranges given by NCCLS (1983) for the same antibiotics is shown in Table 6.3. *Staphylococcus aureus* against the two β-lactam antibiotics are the only instances found to be outside the NCCLS range. In both cases there was no visible tail and a sharp transition from growth to no-growth, i.e., the NIC and FIC endpoints are the same. In all other combinations the spiral gradient MIC's are within, and mostly near the center of the NCCLS MIC range.

The improved sensitivity of the spiral gradient method is particularly useful for the quantitation of relative effects, e.g., measuring the change in the susceptibility of *Campylobacter jejuni* to cadmium chloride due to the presence of iron sulfate (Stern 1985). The effect of combined substances is most conveniently measured by the use of an additional "uniform" cam available with the spiral plater. This cam deposits the liquid sample so as to deliver the same volume per unit length of spiral path. Thus, the primary substance,

Table 6.3 Comparison of NCCLS (1983) and Spiral Gradient MICs

Antibiotic	NCCLS standard strain	MIC-micrograms/mL NCCLS range	Spiral gradient
Ampicillin	E. coli	2–8	5.6
	S. aureus	0.25–1	0.11[a]
Penicillin	S. faecalis	1–4	2.3
	S. aureus	0.25–1	0.04[a]
Cefoperazone	E. coli	0.12–0.5	0.32
	S. aureus	1–4	2.6
Gentamicin	E. coli	0.25–1	0.77
	S. aureus	0.25–1	0.43
Chloramphenicol	E. coli	2–8	3.6
	S. aureus	2–8	5.7
Tetracycline	E. coli	1–4	2.6
	S. aureus	0.25–1	0.6

[a]Significantly smaller than NCCLS low limit.

e.g., the cadmium chloride, is deposited with the variable cam to produce a gradient of concentrations, while the secondary substance, e.g., the iron sulfate, is deposited at a selected constant concentration. The effect of the iron, for example, on quantitative (MIC/MBC) and qualitative features of cadmium chloride susceptibility can thus be determined.

Biocidal Endpoint Determination

Biocidal, as distinct from inhibitory, endpoint measurement requires continuing the incubation of the bacteria in a nutrient medium free of the antimicrobic to which it was previously exposed. For the spiral gradient test this can be done either by replicating the plate onto an inhibitor-free agar plate or by performing the test initially with the use of a membrane filter.

Replication can be done by stretching a sterile paper towel (in lieu of velvet cloth) over a block slightly smaller than the petri dish, lightly touching the surface of the agar containing the grown streaks to the towel, and than touching an inhibitor-free plate to the towel (Maas 1985). Reincubation of the replica plate will show whether or not additional growth occurs in the previously growth-free part of the streak. This method has the advantage of deferring a decision as to whether or not to replicate until after the initial incubation period. However, since not all of the initially deposited population is necessarily replicated from the no-growth region, quantitation of the new biocidal endpoint is more uncertain.

Quantitation of a Minimum Biocidal Concentration (MBC) can be done by initially placing a membrane filter on top of the agar after the antimicrobic has been deposited by the spiral plater, and doing the streaking on the filter. After quantitation of the MIC, the membrane filter is transferred to an inhibitor-free agar plate (preferably twice—to minimize carry over) and reincubated. For a biostatic interaction, there will be growth throughout the previously growth-free region. For a biocidal interaction the NIC/FIC points may advance toward the center but would leave a growth-free region. The new endpoint can be used to compute an MBC value. This method can also be used to study the effect of exposure time to the antimicrobic by making repeat streaks with different time delays.

ACKNOWLEDGMENTS

Raw milk plates and test data were provided by J. Ballash at the Johanna Dairy, Farmington, NJ. Test data and spiral plates of mixed cultures were provided by J. E. Campbell, Spiral Systems, Inc., Cincinnati, OH. E. J. Nath of Ontario, Canada, supplied the skim milk spiral plates and data for these plates as well as for parallel pour plates. These contributions are greatly appreciated but their utilization does not necessarily imply the contributors' endorsement of the conclusions or opinions expressed by the author based on their data.

Spiral gradient endpoint test development was carried out by the author in collaboration with Ellen Schalkowsky and J. E. Campbell. This work was supported in part by NIH grant number SSS-D 3 R43 AI20805-O1S1.

REFERENCES

APHA. 1978. *Standard Methods for the Examination of Dairy Products.* 14th ed. American Public Health Assoc., Washington, DC.
AOAC. 1984. *Official Methods of Analysis.* 14th ed. Sec.t 46.181, 981–982. Assoc. Official Analytical Chemists, Arlington, VA.

BRODSKY, M.H., CIEBIN, B.W., and SCHIEMANN, D.A. 1979. A critical evaluation of automatic bacterial colony counters. *J. Food Prot.* 42(2): 138–143.

COUSE, N.L. and KING, J.W. 1982. Quantitation of the spiral plating technique for use with the Salmonella/Mammalian microsome assay. *Environ. Mutag.* 4: 445–455.

DEAN, A.C.R. and HINSHELWOOD, Sir CYRIL. 1955. The rate of development of colonies of *Bacterium lactis aerogenes* on agar plates containing drugs. *Proc. Royal Soc. B.* 144: 297–314.

DE FLORA, S. 1981. A 'spiral test' applied to bacterial mutagenesis assays. *Mutat. Res.* 82: 213–227.

DEVENISH, J.A., CIEBIN, B.W., and BRODSKY, M.H. 1984. Automated counting of bacterial colonies on spread agar plates and non-gridded membrane filters. *J. Food Prot.* 47(4): 284–287.

DONNELLY, C.B., GILCHRIST, J.E., PELLER, J.T., and CAMPBELL, J.E. 1976. Spiral plate count method for examination of raw and pasteurized milk. *Appl. Environ. Microbiol.* 32(1): 21–27.

FOOD AND DRUG ADMINISTRATION. 1984. *Bacteriological Analytical Manual.* Assoc. Official Analytical Chemists, Arlington, VA.

GAMAY, A.Y., RICHARDSON, G.H., and BROWN, R.J. 1984. Simplified pairing of lactic strains for cheese manufacture. *J. Dairy Sci.* 67: 1181.

GILCHRIST, J.E., CAMPBELL, J.E., DONNELLY, C.B., PEELER, J.T., and DELANY, J. M. 1973. Spiral plate method for bacterial determination. *Appl. Microbiol.* 25(2): 244–252.

GILCHRIST, J.E., DONNELLY, C.B., PEELER, J.T., and CAMPBELL, J.E. 1977. Collaborative study comparing the spiral plate and aerobic plate count methods. *J. Assoc. Off. Anal. Chem.* 60(4): 807–812.

HEDGES, A.J., SHANNON, R., and HOBBS, R.P. 1978. Comparison of the precision obtained in counting viable bacteria by the spiral plate maker, the droplette and the Miles and Misra methods. *J. Appl. Bact.* 45: 57–65.

JARVIS, B., LACH, V.H., and WOOD, J.M. 1977. Evaluation of the spiral plate maker for the enumeration of microorganisms in foods. *J. Appl. Bact.* 43: 149–157.

MAAS, W.K. 1985. Mutations to antibiotic resistance. In *Antibiotics in Laboratory Medicine.* Lorian, V. (Ed.). Williams and Wilkins, New York.

NCCLS. 1983. Methods for dilution antimicrobial susceptibility tests for bacteria that grow aerobicially—tentative standards, 3(2). National Committee for Clinical Laboratory Standards, Villanova, PA.

PEELER, J.T., GILCHRIST, J.E., DONNELLY, C.B., and CAMPBELL, J.E. 1977. A collaborative study of the spiral plate method for examining milk samples. *J. Food Prot.* 40(7): 462–464.

PIRT, S.J. 1975. *Principles of Microbe and Cell Cultivation.* John Wiley, New York.

SCHALKOWSKY, S., SCHALKOWSKY E., and TAWFIQ, S. 1985. Reference data for determination of antimicrobial endpoints by the spiral gradient agar dilution method. Report No. TR 85/1. Spiral System Instruments, Inc., 4853 Cordell Ave., Bethesda, MD.

SHELAIH, M.A., WINKEL, S.A., OKIGBO, O.N., and RICHARDSON, G.H. 1985. Quantitation of bacterial interactions using the spiral plater and membrane filter. *J. Dairy Sci.* 68: 609–612.

STERN, N.J. 1985. Personal communication. Manuscript in preparation. USDA, Meat Science Research Lab., Beltsville, MD.

WILSON, G.S. 1935. The bacteriological grading of milk. Medical Research Council Special Rept. 206, p. 370. H.M. Stat. Office, London.

ZIPKES, M.R., GILCHRIST, J.E., and PEELER, J.T. 1981. Comparison of yeast and mold counts by spiral, pour and streak plate methods. *J. Assoc. Off. Anal. Chem.* 64(6): 1465–1469.

7

Electrical Impedance for Determining Microbial Quality of Foods

Ruth Firstenberg-Eden

Bactomatic, Inc.
Princeton, New Jersey

INTRODUCTION

Impedance microbiology is a rapid methodology in which microbial metabolic activities are monitored by the mediation of electrical impedance. Impedance is the resistance to flow of an alternating current through a conducting material (e.g., growth medium). It is a complex entity composed of a vectorial combination of a conductive element and a capacitive element. Changes in impedance (and its components) due to microbial growth can be measured by placing an inoculated growth medium into a container equipped with two stainless steel electrodes. The bulk of the ionic solution can be characterized by a conductive element, while a model resembling a capacitor can be given to the electrode solution interface region (Fig. 7.1). Therefore, in monitoring microbial growth, conductance measurements can be indicative of changes taking place in the bulk solution, while capacitance measurements can be associated with changes in close proximity to the electrodes.

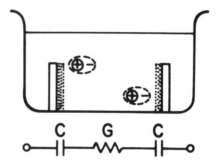

FIG. 7.1   A simplified model of an electrochemical well and the equivalent circuit. C, capacitive element associated with changes near the electrodes; G, conductive element associated with changes in the bulk ionic medium; Z, impedance is the vectorial combination of these components. (*From Firstenberg-Eden and Eden 1984.*)

How Microorganisms Change Impedance Parameters

Impedance changes occur in a medium as its chemical composition changes due to the metabolic activity of microorganisms. During growth, large molecules are converted into smaller, more active metabolites. Figure 7.2 shows the relationship between the growth curve (Fig. 7.2a), the ionic concentration (Fig. 7.2b), and the conductance curve (Fig. 7.2c). At some instant the concentration of ions generated by the bacteria reaches a magnitude similar to the initial ionic concentration of the growth medium (C_S in Fig. 7.2b) and a measurable increase in conductivity can be detected. This time is called detection time (DT). The microbial level associated with this change in conductance is called the microbial threshold level. The bacterial threshold level for both conductance and capacitance was found to be 10^6–10^7 cells/mL. The threshold for yeast was determined for capacitance and found to be 10^4–10^5 cells/mL. Further explanation of the theoretical and mathematical considerations of impedance microbiology are discussed by Eden and Eden (1984) and Firstenberg-Eden and Eden (1984).

Rapidity Ratio

In order to determine the time savings accomplished with the impedance assay relative to the plate count method it is convenient to define a rapidity ratio. Rapidity ratio is the incubation time required for the plate count method divided by the impedance detection time (Firstenberg-Eden and Eden 1984). The rapidity ratio for yeast counts as a function of contamination

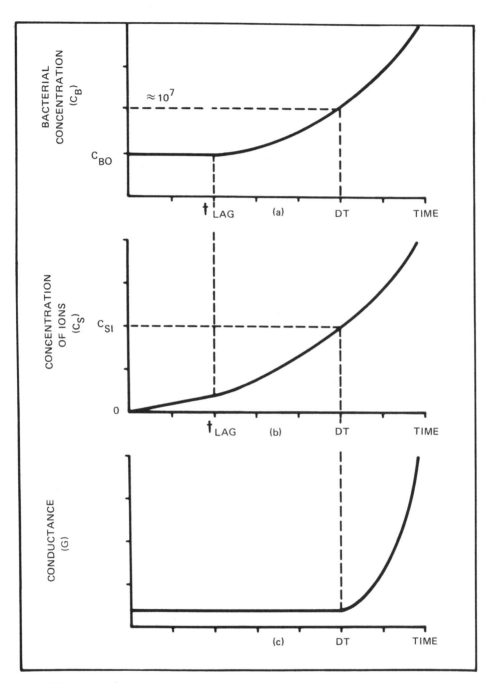

FIG. 7.2   Relationship between bacterial growth curve, ionic concentration and conductance curve. (a) Bacterial growth curve. C_{BO} initial bacterial concentration; (b) Ionic concentration. C_{SI} the initial ionic concentration of the growth medium; (c) Measured conductance. (*From Firstenberg-Eden and Eden 1984.*)

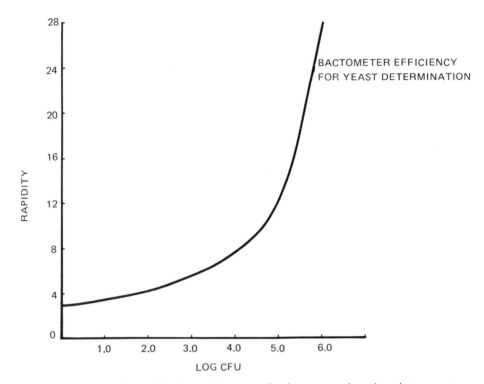

FIG. 7.3   Rapidity of the impedance method compared to the plate count method as a function of the initial yeast concentration.

levels is shown in Fig. 7.3. For very low yeast concentrations the rapidity ratio is mostly determined by the difference between the continuous monitoring of impedance as opposed to the constant incubation time allowed by the plate count method. It increases with increasing initial concentrations reaching a ratio of 12 for 10^5 CFU/mL. This means that with grossly contaminated samples the impedance assay will always result in much faster warnings than the plate count method.

CONSIDERATIONS IN THE DEVELOPMENT OF IMPEDANCE METHODOLOGY

The impedance method relies on the detection of metabolic activity in a growth medium, whereas the plate count methodology depends on the production of visible biomass. Therefore, the impedance method can be viewed as a dynamic method vs the static plate count methodology. As a result of this basic difference, the preparation procedures and growth conditions (e.g. medium, temperature, pH, etc.) utilized with the plate count method might not be appropriate for the impedance assay. A detailed review of the approaches for the development of procedures for impedimetric detection of microorganisms is given elsewhere (Firstenberg-Eden and Eden 1984). Some of the most important considerations are listed below.

Quality of Impedance Curves

The addition of certain ions to a solution yield stronger impedance changes than others. Therefore, some metabolic pathways yield better impedance signals than others. As a result, media specially engineered for impedance produce better impedance curves than traditional media (Firstenberg-Eden and Klein 1983; Zindulis 1984; Kahn and Firstenberg-Eden 1985).

In order to define a "good" impedance curve it is necessary to discuss the significance of specific portions of the impedance curve. The important sections of an impedance curve are shown in Fig. 7.4 and are defined as follows:

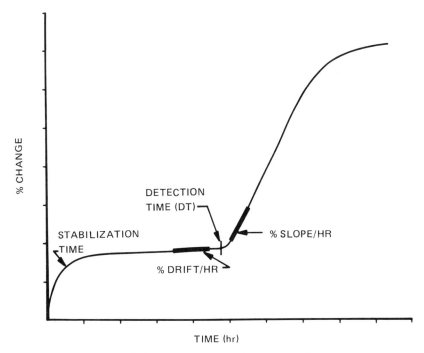

FIG. 7.4   Parameter definitions associated with impedance curves.

Stabilization time. This is the period of time required after the sample is placed in the incubator and before the base line is established. It depends on the temperature difference between sample and incubator, the volume of the sample, and the medium-electrode electrochemical properties.

Baseline. This is the region of the impedance curve between the end of stabilization period and the onset of its acceleration phase.

Drift. This describes the relative change of the impedance curve during the baseline phase. Ideally drift is zero (i.e., impedance does not change). In practice the signal usually drifts upward or downwards. Drift is measured as percent change/hour.

Slope. The "active" segment of the curve starts where the impedance curve accelerates. A portion of this segment is linear, and there, the slope is defined as relative change (percent/hour).

Detection time (DT). The detection time is defined as the point (in hours) where the baseline ends and the acceleration begins.

Those curves characterized by minimal drift and maximum slope produce more distinctive deflections, and minimize differences in calculated DT's among observers. Figure 7.5 compares a few curves in which it is difficult to find the detection point to a good quality curve. Good quality curves can be obtained by proper media engineering.

Choosing Between Capacitance and Conductance

Both signals are found to be useful in monitoring microbial growth, when using stainless steel electrodes (Firstenberg-Eden 1984; Zindulis 1984; Hause et al. 1981). In low conductivity media, such as Plate Count Agar, the change in conductance (G) is indicative of bacterial growth. In more conductive media, such as Brain Heart Infusion, the changes in G, due to bacterial growth are smaller than the changes in Capacitance (C). In high conductivity media, changes in C are a better indication of bacterial growth. Yeast growth results in large changes in C while the changes in G are very small. Furthermore, while the growth of some yeasts and molds result in an increase in G, others are associated with a decrease in G making the direction of the conductance curve unpredictable. On the other hand the capacitance signal obtained with yeasts and molds always increases.

Minimization of Generation Times

The effect of generation times (tg) on the relationship between DT and CFU on plates is shown in Fig. 7.6. This figure illustrates that in order to achieve the best possible correlation between the plate count method and DT, the

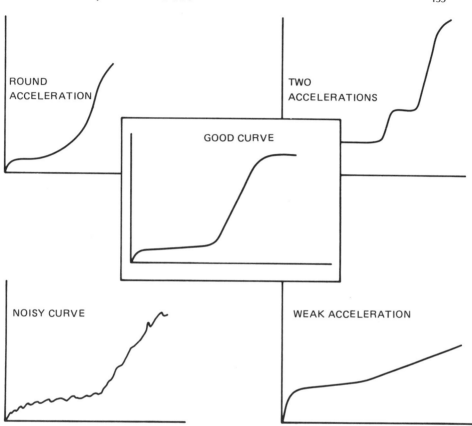

FIG. 7.5 A good impedance curve (center) is compared to four curves in which it might be difficult to define the point of detection.

generation times of all organisms under investigation should be brought as close together as possible under the experimental conditions employed. Therefore, in the development of methodology for the impedimetric estimation of numbers of microorganisms, an effort must be made to minimize differences in tg. By choosing the appropriate temperature, pH, and inhibitor/stimulant concentrations, tg can be minimized.

Inhibitors

The impedance method depends on the kinetics of microbial growth. Therefore, levels of inhibitors that might not affect the plate count method may affect the impedance assay by prolonging the lag phase or increasing the generation times. If the levels of inhibitors in a product are not constant

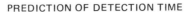

PREDICTION OF DETECTION TIME

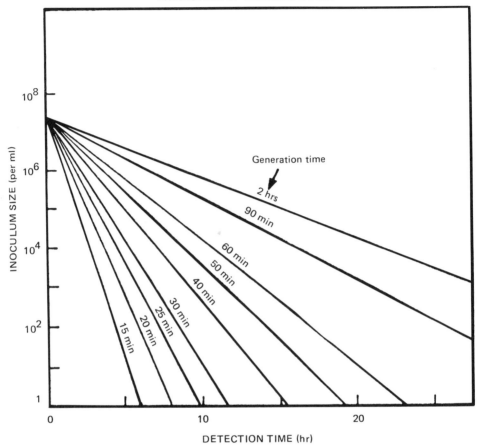

FIG. 7.6   Effect of generation times on detection times. (*From Firstenberg-Eden and Eden 1984*)

their presence might result in a poor correlation between DT and CFU. In such cases a dilution or separation procedure might be required. However, this sensitivity to inhibitors can also be viewed as an advantage of the impedance method when it is desired to predict shelf-life, detect levels of inhibitors, or study microbial growth kinetics.

Time

Since time is a measured parameter in an impedance assay any time elapsed after mixing the food with the medium must be accounted for. This might affect the sample preparation procedure used in the impedance assay.

APPLICATIONS

One of the major advantages of the impedance method is its versatility. It can be used to perform most of the tests needed by the microbiological QC laboratory. Impedance assays can be used to assess the quality of incoming raw material, evaluate and control the process, assess the quality and shelf-life of finished goods as well as to determine line sanitation. In the next section, some of the applications of the impedance assay will be discussed.

Estimation of Contamination Levels

One of the most commonly used applications of the impedance assay is to determine whether a sample contains above or below a predetermined concentration of microorganisms. Prior to adopting an impedimetric method to estimate numbers of organisms a calibration curve must be generated. This curve defines the relationship between DT and a parameter of a standard method, usually log CFU on plates. Since a calibration curve can be prepared for almost any application, the impedance assay can be used to estimate numbers of organisms in many different products. However, proper development of the analytical protocol (as discussed above) is a key to success.

The calibration curve. The reliability of the calibration curve can be assessed by the use of the correlation coefficient. However, the correlation coefficient obtained depends not only on the relationship between the two methods but also upon the number of samples analyzed, the range of concentrations of organisms tested, accuracy of counts and DT, etc. As the number of samples analyzed increases, the calibration curve describes more reliably the relationship between the two methods. In determining the number of samples required to construct the calibration curve, a balance must be struck between the high number of data points desired for a reliable calculation of the curve, and the amount of time and effort required to obtain such data. The samples chosen should have a wide range of microbial concentrations (4–5 log cycles). A narrow range of concentrations (1–2 log cycles) will result in low correlation coefficients and an unreliable line equation. In such a case all statistical parameters can change markedly with the addition of one or two new data points.

Uses of the calibration curve. The calibration curve can be used to (1) classify samples above and below a certain specified level (permissible level); (2) approximate plate count determinations; and (3) determine the generation times of the detecting populations. A calibration curve can be obtained by the use of linear or nonlinear (quadratic) regression technique. The following gives examples of these uses.

1. Figure 7.7 shows an example of a calibration curve obtained for mesophiles in raw milk using a quadratic line equation. If a permissible level of 10^5 CFU/mL is chosen, the corresponding DT will be 4.3 hours. By adding one standard deviation to each side of this DT the time axis can be divided into three areas: (1) red zone where all samples should have levels of organisms above the permissible level (10^5 CFU/mL); (2) yellow zone includes the marginal samples. In this zone the samples cannot be classified with confidence as having microbial levels above or below the 10^5 CFU/mL; (3) green zone where the samples should have levels below 10^5 CFU/mL. Using this scheme only one sample out of 135 was misclassified.

2. A detection time of two hours (arrow line, Fig. 7.7) for example, will result in an estimated count of 7×10^6 CFU/mL.

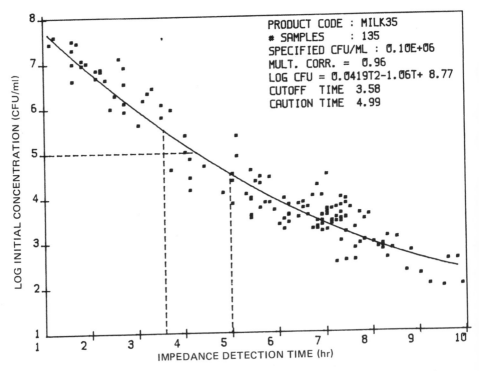

FIG. 7.7   The calibration curve obtained for the relationship between log CFU on plates (32°C, 48 hr) and DT (35°C) in raw milk. The dotted lines are used to classify the samples above and below 10^5 CFU/mL. The arrow dotted line is used to obtain an approximated count of a sample detection in 2.0 hours.

3. If a linear regression analysis is applied to this data set (Fig. 7.7) the line equation obtained will be:

$$\text{Log CFU} = A - B \times DT = 7.84 - 0.62 \, DT$$

It has been shown (Eden and Eden 1984) that:

$$\text{Generation Time (Min)} = (\log 2 \times 60)/B$$

For our example: $tg = 29$ min.

Total counts. The impedance assay is currently being used to classify samples or to estimate their total bacterial levels in products such as raw meats, poultry, milk, ice cream, frozen vegetables, etc. One of the major advantages of these assays is the simplicity of sample preparation. Typically the sample is diluted 1:10 in the medium, introduced into the measuring well and monitored automatically. Milk samples are pipetted directly on top of an agar medium and monitored. Therefore, this assay not only achieves faster identification of microbial problems (e.g., several hours vs several days) but is also less labor intensive than traditional techniques.

Selective media. A calibration curve can be obtained for the relationship between DT in selective media and standard methods for the detection of a variety of groups of organisms, of importance in food. The medium-temperature combination used in the conventional method might not be appropriate for the impedance assay and protocol development might be required. The following selective assays were developed for the impedance assay:

Coliforms (in a variety of products including milk, cream, ice cream, milk powder, whey, meat, frozen vegetables, etc.)

Lactic acid bacteria (in a variety of fruit juices)

Yeasts (in yogurt, fruit juices, fruit mixes)

Staphylococci (in meat, frozen dinners, potatoes)

Most of these assays are more sensitive to low levels of organisms than the traditional techniques and at least as selective. As with the total count procedures, the sample preparation procedures used are simple.

Shelf-life Predictions

The impedance method measures metabolic activity and as a matter of course integrates the effect of numbers of organisms and their metabolic activity. Therefore, it would seem to be one of the most suitable tools to predict shelf-life. The impedance assay for the prediction of shelf-life usually involves a preincubation step where the product is incubated with a diluent or medium (typically at a 1:1 ratio) at a slightly abused temperature. This step is used to allow growth of organisms that have a potential for spoilage. The preincubation step is followed by further dilution in growth medium and impedance monitoring. The assay developed for shelf-life prediction of pasteurized milk (Bishop et al. 1984) correlated better with the product shelf-life than the Moseley test or any other traditional method. Similar results were obtained for cottage cheese (Bishop and White 1985). An assay is currently being developed to predict shelf-life of cultured products, with live cultures, by measuring the activity of the gram negative organisms present in the finished product.

All of these impedimetric assays can predict the shelf-life of the product within 48 hours. Again the sample preparation procedure is very simple.

Sterility Testing of UHT Products

With the introduction of new UHT products into the market, especially those aseptically packed, there is an increasing need to verify that there are no viable organisms in a given volume (usually large) of product. The impedance assay can conveniently be used for this purpose. In "sterility" testing it is less important to minimize differences in generation times of the microbial population. In the development of the impedance assay it is necessary to identify a medium (or several media) that will assure the detection of all organisms that might appear in such a product. Also, the maximum time necessary to monitor impedance must be determined. Any detection indicates a contamination in the product.

Impedance assays were developed to detect bacterial contamination in UHT dairy products, to detect yeast or lactic acid bacteria contamination in UHT treated fruit juices and in UHT aseptically packed fruit juices. All these procedures involve a preincubation step, where the test container is incubated (with or without added medium) at room temperature or slightly abused temperature. This step is followed by a transfer of a predetermined volume of liquid into the module well where impedance is monitored. Typically the total time required for these tests is 48 hours.

Other Uses

A number of additional potential applications of impedance in food micro-biology have been suggested. All these applications are not fully developed to date but several of them are worth mentioning.

Detection of bacteriophage. In cheese manufacturing a serious failure of acid development due to a phage infection has important economic ramifications. Waes and Bossuyt (1984) developed a simple method to detect, within two hours, serious failure of starter cultures due to bacteriophage. This method is based on the observation that starter cultures attacked by phage result in fewer metabolites in the solution than a normal culture.

Sensitivity to antibiotics. Organisms sensitive to an antibiotic show an increase in DT as the concentration of antibiotic is increased. Changes in impedance curve patterns are also observed with these organisms, as a result of the addition of antibiotics. The impedance assay is capable of detecting lower levels of antibiotics than commonly used standard methods.

Microbial activity and growth kinetics. Theoretically the impedance method has potential for obtaining a better understanding of microbial growth kinetics in complex systems. This knowledge can be used in the development of starter cultures for the dairy, meat, and wine industries. Better under-standing of factors affecting microbial growth kinetics can be utilized in extension of product shelf-life, stability, and acceptability.

INSTRUMENTATION

The Bactometer® Microbial Monitoring System M123 is a modular system capable of accommodating from one to four Bactometer® Processing Units (BPU's) (Fig. 7.8). Each BPU contains two separate air incubator compartments. Each compartment is capable of monitoring up to 64 separate samples. A total of 512 samples can be monitored simultaneously, using up to eight different temperatures. The incubators operate in the range of 10°C below ambient to 55°C. The system also includes (Fig. 7.8) a microcomputer, a color video display terminal, a printer, and a digital plotter. The video terminal displays the system's menus and color coded test results on the current status of each sample.

The test samples are pipetted into individual wells of Bactometer® disposable module (Fig. 7.9). The instrument is able to monitor changes in conductance, capacitance, and total impedance.

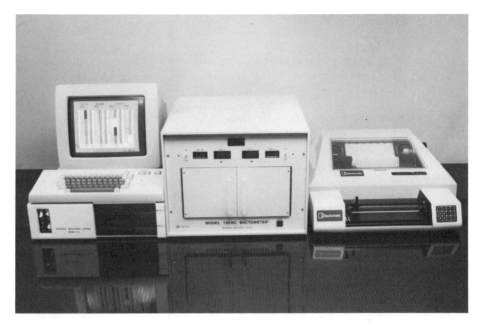

FIG. 7.8   The Bactometer® Microbial Monitoring System consisting of (from left) color video display, microcomputer, Bactometer® processing unit, printer and plotter.

The system's software automatically stores the data, determines the detection time of each sample, and continuously displays the updated results. The system was designed for simplicity of operation and rapid mastery by laboratory personnel with no previous experience in computer controlled systems. Extensive use is made of single keystroke commands. The software allows the user to print reports, view curves, and plot them. The software package includes the statistical analysis required for the creation of calibration curves.

ADVANTAGES OF IMPEDANCE ASSAYS

(1) *Fast identification of microbial problems.* An example of the rapidity of the impedance assay (for yeast) as compared to the plate count method is shown in Fig. 7.3. For low levels of yeasts (10^1–10^2 CFU/mL) the DT will be obtained in 24–35 hours while the plate count method requires 5 days. In addition grossly contaminated samples, which are of most concern, will detect earliest (typically 10^4 yeasts/mL will detect within a few hours). Most

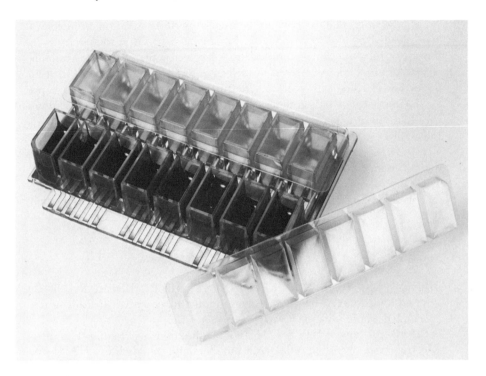

FIG. 7.9   A module containing 16 sample wells for use in the Bactometer®.

impedance assays will identify bacterial contamination within several hours as compared to 1–2 days required by the traditional methodology.

(2) *Reduces costs.* The method usually requires very little sample manipulation prior to its introduction into the instrument. This in turn results in quick and easy set-up. Therefore, the method is less labor intensive than the traditional techniques and many other rapid methods. In addition, due to the small volume of the module well, the method requires less media than the traditional technique.

(3) *Unaffected by opaque sample or small particulate matter.* Small particulate matter or opaque samples might interfere with low counts on plates. Many of the other alternative methods require the separation of such particulates prior to the test. The impedance assay is not affected by these factors.

(4) *Computer controlled.* The system is easy to operate by laboratory technicians. The results obtained are simple to read and interpret. The opportunity for operator error or bias is very small. The system provides automatic recording of data, presentation of data, and reporting of results. The computer allows for the retrieval of old data and sophisticated data analysis.

(5) *Versatile.* The method can be used to perform many microbiological tasks needed by the food industry. It can be used for raw materials, in-process testing, and finished products. A large variety of tests are available: screen for total counts, screen for selective groups of organisms, shelf-life prediction, sterility testing, etc. Currently there are more protocols developed for the impedance method than for any other rapid method. In some industries (e.g., dairy) this method can be used as a total QC tool (Firstenberg-Eden 1984).

(6) *More meaningful results.* By measuring the rate of metabolite production the impedance method integrates numbers of organisms and their activity. Therefore, the results of this method might be more meaningful in the prediction of keeping quality, wholesomeness, etc., than the plate count method.

REFERENCES

BISHOP, J.R., WHITE, C.R., and FIRSTENBERG-EDEN, R. 1984. A rapid impedimetric method for determining the potential shelf-life of pasteurized whole milk. *J. Food Prot.* 47: 471–475.

BISHOP, J.R. and WHITE, C.H. 1985. Estimation of potential shelf-life of cottage cheese utilizing bacterial numbers and metabolites. *J. Food Prot.* 48: 663–667.

EDEN, G. and EDEN, R. 1984. Enumeration of microorganisms by their AC conductance patterns. *IEEE Trans. on Biomed. Eng.* 31: 193–198.

FIRSTENBERG-EDEN, R. 1984. Impedance microbiology as an alternative to standard methods in dairy microbiology. Abst. Fourth International Symp. of Rapid Auto. Methods in Microbiol. and Immunol. W88. Berlin.

FIRSTENBERG-EDEN, R. and EDEN, G. 1984. *Impedance Microbiology.* John Wiley & Sons, Somerset, NJ.

FIRSTENBERG-EDEN, R. and KLEIN, C.S. 1983. Evaluation of a rapid impedimetric procedure for quantitative estimation of coliforms. *J. Food Sci.* 48: 1307–1311.

HAUSE, L. L., KOMOROWSKI, R. A. and GAYON, F. 1981. Electrode and electrolyte impedance in the detection of bacterial growth. *IEEE Trans. Biomed. Eng.* 28: 403–410.

KAHN, P. and FIRSTENBERG-EDEN, R. 1985. An impedimetric estimation of *Staphylococcus aureus* concentration in raw ground beef. Paper #113 presented at the 45th Annual Meeting of the Institute of Food Technologists, Atlanta, GA.

WAES, G.M. and BOSSUYT, R.G. 1984. Impedance measurements to detect bacteriophage problems in cheddar cheese. *J. Food Prot.* 47: 349.

ZINDULIS, J. 1984. A medium for the impedimetric detection of yeasts in foods. *Food Microbiol.* 1: 159–167.

8

The Bioluminescent ATP Assay for Determining the Microbial Quality of Foods

Kathleen A. LaRocco and Kenneth J. Littel

Packard Instrument Company
Downers Grove, Illinois

Merle D. Pierson

Virginia Polytechnic Institute and State University
Blacksburg, Virginia

INTRODUCTION

With the advent of rapid microbial detection systems, instrumentation, reagents, and media, food quality control managers are discovering many time-saving alternatives to the traditional microbiological analysis of incoming ingredients and finished product. The marketplace is currently flooded with companies touting "rapid" microbiological methods. These methods can be grouped into three classes: labor-saving methods in which results are obtained in traditional time frames (laser counting of agar plates); retrospective methods in which results are obtained somewhere between 6 and 24 hours (radiometry, impedance, and microcalorimetry); and very rapid methods in which results are obtained in less than an hour (direct epifluorescence; adenosine triphosphate, ATP; and Limulus lysate assay). These examples are but a few of the many "rapid" assay systems found in the marketplace. When selecting a system for a particular application, quality control managers must carefully compare new methodologies with their needs and this process can often be complicated and confusing. No system, at present, meets every microbiologist's individual application needs or all the attributes of an ideal assay system. Yet the demand for alternative microbiological methodologies continues to intensify. One needs only to read recent national headlines to appreciate the need for rapid microbiological testing. The largest salmonellosis outbreak in United States history might have been limited if rapid screening methodologies had been developed and proven for milk quality control testing.

Although the very rapid and sensitive ATP assay has been used in analytical and clinical research laboratories, it has not yet fulfilled its potential as an alternative to the Standard Plate Count in routine microbiological analysis of food ingredients and finished products. This is largely due to the lack of sample preparation procedures for effective elimination of nonmicrobial sources of ATP found in nearly all food products. In many cases, sample preparation methods must be developed or modified for each food product. This chapter will illustrate how recent developments in sample preparation techniques have made the rapid ATP assay a practical procedure for use with certain food products in the food quality control laboratory. This chapter will also more thoroughly familiarize the food microbiologist with the basic theory of the firefly ATP reaction, and available equipment and reagents for the food quality control laboratory.

FIREFLY BIOLUMINESCENCE

History

Bioluminescent organisms have certainly been observed by man since his beginnings. Remembering the first time we held a firefly in the palm of our hand must evoke memories of wonderment and fascination as we realized that the "glow" was cool and not hot. These same feelings were undoubtedly the inspiration for the studies by renowned natural philosophers and scientists into the nature of bioluminescence.

From the time of Aristotle (384–322 B.C.), the bioluminescence phenomenon has been studied by such famous personages as René Descartes (1596–1650), Robert Boyle (1627–1691), Robert Hooke (1635–1703), Benjamin Franklin (1706–1790), Joseph Priestly (1733–1804), Charles Darwin (1809–1882), and Louis Pasteur (1822–1895) (Johnson and Haneda 1966). In 1887, the French physiologist, Raphael DuBois, coined the term "luciferin" from the noun lucifer, meaning light-bringing. DuBois observed that a hot water extract of the luminescent clam, *Pholas*, produced a material capable of restoring light to a cold water extract obtained from the same clam. He called the cold water extracted material "luciferase," indicating an enzyme. The heat sensitive nature of this enzyme was demonstrated by the inability of a hot water extract to produce light. So significant was his work that his original names for the components of the reaction still remain today.

In nature, bioluminescence is widespread in occurrence among living organisms. In addition to the familiar firefly (*Photuris pyralis*), bioluminescent species appear in marine bacteria, fungi, centipedes, flagellates, corals, crustaceans, sponges, clams, snails, squid, marine worms, and many saltwater fish. E. Newton Harvey (1952), who investigated nearly all aspects of luminescence, more firmly established that light emission in organisms is catalyzed by enzyme systems. While specific luminescent enzyme systems are of several types, generally all bioluminescent systems involve a specific enzyme-substrate system, require oxygen, and usually require the presence of some cofactor (McElroy and Seliger 1962).

The Firefly ATP Reaction

By far, the firefly luminescent reaction has been the most extensively studied of the bioluminescent reactions (Whitehead et al. 1979). William McElroy first proposed a model for this reaction in 1947, and since then much knowledge has been added to the model (McElroy et al. 1969).

The ATP specific luciferin/luciferase reaction in the presence of oxygen produces a bioluminescence having a maximal spectral emission at 560 nm. The optimum temperature range for maximum light production is approximately 15–25°C. The optimum pH range, depending upon the buffer system, usually falls between 7.4–8.2. Cations, including zinc and calcium, and anions, including chloride, iodide, and phosphate, decrease light output. The firefly ATP reaction can be summarized in the following reaction (McElroy et al. 1969):

$$E + LH_2 + ATP \xrightarrow{Mg^{2+}} E \cdot LH_2 - AMP + PP$$

$$E \cdot LH_2 - AMP + O_2 \rightarrow oxyluciferin + CO_2 + AMP + light$$

where E = luciferase; LH_2 = luciferin; $E \cdot LH_2 - AMP$ = enzyme bound luciferyl-adenylate; PP = pyrophosphate. The ATP reacts with luciferase to form a complex. Luciferin reacts with the complex to form the enzyme bound luciferin complex, during which pyrophosphate is eliminated from a molecule of ATP. When the enzyme bound luciferyl-adenylate is exposed to oxygen, a decarboxylation step ensues with the simultaneous emission of light. The final product contains an inhibited luciferase enzyme complex which cannot catalyze another reaction until it is regenerated by the addition of coenzyme A and pyrophosphate (McElroy et al. 1969). Consequently, each light emission from the luciferin/luciferase reaction consists of a single photon of light. The total light output from a sample is directly proportional to the amount of ATP present when luciferin/luciferase are in excess.

EQUIPMENT AND REAGENT CONSIDERATIONS

Instrumentation

Luminescence instrumentation for the food quality control laboratory must meet certain minimal standards. A luminometer must be able to perform reliably under variable temperature and humidity conditions common to many laboratories. In selecting a luminometer for the quality control laboratory, one should consider the following:

1. Signal-to-noise ratio of the luminometer should be as high as possible to allow discrimination of low concentrations of ATP.
2. The luminometer should be constructed of durable material. Light seals should be light-tight to prevent light leakage which could lower signal-to-noise ratios. Maintenance of constant temperature of the reagents, photomultiplier tube, and reaction vials in extreme environmental conditions of humidity and heat is desirable. This will allow the enzymatic reaction to proceed within its optimum temperature range, resulting in a maximum signal-to-noise ratio.
3. The luminometer should be programmable with a minimum of response entries. Software should be available for use with the luminometer providing basic data analysis. Optional provisions should include data output capabilities to allow more detailed data analyses with other commercial software packages (i.e., data base management, report writing, and detailed statistical analyses).
4. The luminometer should have capabilities for automated sample analysis. Automatic injection of reagents coupled with automatic advancing of samples should be standard features if many samples are to be analyzed.

Other considerations include utility and space requirements for the instrument, whether on-site training is offered and by whom, and speed and

availability of technical service representatives. Currently, there are no luminometers commercially available which meet the individual needs of each
quality control laboratory. Therefore, it is necessary to make reasonable
compromises for particular applications. Several companies manufacture both
manual and automated luminometers for the food industry. The equipment
is state of the art and software packages are available for data reduction in
some cases. Table 8.1 is a partial list of currently available automated and
manual luminometer models.

Reagents

Most of the luminometer manufacturers listed in Table 8.1 make a full line
of high quality reagents and reagent kits. While reagents can be purchased
from a specific manufacturer and used with any luminometer, most manufacturers have developed their ATP assays and other applications using their
own reagents and equipment, recommending that the customer do the same.
Lundin (1982) has thoroughly reviewed those technical and biochemical
considerations needed for suitable ATP monitoring.

ATP ASSAY APPLICATIONS

ATP Assay Premises for Microbiological Biomass Measurements

The use of ATP measurements as an index of microbial biomass is generally
based on three premises: (1) All living organisms contain ATP, an unequiv-
ocally accepted fact; (2) with highly purified reagents and a sensitive luminometer, ATP can be selectively measured in very low concentrations; (3)
intracellular concentrations of ATP are maintained in a constant range in
all microorganisms. State of the art equipment and highly purified reagents
have made it possible to detect less than 0.1 picograms (1 pg $= 10^{-12}$g) of
ATP in a controlled laboratory environment. This corresponds to approximately 100 bacterial cells. Consequently, quantitation of intracellular microbial ATP can be conveniently accomplished using rapid and simplified
extraction and assay procedures.

The third premise has been reviewed thoroughly (Chapman and Atkinson
1977; Karl 1980). Correlations between ATP and biomass measurements
could not be drawn if intracellular ATP levels changed radically throughout
the growth cycle. The turnover time of ATP in growing microorganisms is
reported to be one second or less (Chapman and Atkinson 1977) and reactions

Table 8.1 Luminometer Systems

Manufacturer	Model	Comments[a]
Analytical Luminescence Laboratory San Diego, CA	Monolight 2001 analyzer for testing applications in microbiology	Injection system: 2 modes, manual, automatic dispensing with start button. Single sample chamber: single sample analysis. Software: ATP determinations, 4 programs including absolute ATP quantities using internal standardization. Measuring chamber: variable temperature control[b] (25, 30, or 37°C).
Berthold Wildbad, W. Germany	Biolumat LB9500 analyzer for microbial and somatic ATP	Injection system: 2 modes, manual and automatic dispensing with start button. Single sample chamber: single sample analysis. Software: for absolute ATP determination using internal standardization. Measuring chamber: variable temperature control[b] (25, 30, or 37°C).
LKB-Wallac Turku, Finland	1251 Luminometer	Injection system: 2 modes, manual and automated with push-bottom control. Multiple sample chamber: 25 sample carousel. Software: absolute ATP determination using internal standardization. Measuring chamber: variable temperature control[b] (20–45°C).

Manufacturer	Instrument	Comments
Lumac (3M) St. Paul, MN	Biocounter M2010	Injection system: 2 modes, manual and automated push-button control. Single sample chamber: single sample analysis. Software: absolute ATP determination in relative light units. Measuring chamber: variable temperature control[b] (25, 30, or 37°C).
Packard Instrument Company Downers Grove, IL	Auto PICOLITE 6200 Luminometer	Injection system: fully automated, computer controlled. Multiple sample chamber: 48 sample carousel. Software: absolute ATP or CFU determination using internal standardization. Measuring chamber: no temperature control.
Turner Designs Mountain View, CA	Model 20e Luminometer	Injection system: automatic syringe dispenser or manual options. Single sample chamber: single sample analysis. Software: ATP determination using internal standardization. Printer or computer interfaces are optional purchases. Measuring chamber: no temperature control.

[a]Instrument sensitivity has been deliberately omitted from comments because conditions of the testing from manufacturer to manufacturer are not standard and thus direct comparisons are not possible.
[b]If chamber temperatures below 20°C are desired, external cooling devices must be purchased.

in which ATP is utilized and regenerated in the cell are numerous. There is, however, much evidence that a steady-state balance for intracellular ATP exists to provide sufficient energy for maintenance of enzyme systems and for biosynthesis of macromolecular cellular constituents during all phases of growth (D'Eustachio and Levin 1967; Chapman and Atkinson 1977; Karl 1980). This is accomplished through precise regulation of the metabolic energy stored in the adenine nucleotide pool. Therefore, given equipment and reagents, correlating intracellular ATP concentrations with biomass measurements is a relatively simple matter. Growth curve studies involving ATP measurements and conventional yeast colony forming units (CFU) illustrate that ATP levels increase in parallel with CFU during the logarithmic phase of growth (Fig. 8.1, Galligan et al. 1984). Fig. 8.2 demonstrates linear relationships between cellular ATP levels and conventional CFUs of a *Pseudomonas* species grown in Trypticase Soy Broth (TSB) and mixed hamburger spoilage flora. Femtograms of ATP/CFU (1 fg = 10^{-15}g) generally remain constant at various cell concentrations (Littel et al. 1984).

There have been numerous studies on the quantitation of the steady-state ATP levels of a variety of microorganisms (D'Eustachio and Levin 1967; Sharpe et al. 1970; Holms et al. 1972; Chapman and Atkinson 1977; Karl 1980; Theron et al. 1983). Even though assay conditions, reagent purity, and equipment differed in each study, fg ATP/CFU were found to range from approximately 0.1–4.0 with an average of approximately 1 fg ATP/CFU for bacteria and 10–100 fg ATP/CFU for yeast. It has also been reported that suboptimal conditions involving injury may depress intracellular ATP levels (Karl 1980; Patel and Wood 1983; Stannard and Wood 1983; Theron et al. 1983). Incorporating a resuscitation period involving incubation in a nutritionally rich medium will often replenish intracelleular ATP to normal levels (Patel and Wood 1983; Theron et al. 1983).

The ATP Assay in Food Applications

Early ATP assay applications included the development of biomass determinations from both marine and fresh water (Holm-Hansen and Booth 1966; Riemann 1979), soils and sediments (MacLeod et al. 1969; Karl and LaRock 1975), drinking water and wastewater (Daly 1974; Levin et al. 1975), and fermentation studies (Hysert et al. 1976). These studies have shown that the ATP assay can be used successfully in biomass determinations where relatively little interference from other ATP sources may occur. However, problems were encountered when these methods were applied to foods because many food products contain large amounts of intrinsic or somatic ATP which

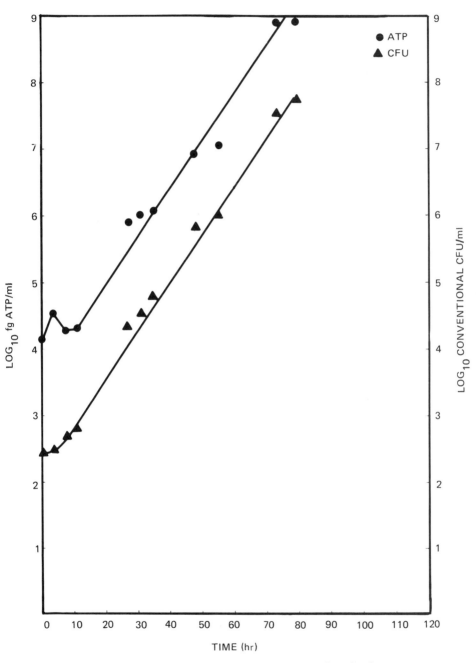

FIG. 8.1 Growth of *Saccharomyces rouxii* in a stimulated cola environment under ambient conditions. *(From Galligan et al. 1984.)*

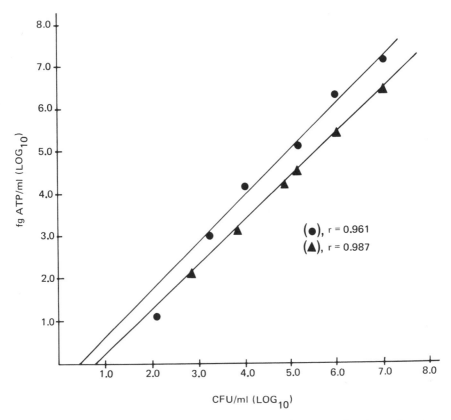

FIG. 8.2   Linear relationship between bacterial ATP and colony forming units for fresh beef isolates: ● *Pseudomonas* sp; ▲ Mixed spoilage flora from retail hamburger.

often exceed microbial ATP levels. Since the firefly luciferin/luciferase reagent reacted with ATP regardless of its source, it was surmised that all nonmicrobial sources of ATP must in some way be eliminated from food samples if bacterial ATP was to be measured (Sharpe et al. 1970).

More recently, ATP applications have been developed and successfully used in determining the microbial quality of a variety of foods (Baumgart et al. 1980; Bossuyt 1982; Stannard and Wood 1983; Galligan et al. 1984; Littel et al. 1984; Graumlich 1985). The key to these applications lies in sample preparation, more specifically, the elimination of intrinsic nonmicrobial ATP sources from food samples. These methodologies will be discussed in the following section.

SAMPLE PREPARATION METHODOLOGIES

Factors to Consider

Development work involving sample preparation procedures for ATP assays is often needed to estimate microbial contamination levels in food products. In some cases there are preparation procedures commercially available. These will be discussed in the next section. In order to develop a sample preparation method for any food product, the following factors should be addressed:

1. intrinsic ATP
2. minimum microbial detection limits
3. reference procedures

Intrinsic ATP is all the ATP from nonviable microbial or nonmicrobial origins in a food sample. Many food products, including beef, poultry, and shellfish, contain a certain amount of intrinsic ATP. For example, fresh meat samples contain highly variable amounts of intrinsic ATP depending upon the cut and age of the meat (Hamm 1982). The ATP background levels in a meat sample, assuming 1 fg ATP/bacterial CFU, may be equivalent to 1 $\times$ 10^5 to 1 $\times$ 10^8 CFU/g. Other products such as carbonated beverages contain small or undetectable levels of intrinsic ATP. It becomes apparent that with certain products, intrinsic ATP values need to be evaluated and sample preparation procedures designed in order to quantitate microbial numbers below gross contamination levels.

When developing a sample preparation method, the minimum threshold level of microbial detection is determined by the steps required to prepare a sample for the assay including dilution or concentration steps and, as previously discussed, any extreme environmental conditions in the laboratory which can affect enzyme activity and signal-to-noise ratio of the luminometer system. The sample preparation procedure should be designed to measure microbial numbers within the microbial specification levels of the food product.

In quantitating microbial ATP levels from food products, a reference method of comparison should be considered. At present, conventional CFU measurements are routinely used in the interpretation of ATP results because food quality control laboratories use the CFU as a standard method of reference. However, there has been much discussion on the usefulness of such a comparison (Sharpe et al. 1970; Patel and Wood 1983; Patel and Williams 1983; Stannard and Wood 1983). Numbers of microbial cells comprising a CFU, clumping of cells, and injured populations are several contributing factors to the inherent variability of the CFU estimate. It has been suggested, therefore, that the ATP biomass measurement may indeed be a better indicator of microbial activity than the standard CFU (Sharpe et al. 1970; Patel and Williams 1983). Perhaps a more useful reference method for the comparison and interpretation of ATP results is an assay technique measuring some cellular metabolic activity such as electrical impedance, radiometry, or microcalorimetry. Correlating ATP results to one of these metabolic measurements may in fact generate a most useful standard curve for predicting microbial activity during shelf-life studies.

Methodologies

In food products where intrinsic nonmicrobial ATP is of little consequence, sample preparation methodologies are relatively simple. A direct type assay would be applicable when contamination levels are high, greater than 1×10^5 bacterial cells or 1×10^3 yeast cells per unit measure. In a direct assay, a small volume of sample is directly exposed to the extractant followed by ATP measurement. Sample properties, however, can limit the usefulness of a direct assay. Extreme pH values, intense colors, or inhibitory compounds can inhibit or quench the firefly ATP reaction to such an extent that no sample ATP would be detected.

Figure 8.3 pictorially describes a vacuum filtration procedure developed for easily filterable products that contain little or undetectable levels of intrinsic ATP and low levels of microbial contamination (Galligan et al. 1984). The filtration procedure involves passing a sample of product through a vacuum filtration apparatus containing a membrane filter (MF, typically polycarbonate, Nuclepore, Pleasanton, CA) of sufficient pore size to collect the common spoilage flora that may be present in the sample. Following microbial collection the filter is rinsed to remove any inhibitory substances and ensure complete microbial deposition on the MF. The MF is then removed and microbial ATP is extracted from the microbial cells using an appropriate extractant. Potential applications include monitoring the microbial quality of readily filterable carbonated, still, and fermented beverages and water.

Samples that contain intrinsic ATP require that sample preparation methodologies be designed to reduce or eliminate intrinsic ATP. There are several approaches used in removing nonmicrobial sources of ATP from a sample. These include enzymatic degradation of interfering ATP sources or physical separation of intrinsic ATP from the microbial population, thereby allowing the measurement of microbial ATP.

Apyrase, isolated from potatoes, is the most commonly used enzyme for the degradation of intrinsic ATP. Typically, apyrase is combined with a

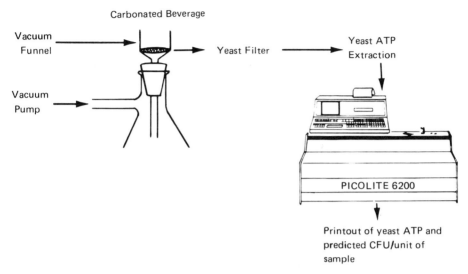

FIG. 8.3   Vacuum filtration procedure for samples with little or undetectable levels of intrinsic ATP. A single filter of sufficient pore size retains yeast and mold while allowing bacteria and nonmicrobial ATP to pass through. (*From Spurgash et al. 1985.*)

chemical ATP extractant that is specific for somatic cell membranes. The somatic ATP extractant makes the cell membrane permeable to ATP. This increases the overall effectiveness of the apyrase degradation of intrinsic ATP. A direct assay utilizing an enzymatic degradation technique was developed by Bossuyt (1982) and Waes and Bossuyt (1982) to test the bacteriological quality of milk. A raw milk procedure involved treating samples with an apyrase-somatic ATP extractant reagent prior to microbial ATP extraction. Keeping quality of pasteurized milk was estimated using a similar procedure which involved the incubation of pasteurized milk samples supplemented with gram (+) bacterial growth inhibitors for 24 hours at 30°C. In addition, the enzymatic approach has been used to analyze fresh beef (Baumgart et al. 1980; Kennedy and Oblinger 1985).

Common methods for separating biological agents are selective filtration and centrifugation. A procedure developed by Stannard and Wood (1983) utilizes both centrifugation and filtration to separate the intrinsic ATP from the bacterial population in fresh beef samples. An initial centrifugation ($2000 \times g$, 10 sec) is used to remove large debris from a meat/buffer homogenate. The supernatant liquid is then mixed with a cation exchange resin (Bio-Rex 70, equilibrated to pH 5.8). The exchange resin absorbs protein and other nonmicrobial materials from the homogenate to allow easy sample filtration. A sample of the treated homogenate is passed through a membrane filter to collect the bacterial cells. The filter is washed to remove any remaining intrinsic ATP and finally the bacterial ATP is extracted and measured. An alternative separation procedure developed by Patel and Wood (1983) uses an anionic polyelectrolyte flocculant (a soluble form of the cation exchange resin used by Stannard and Wood 1983) to remove meat particles, followed by centrifugation (2000 × g, 20 min) to collect the bacterial cells from fresh beef samples.

Depending upon the food product tested, separation and enzymatic degradation procedures alone may not sufficiently eliminate or reduce intrinsic ATP levels in the sample to allow for efficient measurements of microbial numbers. Combinations of both techniques, therefore, have been devised and incorporated into sample preparation methods. Stannard and Wood (1983) developed a dual treatment procedure for fruit juices. Centrifugation was used to separate the yeast flora from soluble ATP while the enzyme reagent containing apyrase degraded ATP that was associated with the yeast cell pellet. Another dual treatment procedure utilizes selective membrane filtration and an enzyme degradation step to assay fresh beef samples (Littel et al. 1984). The filtration step involves passing a meat homogenate through two disposable filters fitted in tandem. A large pore size filter retains large debris while allowing the bacterial flora to pass through to be collected on the smaller pore diameter filter. The bacterial filter is then treated with an enzyme reagent to eliminate any intrinsic ATP present on the filter. Following a wash of the bacterial filter, the bacterial ATP is extracted and assayed. This sample preparation method, as summarized in Fig. 8.4, is relatively easy to perform and utilizes disposable filtration equipment.

ATP ASSAY

Microbial ATP Extraction

The sample preparation methodologies described above ensure partial if not complete separation of intrinsic ATP from the microbial population for specific food products. To measure microbial ATP, the cells must first be treated so that intracellular ATP is released and available for reaction with firefly luciferin/luciferase. As described previously, ATP pools in microbial cells turn over very rapidly, therefore the extractant must promote the rapid release of ATP if true estimates of microbial ATP are to be made. Other factors to consider in choosing an extractant are efficiency of ATP release and the stability of ATP in the extract. Nearly all luminometer companies produce or distribute a full line of reagents for microbial ATP measurements including extracting reagents (Table 8.1). These commercial extractants use

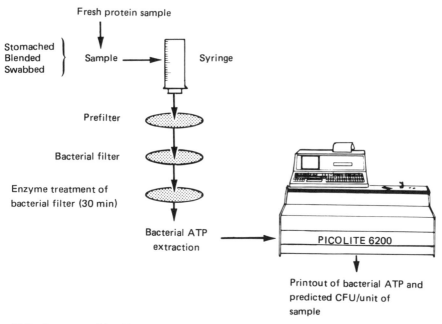

FIG. 8.4   Double filtration procedure for determination of bacterial ATP. Two filters, a prefilter and bacterial filter, are fitted in tandem. Pore size of prefilter is sufficient to allow bacteria to pass through while retaining large particulate matter. The bacterial filter retains the bacterial population and is subsequently treated with an enzyme reagent to eliminate any remaining nonmicrobial ATP. (*From Spurgash et al. 1985.*)

proprietary materials that promote rapid ATP release at high efficiency levels. The efficiency of an extractant is determined by comparing the ATP results obtained when samples are extracted with the commercial extractant and a total cell disruptive procedure such as exposure to boiling tris buffer for five minutes. Most commercial extractants contain chemical agents to inhibit enzymatic conversions of ATP during the extracting procedure. Ethylenediamine tetraacetic acid (EDTA), an ion chelator, is commonly used to inactivate converting enzymes (Lundin and Thore 1975). Commercial extractants are particularly attractive because formulations are designed specifically for the firefly reaction, often containing little or no inhibiting ions and requiring no special dilutions or processing steps. The microbial cells, either in solution or on filters, are exposed to the ATP releasing agent for some period of time (typically 15 sec) to complete the sample preparation procedure.

Microbial Measurement

When food products are assayed for microbial ATP, the cell extracts contain compounds in addition to ATP. These compounds may inhibit firefly luciferase as well as quench the light output of the reaction. An internal standardization technique is often recommended by reagent manufacturers to account for the effects these compounds may have on the ATP assay. To measure ATP present in a sample using an internal standard procedure, the sample is first reacted with firefly luciferin/luciferase and the light produced is measured. Following this initial count, a known amount of ATP is injected into the sample. The sample is recounted to quantitate the additional light produced (Stanley 1982). The sample count and ATP standard counts are then used to calculate the ATP concentration in the sample. The ATP concentration is calculated differently depending on the instruction inserts often supplied by the manufacturer of the instrument and reagent system. Figure 8.5 summarizes an example of the formula used to calculate the amount of ATP in a sample (Packard Instrument Company, Downers Grove, IL). The ratio value obtained from sample counts and internal standard counts is transformed to a final sample ATP concentration by interpolation from a standard curve relating known ATP levels to their ratio values (Littel 1985).

Interpretation of ATP Data

Automated luminometer systems will report light response in terms of ATP per unit measure and, in some cases, transform ATP results into CFUs per unit measure. Typically, it is the user's responsibility to change the data format in order to accommodate specific needs. Furthermore, it is the user's responsibility to recognize the success or failure of specific sample preparation

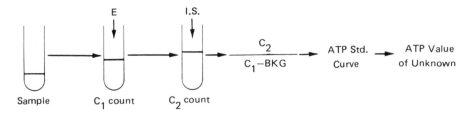

FIG. 8.5   ATP assay and calculation procedure used for the Packard system. E, Picozyme F, purified firefly enzyme; I.S., ATP internal standard; C_1, sample ATP count; C_2, sample + internal standard count; BKG, background is the C_1 count of an ATP free sample buffer blank. (*From Littel 1985.*)

methods in separating microbial ATP from nonmicrobial sources through ATP data analysis. Representative ATP results from studies describing sample preparation procedures for meat, carbonated beverages, and fruit juice will serve as examples of ATP data reduction and interpretation.

Fresh meat products. The sample preparation procedures previously described have been used to estimate bacterial spoilage levels in fresh meat such as beef, lamb, pork, poultry, and fish. In general, measured ATP levels are correlated with actual aerobic plate counts and, in some cases, these data plots are used as standard curves to predict CFU levels in fresh samples.

Cook et al. (1984) aged retail beef samples at 7°C and then obtained periodic ATP and conventional CFU results. A differential filtration approach was used to physically separate the microorganisms from somatic beef cells. Results demonstrated that above 1×10^6 CFU/g, the correlation between microbial ATP and conventional CFUs was high ($r > 0.90$, Fig. 8.6). Below 1×10^6 CFU/g, the linear relationship was not maintained, apparently due to the presence of intrinsic ATP. Consequently, a standard curve relating ATP levels with conventional CFUs could not accurately predict CFU levels from samples containing less than 1×10^6 CFU/g (Cook et al. 1984).

While differential filtration alone may not effectively remove intrinsic ATP from beef samples, Stannard and Smith (1982) and Stannard and Wood (1983) demonstrated that a combination of exchange resin and filtration to physically separate microorganisms from somatic meat cells produced linearity between ATP and conventional CFUs down to an approximate range of 5×10^5 to 1×10^6 CFU/g. Patel and Wood (1983), using a similar dual physical separation technique employing a soluble form of the exchange resin and centrifugation, demonstrated assay sensitivity of approximately 1×10^5 CFU/g. These sensitivity levels may be acceptable to the user, especially where fresh meat products are concerned; however, there are no commercially available "resin kits" and all supplies must be purchased separately, often from specific manufacturers.

Procedures for the enzymatic destruction of intrinsic ATP have been marketed by Lumac (Medical Products Division/3M, St. Paul, MN) and reagent kits are currently available for specific food applications. Using commercial reagents from Lumac for the determination of microbial levels in ground beef, Kennedy and Oblinger (1985) demonstrated that the sensitivity of this method was approximately 1×10^6 CFU/g. This was evidenced by large and highly variable ATP per CFU levels below 1×10^6 CFU/g.

A dual treatment procedure using differential filtration and enzymatic destruction of intrinsic ATP, developed by Packard Instrument Company, has been used to determine microbial levels from beef, poultry, and fish (Littel et al. 1984; Spurgash et al. 1985). Results from a study on ground beef are summarized in Fig. 8.7 and Table 8.2. Preliminary experiments were

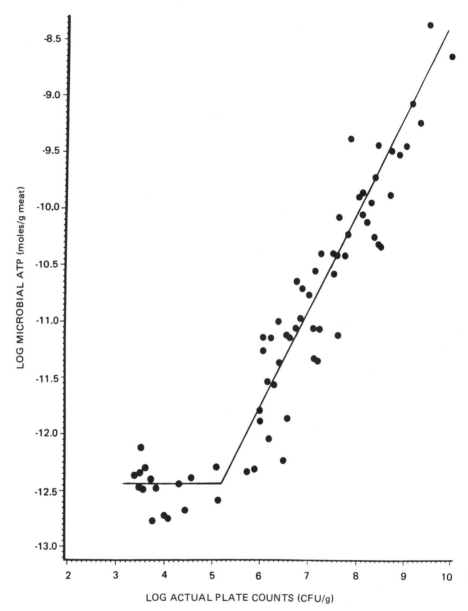

FIG. 8.6   Microbial ATP concentrations and plate counts of retail and laboratory-prepared ground beef stored at 7°C. (*From Cook et al. 1984.*)

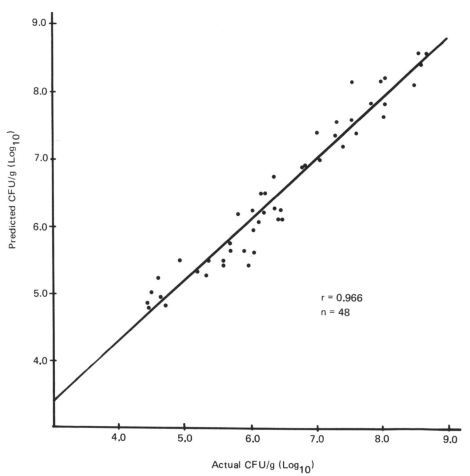

FIG. 8.7   Linear relationship between predicted and actual colony forming units for ATPase-treated fresh ground beef samples. *(From Littel et al. 1984.)*

performed to characterize the relationship between microbial ATP and conventional CFUs in fresh beef. Finally, a standard curve from a previous study was used to transform bacterial ATP from fresh beef samples aged at 5°C to predicted CFU/g (Fig. 8.7). When predicted CFUs were plotted against the actual CFU levels (aerobic plate counts), a high linear correlation was obtained ($r = 0.966$) over a range from 5×10^4 to 2×10^8 CFU/g. When comparing the effectiveness of this dual treatment in removing intrinsic ATP (Fig. 8.7) to a physical separation involving differential filtration (Fig. 8.6),

Table 8.2 Summary of Bacterial ATP Levels with a Comparison Between Aerobic Plate Counts and Transformed ATP Values Determined from Fresh Beef Samples

Sample CFU range[a] ($\log_{10}$)		n^b	ATP/CFU[c]	Difference[d] ($\log_{10}$)	Percent agreement[e]
4.00–4.99	mean	7	1.68	−0.38	86%
	range		(0.89–2.69)	(−0.6 −−0.1)	
5.00–5.99	mean	13	0.67	+0.01	100%
	range		(0.20–1.55)	(−0.40−+0.47)	
6.00–6.99	mean	12	0.77	−0.12	100%
	range		(0.29–1.38)	(−0.45−+0.29)	
7.00–7.99	mean	13	0.67	−0.09	92%
	range		(0.15–1.02)	(−0.68−+0.49)	
8.00–8.99	mean	3	0.42	+0.03	100%
	range		(0.25–0.58)	(−0.16−+0.23)	

[a]Expressed as CFU/g of aerobic plate count (25°C).
[b]Number of samples for CFU range.
[c]fg ATP level per CFU (1 fg = 10^{-15} g).
[d]Actual plate count less predicted plate count. Differences calculated from $\log_{10}$ transformed values.
[e]Percent of samples with difference less than ±0.5 $\log_{10}$.

the sensitivity of the assay increases by more than one $\log_{10}$ cycle. The additional step of treating filters with an enzyme reagent prior to microbial ATP measurement removes intrinsic ATP from the sample more effectively than a filtration procedure alone. This is further evidenced by the fact that fg ATP/CFU levels remained relatively constant throughout the range of linearity (Table 8.2). The overall efficacy of the standard curve in predicting CFU levels from new meat samples can also be evaluated from calculation of $\log_{10}$ differences between the two estimates of bacterial levels (actual CFU less predicted CFU, Table 8.2). These differences range from −0.68 to +0.47 $\log_{10}$ with a mean value of −0.11 $\log_{10}$ indicating that predicted values are well within a 0.5 $\log_{10}$ of actual CFU values throughout the range of linearity. A summary of ATP analyses of beef, poultry, and fish samples in three studies is presented in Fig. 8.8. High correlations ($r > 0.97$) between ATP and CFUs were obtained for all three products. When individual standard curves were constructed from these data, high linear correlations were again demonstrated ($r > 0.90$) between predicted and conventional CFUs for all three products (data not presented).

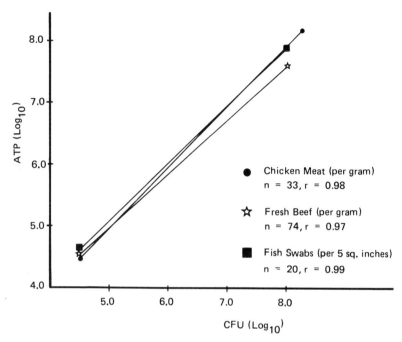

FIG. 8.8   Relationship between CFU and ATP for three types of fresh protein products. (*From Spurgash et al. 1985.*)

Carbonated beverages.   Many carbonated beverages are readily filterable and often contain low or undetectable levels of intrinsic ATP (Galligan et al. 1984). These observations led to the development of a simple versatile vacuum filtration procedure to detect low levels of yeast in a cola beverage (Galligan et al. 1984). Acclimated yeast species were individually spiked into a cola beverage, dilutions made, and ATP levels and conventional yeast CFUs determined. Figure 8.9 demonstrates the linear relationship ($r > 0.945$) between yeast ATP and conventional yeast CFUs. A standard curve relating yeast ATP to conventional yeast CFUs, from a previous study, was used to transform the yeast ATP results of all three yeast types into predicted yeast CFU values. Figure 8.10 illustrates the linear relationship ($r = 0.946$) between predicted yeast CFUs and conventional yeast CFUs for the individual yeast types. The accuracy of this standard curve is further demonstrated when the regression line passes through the y-axis near or through the origin indicating a unitary relationship between predicted yeast CFUs and conventional yeast CFUs.

From the study of Galligan et al. (1984), which demonstrated that carbonated beverages contain little intrinsic ATP, an ATP screening procedure

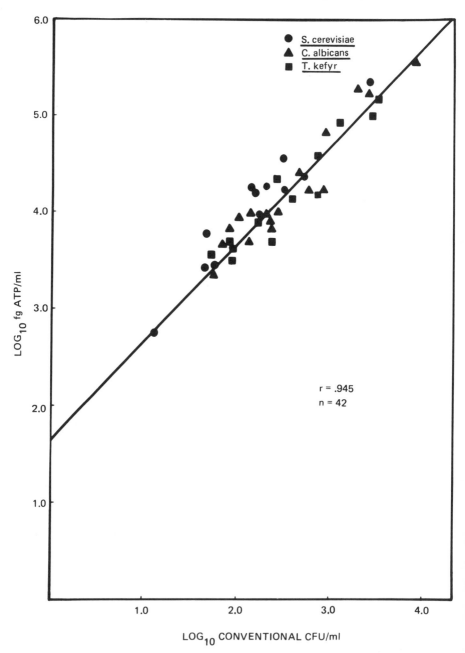

FIG. 8.9   Linear relationship between ATP and CFU levels of three yeasts individually spiked in a cola beverage. (*From Spurgash et al. 1985.*)

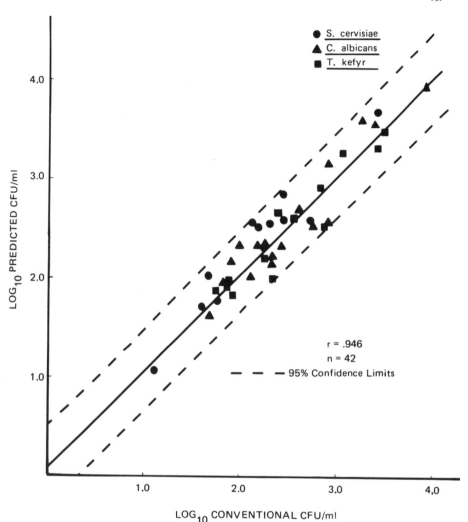

FIG. 8.10   Linear relationship between predicted and conventional CFU levels of three yeasts individually spiked in a cola beverage. (*From Spurgash et al. 1985.*)

was devised by Littel et al. (1985). In this application, the vacuum filtration technique was used to measure background ATP and conventional yeast levels from cola beverage samples. Those samples which contained less than one yeast per 100 mL of product were considered sterile, and the ATP results from these samples were used to determine an ATP screen level. Figure 8.11 summarizes the distribution of 240 cola samples. Ninety-five percent of the sample population ATP levels were below 200 fg ATP/mL. The screening value was set at this level and used for both the ATP screening of additional commercial cola samples (Fig. 8.12) and for ATP screening in yeast spiked studies (Fig. 8.13).

The utility of the screening method is demonstrated in Fig. 8.13. For those spiked samples falling above the ATP screening value, a linear relationship ($r = 0.85$) between yeast CFU and ATP values was demonstrated. When an arbitrary product specification of 5.0 CFU/mL was selected (as shown by the vertical line in Fig. 8.13), more than 90% of the samples were correctly identified as presumptive positive for yeast. The reported sensitivity range

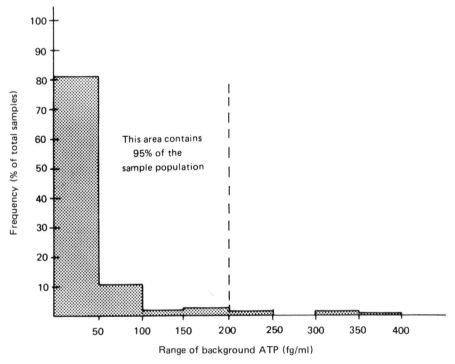

FIG. 8.11   Frequency distribution of background ATP in 240 microbiologically negative cola samples. (*From Littel et al. 1985.*)

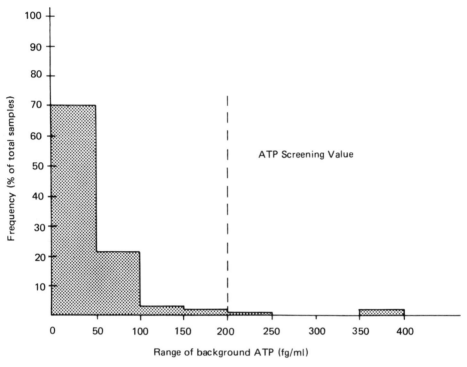

FIG. 8.12   Frequency distribution of background ATP in 182 retail cola samples. *(From Littel et al. 1985.)*

of the vacuum filtration procedure for easily filterable carbonated beverages is between 1 and 10 yeast/mL and could be increased by analyzing larger volumes of beverage (Littel et al. 1985).

Fruit juices.   To date, estimating levels of yeast contaminants in fruit juices via the ATP assay has been only marginally successful. In preliminary studies using a commercial fruit juice kit, Stannard and Wood (1983) showed that enzymatic treatment of fruit juice samples was not successful in removing sufficient quantities of intrinsic nonmicrobial ATP. The lower sensitivity limit of this assay was approximately 1×10^5 yeast CFU/mL for spiked samples. When a dual centrifugation/enzyme treatment procedure was adapted for fruit juices, however, the sensitivity of the assay was increased to approximately 1×10^4 yeast CFU/mL. In order to further increase the sensitivity of the procedure for commercial sterility testing, a 24-hour sample incubation period was recommended; however, optimum conditions for the incubation were not determined.

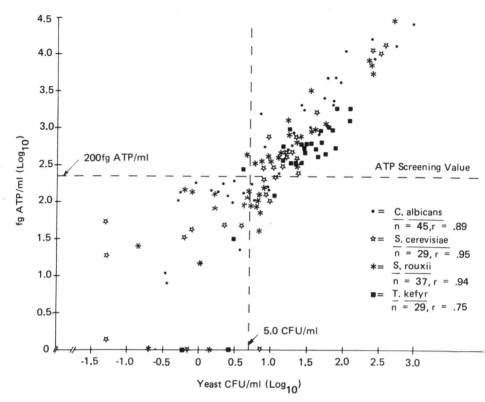

FIG. 8.13   Cumulative data of yeast inoculated cola samples. *From Littel et al. 1985.*)

Graumlich (1985) found that a 24-hour incubation period at 25°C was needed to obtain a linear relationship ($r = 0.92$) between ATP, measured in Relative Light Units (RLU, Lumac) and yeast CFUs. Centrifugation combined with enzymatic treatment of resuspended sample was used to remove intrinsic ATP. The sensitivity of this method appears to be limited to actively growing populations at approximately 10^3 yeast CFU/mL.

SUMMARY

The firefly ATP bioluminescent assay has several distinct advantages when compared with other rapid microbiological detection/enumeration procedures. This methodology is rapid, sensitive, and standardized reagent kits are available to perform the ATP assay. One major concern in using the ATP assay for microbial analysis of foods is the ubiquitous nature of ATP. The sample preparation procedures described in this chapter are representative examples of how the state of the art microbial ATP detection systems can effectively be used in estimating microbial populations in foods.

It is apparent that a dual treatment sample preparation procedure is necessary in reducing intrinsic ATP levels in foods to instrument/reagent backgrounds. Single step sample preparation techniques may be improved, however, to increase sensitivity.

As the market demands for new and proven rapid microbiological technology accelerate, investigators will begin to realize the full potential of the ATP assay. Exciting and new areas of research which will lend themselves well to bioluminescence assays include immunological and DNA hybridization techniques. Firefly luciferin has been covalently linked to a snake venom toxin and was shown to be an extremely sensitive nonradioactive probe in studying nicotinic acetylcholine receptors (Schaeffer and Hsueh 1984). There is no doubt that the conjugation of luciferin to specific immunoglobulins could be used for the detection of food pathogens. These new areas of research should further demonstrate the versatility of bioluminescent assay methods and contribute to improvements in our old "standard" microbiological procedures. In this way, food microbiologists continue to meet the demands of our technologically advanced society.

REFERENCES

BAUMGART, J., FRICKE, K., and HUY, C. 1980. Quick determination of surface bacterial content of fresh meat using a bioluminescence method to determine adenosine triphosphate (ATP). *Fleischwirtsch.* 60: 266–270.

BOSSUYT, R. 1982. A 5-minute ATP platform test for judging the bacteriology quality of raw milk. *Neth. Milk Dairy J.* 36: 355–364.

CHAPMAN, A.G. and ATKINSON, D.E. 1977. Adenine nucleotide concentrations and turnover rates. Their correlation with biological activity in bacteria and yeast. In *Advances in Microbial Physiology*, Vol. 15. Rose, A. H. and Tempest, D. W. (Ed.). Academic Press, New York, NY.

COOK, F.K., KNOX, P.R., and PIERSON, M.D. 1984. Luminometry for the rapid estimation of microbial numbers in ground beef. Presented at the 44th Annual Meeting Institute of Food Technologists, Anaheim, CA, June 10-13.

DALY,K. 1974. The luminescence biometer in the assessment of water quality and wastewater analysis. *American Laboratory* Dec.: 38–44.

D'EUSTACHIO, J.W. and LEVIN, G.V. 1967. Levels of adenosine tri-phosphate during bacterial growth. *Bacteriol. Proc.* 121–122.

GALLIGAN, P., LA ROCCO, K., TSAI, T., and SPURGASH, A. 1984. A rapid bioluminescent screening method for determining yeast contamination in a carbonated beverage. Presented at the 44th Annual Meeting Institute of Food Technologists, Anaheim, CA, June 10–13.

GRAUMLICH, T.R. 1985. Estimation of microbial populations in orange juice by bioluminescence. *J. Food Sci.* 50: 116–117.

HAMM, R. 1982. Postmortem changes in muscle with regard to processing of hot-boned beef. *Food Technol.* 36(11): 105–115.

HARVEY, E.N. 1952. *Bioluminescence.* Academic Press, NY.

HOLM-HANSEN, O. and BOOTH, C.R. 1966. The measurement of adenosine triphosphate in the ocean and its ecological significance. *Limnol. Oceanogr.* 11: 510–519.

HOLMS, W.H., HAMILTON, I.D., and ROBERTSON, A.G. 1972. The rate of turnover of the adenosine triphosphate pool of *Escherichia coli* growing aerobically in simple defined media. *Arch. Mikrobiol.* 83: 95–109.

HYSERT, D.W., KOVECSES, F., and MORRISON, N. 1976. A firefly method for rapid selection and enumeration of brewery microorganisms. *J. Amer. Soc. Brew. Chem.* 34: 144–150.

JOHNSON, F.H. and HANEDA, Y. 1966. *Bioluminescence in Progress.* Princeton University Press, Princeton, NJ.

KARL, D.M. and LA ROCK, P.A. 1975. Adenoise triphosphate measurement in soil and marine sediments. *J. Fish Res. Bd. Can.* 32: 599–607.

KARL, D.M. 1980. Cellular nucleotide measurements and applications in microbial ecology. *Microbiological Rev.* 44: 739–796.

KENNEDY, J.E. and OBLINGER, J.L. 1985. Application of bioluminescence to rapid determination of microbial levels in ground beef. *J. Food Prot.* 48: 334–340.

LEVIN, G.V., SCHROT, J.R., and HESS, W.C. 1975. Methodology for application of adenosine triphosphate determination in wastewater treatment. *Environ. Sci. Technol.* 10: 961–965.

LITTEL, K.J., PIKELIS, S., TSAI, T., and SPURGASH, A. 1984. Rapid bioluminescent screening method for estimating the microbial quality of fresh beef and chicken. Presented at the 44th Annual Meeting, Institute of Food Technologists, Anaheim, CA.

LITTEL, K. 1985. PICOLITE® calibration for ATP analysis. Application Communication: Luminescence report no. 4. Packard Instrument Company, Downers Grove, IL.

LITTEL, K., LA ROCCO, K., and SPURGASH, A. 1985. ATP screening method for presumptive detection of yeast in carbonated beverages. Presented at the 45th Annual Meeting, Institute of Food Technologists, Atlanta, GA, June 9–12.

LUNDIN, A. 1982. Analytical applications of bioluminescence: The firefly system. In *Clinical and Biochemical Luminescence*. Kricka, L., and Carter, T. J. N. (Ed.). Marcel Dekker, Inc., New York, NY.

LUNDIN, A. and THORE, A. 1975. Comparison of methods for extraction of bacterial adenine nucleotides determined by firefly assay. *Appl. Microbiology* 30: 713–721.

MAC LEOD, N.H., CHAPPELLE, E.W., and CRAWFORD, A.M. 1969. ATP assay of terrestrial soils: A test of an exobiological experiment. *Nature* 223: 267–268.

McELROY, W.D. 1947. The energy source for bioluminescence in an isolated system. *Proc. Natl. Acad. Sci. USA* 33: 342–345.

McELROY, W.D. and SELIGER, H.H. 1962. Biological Luminescence. *Scientific American* Dec. 2–14.

McELROY, W.D., SELIGER, H.H., and WHITE, E.H. 1969. Mechanism of bioluminescence, chemiluminescence, and enzyme function in the oxidation of firefly luciferin. *J. Photochem. Photobiol.* 10:153–170.

PATEL, P.D. and WILLIAMS, A.P. 1983. Estimation of food spoilage yeast by measurement of adenosine triphosphate (ATP) after growth at various temperatures. Leatherhead Fd. R.A. *Res. Rep. No.* 419.

PATEL, P.D. and WOOD, J.M. 1983. Separation of microorganisms from raw meats and their rapid estimation by measurement of microbial ATP. Leatherhead Fd. R.A. *Res. Rep. No.* 420.

RIEMANN, B. 1979. Interference in the quantitative determination of ATP extracted from freshwater microorganisms. In *Proceedings from the International Symposium on Analytical Applications of Bioluminescence and Chemiluminescence*. Schram, E. and Stanley, P. (Ed.). State Printing and Publishing, Westlake Village, CA.

SCHAEFFER, J.M. and HSUEH, A.J. 1984. α-Bungarotoxin-luciferin as a bioluminescent probe for characterization of acetylcholine receptors in the central nervous system. *J. Biol. Chem.* 259: 2055–2058.

SHARPE, A.N., WOODROW, M.N., and JACKSON, A.K. 1970. Adenosine triphosphate (ATP) levels in food contaminated by bacteria. *J. Appl. Bacteriology* 33: 758–767.

SPURGASH, A., LITTEL, K.J., GALLIGAN, P., PIKELIS, S., and LA ROCCO, K. 1985. Rapid bioluminescent methods for the detection of microbiological contamination in food products. Presented at the 3rd European Conference on Food Chemistry, Antwerp, Belgium, March 26–29.

STANLEY, P.E. 1982. Rapid microbial counting using ATP technology. *Fd. Flavour Ingred. Process. Packag.* 4: 29–34.

STANNARD, C.J. and SMITH, J. 1982. Factory trial of the ATP assay method for estimation of microbial numbers on meat. Leatherhead Fd. R.A. *Technical circular No.* 773.

STANNARD, C.J. and WOOD, J.M. 1983. The rapid estimation of microbial contamination of raw meat by measurement of adenosine triphosphate (ATP). *J. Appl. Bacteriol.* 55: 429–438.

STANNARD, C.J. and WOOD, J.M. 1983. Rapid estimation of yeast in fruit juices by ATP measurements. Leatherhead Fd. R.A. *Res. Rep. No.* 443.

THERON, D.P., PRIOR, B.A., and LATEGAN, P.M. 1983. Effect of temperature and media on adenosine triphosphate cell content in *Enterobacter aerogenes*. *J. Food Protec.* 46: 196–198.

WAES, G.M. and BOSSUYT, R.G. 1982. Usefulness of the benzalkoncrystal violet-ATP method for predicting the keeping quality of pasteurized milk. *J. Food Prot.* 45: 928–931.

WHITEHEAD, T.P., KRICKA, L.J., CARTER, T.J., and THORPE, G.H. 1979. Analytical luminescence: Its potential in the clinical laboratory. *Clin. Chem.* 25: 1531–1546.

9

New Methods
for Indicator Organisms

Paul A. Hartman, James P. Petzel, and Charles W. Kaspar

Iowa State University
Ames, Iowa

This review encompasses recent modifications of conventional most probable numbers (MPN) and plating methods and new ideas and concepts for the recovery and recognition of indicator organisms. Emphasis is placed on studies published within the past five years. For access to earlier literature, the reader is referred to excellent reviews on indicator organisms in food (Mossel 1978, 1982a; Stadhouders et al. 1982) and water (Hoadley and Dutka 1977; Pipes 1978; McFeters and Camper 1983). Summaries of membrane filtration (Entis), spiral plating (Schalkowsky), impedance (Firstenberg-Eden), bioluminescence (LaRocco et al.), and *Limulus* assays (Jay) appear elsewhere in this book; those topics will not be repeated in this review. Philosophies behind the use of indicator organisms (Mossel 1982b) and their numbers and importance in foods (Berg 1978; Mossel 1978, 1982a; Splittstoesser et al. 1983), water, and wastewater (Metcalf 1978; Bordner 1983; Geldreich 1983; Reasoner 1983) are also beyond the scope of this presentation. Many

Journal Paper No. J-11883 of the Iowa Agriculture and Home Economics Experiment Station, Ames, IA. Project 2678.

methods include a resuscitation step to permit repair of injured organisms before exposure to inhibitory dyes, elevated temperature, or other selective agent. The topic of cellular injury and repair will not be elaborated upon here. For thorough discussions, see Ray and Speck (1973), Busta (1976), van Schothorst (1976), Perlman (1978), Ray (1979), Hartman (1979), Andrew and Russell (1984), and Hurst and Nasim (1984). This review is strictly on MPN and plating methods and on techniques proposed to confirm the presence of indicator organisms. Liberal reference will be made to methods used in clinical and water microbiology because many of the same principles are applicable to food microbiology.

For an indicator organism to reliably reveal a health risk, it must meet five criteria (Dutka 1973; Mossel 1982b). First, it should be consistently and exclusively associated with the source of the intestinal pathogen. Second, it should occur in greater numbers than any of the various intestinal pathogens. Third, it should be more resistant than intestinal pathogens to a wide variety of environmental stresses. Fourth, it should not proliferate to any great extent in the environment. Fifth, simple, reliable, and inexpensive methods should be available to detect, enumerate, and identify the indicator. No indicator organism or method meets all these criteria, and correlations between the presence of an indicator organism and pathogens are often poor. However, with improved methodologies and technologies, it should be possible to obtain improved correlations between indicator organisms and actual health hazards.

COLIFORMS, FECAL COLIFORMS, AND *ESCHERICHIA COLI*

The concept of using an indicator organism was proposed almost 100 years ago (Schardinger 1892, cited in Mossel 1967), shortly after the discovery (Escherich 1885) of a bacterium almost universally present in human excreta. This indicator organism acquired the name *Escherichia coli* after the person who discovered it. Soon thereafter it was discovered that *E. coli* was only part of a group of morphologically and physiologically similar bacteria (the coliform or coli-aerogenes bacteria) that originate from feces. At that time, it was difficult to distinguish these bacteria from *E. coli*. Coliforms soon supplanted *E. coli* as the indicator of choice (Clemesha 1912; Levine 1961), despite the fact that the coliform group included species found outside the intestine (Prescott 1902; Metcalf 1905). Eijkman (1913) proposed production of gas from glucose at 46°C as a test for fecal coliforms. Various modifications of the "Eijkman" or "EC" test have been used for the detection of "fecal coliforms," and many people were led to believe that the EC test detected only fecal coliforms or only *E. coli*. Because of such high expectations, "short-comings" of the EC test were observed. Attempts were made to make the EC test more specific and to devise alternative tests to estimate the presence of *E. coli*. Thus, in the past 100 years, we have gone full circle insofar as the indicator organism of choice is concerned: from *E. coli* to coliforms to fecal coliforms and back to *E. coli*.

Most-Probable-Numbers Methods

The MPN method (APHA 1984, 1985a,b,c) is one of the older and more involved methods used to determine "*E. coli*" (Fig. 9.1). Coliform numbers are estimated first, and then the possible presence of *E. coli* is determined. Advantages of the method are that it is easy to perform and it has been around a long time, so we know much about it. Disadvantages are many. It can take 10 days to perform the five steps shown (Fig. 9.1), although shortcuts have been proposed, such as incubating the LT and/or EC broths for only 24 hr (Dexter 1981; Hastback 1981). MPN estimates are imprecise unless many replicates are made (de Man 1975, 1983). Noncoliform bacteria, when

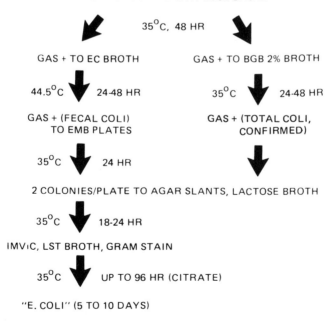

LAURYL SULFATE TRYPTOSE BROTH

35°C, 48 HR

GAS + TO EC BROTH   GAS + TO BGB 2% BROTH

44.5°C 24-48 HR   35°C 24-48 HR

GAS + (FECAL COLI)   GAS + (TOTAL COLI,
TO EMB PLATES   CONFIRMED)

35°C 24 HR

2 COLONIES/PLATE TO AGAR SLANTS, LACTOSE BROTH

35°C 18-24 HR

IMViC, LST BROTH, GRAM STAIN

35°C UP TO 96 HR (CITRATE)

"E. COLI" (5 TO 10 DAYS)

FIG. 9.1   A typical MPN procedure.

present in high numbers, can interefere (Goepfert 1976; Geldreich et al. 1978), especially in the first (presumptive) step of the test (Hussong et al. 1980, 1981; Evans et al. 1981c). Colicin-like substances present in water samples (Means and Olson 1981) may also interfere with test results. Anaerogenic *E. coli* would not be detected, and to obtain reliable estimates in some instances, all presumptive tubes that show growth but no gas should be confirmed (Olson 1978; Evans et al. 1981a,c); this would be expensive. Also, if the *E. coli* did not ferment lactose or it produced an atypical colony, the wrong colony might be selected for confirmation (Henriksen 1955). Many bacteria isolated from completed MPN tests are not coliforms (Austin et al. 1981). The absence of recoverable coliforms in tubes with gas formation is a severe problem when dried milk products are examined (Bindschedler et al. 1981).

Fluorogenic methods to detect the presence of *E. coli* in mixed populations for food and water analyses were recently described by Feng and Hartman (1982). According to one report (Kilian and Bülow 1976), about 97% of *E. coli* produce β-glucuronidase, an extracellular enzyme that hydrolyzes the glucuronosyl-O-bond (Levvy and Marsh 1960) of glucuronide conjugates such as 4-methylumbelliferyl-β-D-glucuronide (MUG). Among the *Enterobacteriaceae*, only *Escherichia coli*, some shigellae and salmonellae (Feng and Hartman 1982), and a few yersiniae (Petzel and Hartman 1985) hydrolyze MUG. To detect the enzyme, MUG is added to media selective for *Enterobacteriaceae*. After incubation, the tubes are placed under a long-wave ultraviolet lamp. Tubes in which β-glucuronidase was produced (Fig. 9.2) exhibit a distinct bluish fluorescence. In tests on water and food samples, the false-positive rate was only 2% (Feng and Hartman 1982) to 5% (Robison 1984). False-negative tests were infrequent. In contrast, up to 16% false negatives are obtained from foods with other methods (Van Wart and Moberg 1984).

Feng and Hartman (1982) described MPN tests with lauryl tryptose-MUG broth (LTB-MUG), plate counts on violet red bile-MUG (VRB-MUG) agar, a membrane-filter mEndo-MUG technique, and rapid mini-tests conducted in microtitration plates to confirm the presence of *E. coli*. Alvarez (1984) confirmed the value of the LTB-MUG-MPN, VRB-MUG, and mEndo-MUG procedures in discriminating seafood samples with high total coliform and/or *E. coli* counts. Robison (1984) adapted the test for presence-absence (P-A) (Clark 1968, 1980; APHA 1985c) estimations of *E. coli* in 11-g samples of raw ingredients and powdered foods by using an 18- to 24-hr preenrichment in nutrient broth followed by a 24-hr confirmatory test in LTB-MUG.

Various investigators conducted confirmatory tests to determine the efficiency of *E. coli* detection using MUG, and several conclusions can be reached. One conclusion is that results of MUG tests for *E. coli* will not correlate

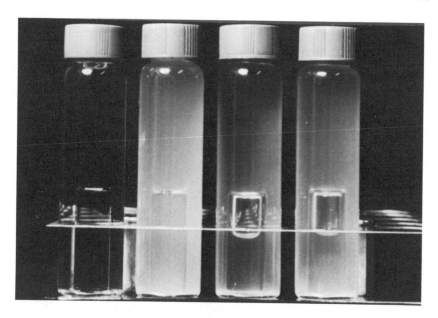

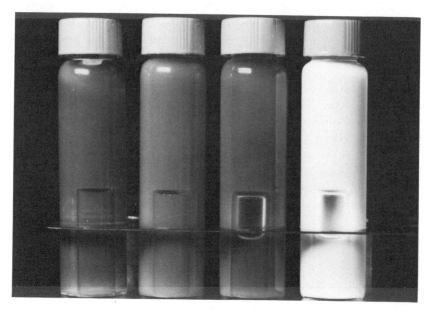

FIG. 9.2 LTB-MUG tubes photographed under white light (top) and long-wave ultraviolet light (bottom). From left to right: uninoculated, *Proteus* sp., *Enterobacter* sp., and *E. coli. (Photographs courtesy of Hach Co., Ames, IA.)*

100% with EC tests for fecal coliforms. Positive EC tests are closely associated with coliforms from animal wastes (Table 9.1), but substantial numbers of nonfecal coliforms also produce a positive EC test. The problem becomes complex when foods that contain an indigenous flora derived from a variety of sources are examined. Bacteria produce a positive EC test in the absence of fluorescence in 3.5 to 14.8% of LTB-MUG-MPN tubes, depending on the type of sample examined (Feng and Hartman 1982; Alvarez 1984; Van Wart and Moberg 1984). These might be considered false-negative MUG reactions; however, we prefer to consider that many of them are false-positive EC reactions produced by bacteria not of fecal origin. Also, some tubes became fluorescent, and confirmatory tests did not indicate the presence of typical *E. coli;* these might be considered false-positive tests. Feng and Hartman (1982) isolated anaerogenic *E. coli* from 2 of 17 such tubes and a *Salmonella* sp. and a *Shigella* sp. from other tubes; the remaining 13 tubes may or may not have contained *E. coli* or a pathogen that could not be isolated. Rippey and Chandler (1985) reported MUG-positive tubes at 44.5°C from which *E. coli* could be isolated after 24 hr of incubation but not after 48 hr of incubation. Their results demonstrate that *E. coli* can produce a positive MUG reaction before being overgrown. However, false-positive MUG reactions caused by streptococci (Robison 1984) and staphylococci (Van Wart and Moberg 1984) have been described. These are usually in gas-negative LTB-MUG tubes, and generally, growth is relatively sparse. Soy products and foods containing them were the main offenders of the commodities tested. When a less selective medium is used (Petzel and Hartman 1985), substantial numbers of MUG-positive pseudomonads and flavobacteria will grow from some sample types. Thus, selectivity of the medium, food composition, and flora specific to different commodities can influence the occurrence of false-positive and false-negative MUG reactions.

Table 9.1. Percentage Distributions of IMViC and EC Reactions from Five Sample Types

IMViC	Animals	Insects	Plants	U. Soil[a]	P. Soil[a]
+ + − −	91.8	12.4	10.6	5.6	80.6
− − + +	2.8	10.4	19.7	18.8	2.0
− + − +	0.6	30.6	14.0	48.1	13.0
+ + − +	0.8	10.9	9.6	3.7	3.3
+ + + +	0.1	23.4	24.2	6.8	0.0
EC +	96.2	14.9	14.1	9.2	82.9

[a]P = polluted, U = unpolluted.
(*Data from Geldreich 1966*)

Feng and Hartman (1982) recommended the use of MUG at a level of 100 μg/mL of culture medium, but Van Wart and Moberg (1984) discovered that 50 μg/mL provided a sufficient intensity to detect fluorescence. We have confirmed this observation (P. A. Hartman, unpublished data). Selection of the long-wave ultraviolet lamp used to detect fluorescence is very important when dye-containing media, such as brilliant green bile 2% (BGB) broth, are used with MUG. Fluorescence can be detected in glass tubes containing LTB-MUG but not in tubes containing BGB-MUG broth when an inexpensive, low-output UV lamp is used. Observation under a 15-watt blacklight blue UV lamp is satisfactory. Model UVL-56 Blak-Ray long-wave UV lamps are the best of those tested for observing tubes and plates.

A problem can arise when large inocula of certain animal products are examined by using MUG. Shellfish guidelines, for example, specify a limit of 230 MPN fecal coliforms/100g or 230 MPN *E. coli*/100g (Kilgen et al. 1985). Since urease-negative klebsiellae often outnumber *E. coli* 1,000 to 1 in shellfish (Kilgen et al. 1985), false-positive presumptive tests delay many shellfish shipments at a cost of millions of dollars a year. Therefore, rapid *E. coli* tests are being investigated. At high shellfish-sample concentrations needed to detect 230 *E. coli*/100g, all lower dilution tubes fluoresce because the shellfish contain endogenous glucuronidase. Koburger and Miller (1985) proposed using standard MPN procedures for 24–48 hr at 35°C and confirming for *E. coli* by transfer to EC-MUG medium for the EC test (Table 9.2). No false-negatives and only one false-positive was obtained. The false-positive tube yielded a *Klebsiella* sp., which was negative when retested in EC-MUG. An EC-MUG test was used for shellfish by Kilgen et al. (1985), who also recovered klebsiellae from fluorescent EC-MUG tubes that apparently did

Table 9.2.   Analyses of Shellfish for *E. coli* with EC-MUG

Parameter	Investigators[a] A	B
Number of samples	25	40 +
Total positive EC tubes	127	368
Total fluorescent tubes	103	215
Fluorescent +, *E. coli* +	102	205
Fluorescent +, *E. coli* −	1	10
Fluorescent −, *E. coli* −	24	153
Fluorescent −, *E. coli* +	0	19

[a]A = Koburger and Miller 1985; B = Rippey and Chandler 1985.

not contain *E coli*. Most of these were from tubes with high fecal coliform: *E. coli* ratios, which indicates that *E. coli* was or had grown in the tubes but could not be recovered on streak plates because of a high background flora. Rippey and Chandler (1985) also investigated an EC-MUG test for shellfish analysis (Table 9.2). They isolated *E. coli* from 10.5% of fluorescence-negative tubes, so caution should be exercised before assuming that tubes do not contain *E. coli*. The assay might be improved further by adding an indole test or other supplementary procedure to EC-MUG assays for shellfish (see later discussion).

The significance of *Klebsiella* spp. in shellfish and other foods, as well as potable waters (Dyck and Quinley 1984), recreational waters (Caplenas and Kanarek 1984), and soil (Hiraishi and Horie 1982) is unknown. Selective media for klebsiellae (Kregten et al. 1984; Wong et al. 1985; APHA 1985c) might be used to study this problem.

The glucuronide conjugate used to detect glucuronidase activity is important. Various conjugates are available for both colorimetric and fluorimetric tests. Kilian and Bülow (1976) and Hansen and Yourassowsky (1984) used *p*-nitrophenyl-β-D-glucuronic acid for colorimetric glucuronidase determinations and obtained results similar to those reported for MUG. *Klebsiella* spp. are generally considered MUG-negative, but Sherrill (1985) reported that *Klebsiella pneumoniae, Enterobacter aerogenes, Citrobacter* sp., and *Proteus mirabilis* possessed β-glucuronidase activity when phenolphthalein-β-glucuronic acid served as the substrate. Furthermore, Gadelle et al. (1985) obtained only two weak-positive reactions of 16 *E. coli* strains isolated from rats; phenolphthalein-β-glucuronide was the substrate. Until comparative studies have been conducted, phenolphthalein substrates should be avoided for use in glucuronidase tests for *E. coli* confirmation in foods.

The A-1 Test

An "A-1" test to recover *E. coli* from estuarine water was reported by Andrews and Presnell in 1972. The test was later modified (A-1-M test) by including a 3-hr resuscitation step (Andrews et al. 1979). The A-1-M procedure is a direct MPN test that includes the EC-test principle. Tubes of A-1 broth (Table 9.3) are inoculated as in an ordinary MPN test. The tubes are incubated for 3 hr at 35°C, transferred to a waterbath at 44.5°C, and incubated for 21 hr (Fig. 9.3). Gas production indicates "coliforms of fecal origin" (APHA 1985c).

The A-1 and A-1-M procedures have been tested for use in food microbiology. Results of the A-1 and A-1-M methods compared favorably with

Table 9.3. A–1 Medium

tryptone	20 g/L
lactose	5 g/L
NaCl	5 g/L
salicin	0.5 g/L
Triton X–100	1 ml/L

(From Andrews and Presnell 1972)

those of conventional tests, especially when the resuscitation step was included (Andrews et al. 1981). The A-1-M test is suitable for the analysis of waters (APHA 1985a, c) and chlorinated wastewaters (Standridge and Delfino 1981), but extensive studies on foods revealed that considerable variation in recovery was experienced and that reproducibility of recovery was dependent on the type of food sample (Andrews et al. 1979, 1981). Hunt et al. (1981) obtained significantly higher fecal coliform counts from shellfish with the A-1-M method than with the conventional MPN method; there was no difference in the recovery of *E. coli* by the two methods. Kilgen *et al.* (1985) obtained higher geometric mean counts of both fecal coliforms and *E. coli* from shellfish with the A-1-M test when compared with the APHA (1985a) method. The A-1-M method did not perform as well as two other methods in another study (Yoovidhya and Fleet 1981), and it is not recommended for the routine examination of shellfish (APHA 1985a). With some commodities, sample sediment may inhibit gas formation in fermentation tubes of A-1 medium (Varga and Doucet 1984). In these instances, higher estimates can be obtained

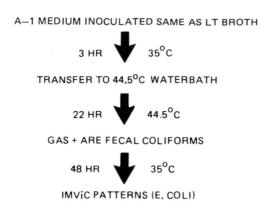

FIG. 9.3 A-1-M procedure. (*From Andrews et al. 1981.*)

by increasing the incubation time at 44.5°C to 45 hr or by using elevated fermentation vials and incubating at 44.5°C for 27 hr. With further improvement, the A-1-M method could become the method of choice for MPN determinations of coliforms, fecal coliforms, and, possibly, *E. coli* in foods.

Anderson and Baird-Parker Membrane-Filter Method

The Anderson and Baird-Parker method (Anderson and Baird-Parker 1975; Holbrook and Anderson 1982; APHA 1984) is another technique that can yield *E. coli* as well as coliform estimates. It takes only one day to perform (Fig. 9.4). A 1.0-mL sample is spread on a membrane resting on the surface of a predried plate of minerals-modified glutamate agar. After the liquid has absorbed into the agar, the plate is incubated for 4 hr at 35°C to permit resuscitation of injured cells (Mackey et al. 1980) and diffusion from the membrane of carbohydrates that might interfere with indole production. The membrane is transferred to a plate of tryptone-bile agar. After incubation at 44°C for 18 hr, the membrane is removed, stained to detect indole, dried under a UV light to fix the color, and observed within 30 min for the presence of indole-positive colonies.

Advantages of the Anderson and Baird-Parker method (Holbrook and Anderson 1982) are the short analysis time (24 hr), ability to detect the *E. coli* strains that do not ferment lactose to acid within 48 hr, and ability to detect the 3 to 12% of strains that are anaerogenic. Disadvantages are that each lot of tryptone-bile agar must be tested to assure that *E. coli* will grow and form indole and that indole-positive klebsiellae will not grow. The method

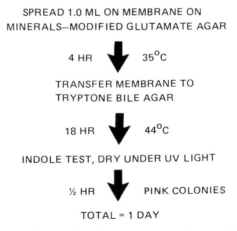

SPREAD 1.0 ML ON MEMBRANE ON
MINERALS—MODIFIED GLUTAMATE AGAR

4 HR   ⬇   35°C

TRANSFER MEMBRANE TO
TRYPTONE BILE AGAR

18 HR   ⬇   44°C

INDOLE TEST, DRY UNDER UV LIGHT

½ HR   ⬇   PINK COLONIES

TOTAL = 1 DAY

FIG. 9.4   Anderson and Baird-Parker procedure. (*From APHA 1984.*)

fails to detect indole-negative *E. coli* (about 1% of nonenteropathogenic strains and a larger percentage of enteropathogenic strains). Another disadvantage is that several labor-intensive timed manipulations must be made, including a stain for indole production.

The Anderson and Baird-Parker method has attracted much interest and has received wide acceptance because of the speed with which results are obtained. Most tests with food samples yield satisfactory results (Rayman and Aris 1981; Sharpe et al. 1983), except bean and alfalfa sprouts that contain high levels of klebsiellae. In recent tests on shellfish (Kilgen et al. 1985), dilutions high enough to have countable colonies on the membrane did not contain detectable *E. coli* because background levels of bacteria far exceeded those of *E. coli*. Motes et al. (1984) obtained lower counts from estuarine waters and shellfish when the Anderson and Baird-Parker method was compared (without preincubation at 35°C) with the APHA (1985a) method, a 24-hr British roll-tube method, and a French brilliant green lactose bile broth MPN method. Yoovidhya and Fleet (1981) obtained equivalent results with the Anderson and Baird-Parker method and a lengthy MPN procedure recommended by the Standards Association of Australia.

MUG has not been tested in conjunction with the Anderson and Baird-Parker method, but such a study would be interesting. Use of both an indole test and a MUG test should increase detection of *E. coli* and differentiation from other coliforms.

Rapid Confirmatory Tests for *E. coli*

A colorimetric β-galactosidase assay, utilizing *o*-nitrophenyl-β-D-galactose in EC medium, was devised by Warren et al. (1978). Numbers of *E. coli* were determined by the time taken (8–24 hr) to reach half-maximum ONPG absorbance. Of 302 isolates from water, 96.7% were *E. coli*, 2.3% *Enterobacter cloacae*, 0.7% *K. pneumoniae*, and 0.3% *Citrobacter freundii*. A fluorogenic substrate for rapid β-galactosidase detection has also been described (Cundell 1981).

In Britain, the production of gas in media incubated at 44°C is taken as strong presumptive evidence for the presence of *E. coli* in water. To provide additional evidence that *E. coli* is present, a tube of tryptone water is inoculated at the same time as a tube of EC medium to demonstrate indole formation within 1 day at 44°C (Joint Committee 1980; Motes et al. 1984). Thus, the indole test has been used for a number of years to confirm the presence of *E. coli*. BGB broth was too inhibitory to use for this test, and LTB gave 53% false-negative results (Joint Committee 1981). Substitution of mannitol for lactose and addition of tryptophan to LTB improves its performance. The use of mannitol instead of lactose permits detection of gas production from mannitol. Of the methods discussed in detail thus far, only the Anderson and Baird-Parker technique incorporates the use of an indole test. Consideration should be given to the addition of an indole test to other protocols that are specifically designed to detect *E. coli*. However, care should be taken because IMViC + + − − strains of *Enterobacter aerogenes* can be present in some samples (Goshko et al. 1984).

Glutamate decarboxylase activity is another parameter that could be used to separate *E. coli* from other enteric bacteria, but detecting the presence of this enzyme is difficult. Glutamate decarboxylase cleaves glutamic acid to γ-amino butyric acid and CO_2. Trinel et al. (1980; see also Moran and Witter 1976) measured CO_2 evolution by using procedures too complex to be of value in routine determinations. Maccani (1979) described an agar-plate method for detecting decarboxylase activity, but we discovered (P.C.S. Feng and P.A. Hartman, unpublished data) that the initial pH of the medium was critical and that the method would not be suitable for routine use. Other rapid decarboxylase tests (Jilly et al. 1984) should be considered because glutamate decarboxylase could be used to confirm the presence of *E. coli* if a suitable detection system was devised.

Verification of total coliforms from water samples was doubled when MPN tests that were negative were subjected to additional manipulations (Evans et al. 1981c) and by 87% when MF tests that were negative (LeChavallier et al. 1983b) were examined thoroughly (Table 9.4). For the MPN confirmations (Evans et al. 1981c), turbid gas-negative tubes were subcultured onto m-LES and EMB, and 1 mL was transferred to tubes of BGLB or EC

Table 9.4. Most Common Coliforms
Recovered from False-Negative Tests of Water

| Organism | Percentage of isolates | |
	MF (A)[a]	MPN (B)[b]
Citrobacter spp.	4	32
Enterobacter spp.	55	57
Escherichia coli	4	6
Klebsiella spp.	11	6
Serratia liquefaciens	1	0
Yersinia enterocolitica	4	0

[a](*From LeChevallier et al. 1983b*)
[b](*From Dyck and Quinley 1984*)

broth; further tests were made if any of these were positive. Colonies on MF membranes were examined by using a 4-hr β-galactosidase test with ONPG and a cytochrome oxidase test (Lupo et al. 1977). It is clear that combinations of tests will detect many anaerogenic *E. coli*, other anaerogenic coliforms, and instances of interference. A cytochrome oxidase test is recommended for the verification of coliforms from shellfish (APHA 1985a). Dyck and Quinley (1984) reported that modifications of US-EPA acceptable coliform procedures for potable water resulted in finding coliforms in 13.4% of water samples officially reported as "coliform not found" (Table 9.4). Enhancements included streaking spent LST broth tubes on MacConkey's agar, followed by an extensive series of additional tests. The results of these and other studies (Olson 1978, Evans et al. 1981c) show that sufficient tubes negative for coliforms or *E. coli* should be verified to determine if false-negative tests are a problem.

Few studies have been conducted to determine which of several tests would be most suitable for the confirmation of *E. coli* (Abbiss and Blood 1982). Varga et al. (1985) compared β-galactosidase (ONPG), β-glucuronidase (MUG), and indole tests on 190 biochemically confirmed *E. coli* isolates (Table 9.5). Of 22 strains that were negative by one or more of the three tests, only 1/22 was ONPG-negative, and 5/22 were indole-negative, whereas 21/22 were MUG-negative. These results might indicate that the MUG test was the least satisfactory of the three tests; however, colonies growing on MacConkey agar were subjected to rapid (30-60 min) tests. Glucuronidase is an adaptive enzyme (Levvy and Marsh 1959), as are galactosidase and tryptophanase. MacConkey agar contains lactose and tryptophan but no glucuronide; thus, the *E. coli* had not been induced for glucuronidase production. When MUG was incorporated into MacConkey agar at a level of 150 μg/mL (Trepeta and Edberg 1984b), 72 of 75 strains of *E. coli* were

Table 9.5.   Galactosidase, Glucuronidase (MUG), and Indole Reactions of 22 *E. coli* Isolates That Were Negative by One or More of the Three Tests[a]

Gal	MUG	Indole	Number
+	−	−	4
−	+	−	1
+	−	+	17

[a]190 biochemically confirmed *E. coli* were tested by Varga et al. (1985).

positive for β-glucuronidase production, whereas only 63 of 75 fermented lactose. Anderson et al. (1980) and Bueschkens and Stiles (1984) demonstrated that gas and indole production at elevated incubation temperatures were unchanged when cells were injured by heat, but when cells were frozen and thawed (Bueschkens and Stiles 1984) indole production by *E. coli* at elevated temperatures was a more stable characteristic than gas production. Indole production was the best test for *E. coli* confirmation of those reviewed by Abbiss and Blood (1982). Clearly, further studies are needed on confirmatory tests for *E. coli*. A combination of tests, such as indole plus galactosidase or glucuronidase (or all three) would be most satisfactory to assure that *E. coli* was present and to recover maximal numbers of this indicator organism.

Tests for *E. coli* and other coliforms can be miniaturized. The wells of microtitration plates can be used as "mini-tubes" for MPN determinations of high-count samples or for confirmatory tests (Fung and Kraft 1969; Fung and Miller 1972; Feng and Hartman1982; Hartel and Hagedorn 1983; Maul and Block 1983). A rapid, 4-hr tube test for gas and indole production at 44°C has also been described (Smith and Rockliff 1982).

On the other hand, one may wish to test large volumes of sample. If the sample is filterable, a membrane filter-MPN test (Presnell and Andrews 1976) might be suitable. A presence-absence (P-A) type of test for water (APHA 1985c), popularized by Clark (1968, 1980; see also Weiss and Hunter 1939) can also be used to detect coliforms in large volumes of water. The P-A test reportedly is more effective than the MF technique for detecting coliforms in samples in which the standard plate count is greater than 1,000/ mL (Clark 1980); however, few samples of potable water with such high counts are found (Pipes et al. 1985). When food samples are examined for coliforms by using a P-A type of test (Robison 1984), bacterial interference with positive results might occur if the background is high (Goepfert 1976).

A few methods have been proposed to detect *E. coli* without measuring enzyme activity. Abshire and Guthrie (1973) used fluorescent antibodies. Crichton et al. (1981) developed a hemagglutination test to detect biochemically atypical strains. Buras and Kott (1972) devised a two-filter MF technique; the difference in counts on a filter treated with 90 strains of coliphage and on an untreated filter was considered *E. coli*. Additional methods were mentioned in two earlier reviews (Hartman 1979; Hartman et al. 1982).

The formulations of commonly used media, some of which have not been improved upon since their original descriptions decades ago, could be improved. Some media should be formulated with increased buffering capacity (Meadows et al. 1980). Standridge and Delfino (1982), when examining membrane filter-verification procedures, observed that some coliforms, primarily *Citrobacter freundii*, produce gas in BGB 2% broth but not in LTB. The source of the discrepancy seems to be the use of different nitrogen sources in the two media; peptone in BGB 2% and tryptose in LTB. Some newer media, such as minerals-modified glutamate medium (Joint Committee 1980; Abbiss et al. 1981) or lactose-glutamate broth (Bindschedler et al. 1981) might be used to replace LTB for improved yields and increased selectivity and specificity.

Sample collection and methodology are important for some samples of water (McFeters et al. 1982; Domek et al. 1984), but not for other samples (Standridge and Delfino 1983). These parameters are also important when examining foods to minimize variations both within and among laboratories (Silliker et al. 1979). For example, procedures recently described for poultry (Lillard and Thomson 1983) and shellfish (Cook and Pabst 1984) demonstrate how coliform recoveries can be affected by sampling method.

One other factor that should be standardized is the temperature used to perform the EC test. Various temperatures (especially 44.0, 44.5, 45.0, and 45.5°C) have been suggested. In general, the lower two temperatures are used to confirm fecal coliforms (*E. coli*) in water samples and the higher two temperatures for foods. New studies are needed to determine if this variety of temperatures is warranted. The results of one study (Weiss et al. 1983) demonstrated that 45.0°C could be used for all tests (Table 9.6). If these results are confirmed, adoption of a single temperature, 45.0°C, would result in more uniformity between various tests and reduce the requirement for a multitude of water baths set at slightly different temperatures.

It would be premature to conclude a discussion of indicator organisms and *E. coli* without mentioning the increasing problem of antibiotic resistance in bacteria. Antibiotic-resistant salmonellae (Holmberg et al. 1984) and other

Table 9.6. Percentages of False+ and False– EC Tubes Incubated at 44.5, 45.0, and 45.5°C

°C	Sample	% false +	% false –
44.5	sewage	3.3	0.1
	milk	20.2	1.2
	meat	1.4	0.6
45.0	sewage	1.1	1.3
	milk	1.0	3.3
	meat	0.7	1.1
45.5	sewage	2.4	8.2
	milk	2.1	4.1
	meat	0.3	16.8

(*Data from Weiss et al. 1983*)

antibiotic-resistant bacteria pose a more serious public health threat than antibiotic-susceptible organisms. Because "birds of a feather tend to flock together," consideration should be given to incorporating antibiotic-resistance tests in protocols for the determination of *E. coli*, fecal coliforms, coliforms, and *Enterobacteriaceae*. Antibiotic-resistance patterns, at least in *E. coli* (Krumperman 1983; Marshall et al. 1983) vary with animal species, feeding regimen, and environmental conditions (Langlois et al. 1983; Hinton et al. 1985). Detection of antibiotic-resistant indicator organisms in water (Armstrong et al. 1981, 1982) or a food (Krumperman 1983; Chaslus-Dancla and LaFont 1985) might signal greater health risks than the finding of antibiotic-susceptible indicator organisms.

PLATING METHODS

Violet red bile agar is used for coliform determinations of dairy products (APHA 1985b) and other foods (APHA 1984). Generally, VRB agar is heated to boiling just before use to dissolve the agar and pasteurize the medium (APHA 1984). The medium may be prepared ahead of use and sterilized with modest sacrifice in productivity (Hartman and Hartman 1976; APHA 1985b), provided that the pH at time of use is 7.0 to 7.2. Conventionally, a base layer is mixed with the sample and allowed to solidify. An overlay of the same medium is poured to prevent growth of atypical surface colonies. VRB agar is inhibitory to injured cells, however, and it probably should not be used without a resuscitation step to permit cellular repair.

Almost identical resuscitation-overlay methods for use with VRB agar were reported in 1975 (Speck et al. 1975; Hartman et al. 1975). In one method (Speck et al. 1975), a base layer of tryptic soy agar was used; in the other method (Hartman et al. 1975), the base layer consisted of all the constituents of VRB agar except bile and dyes (Fig. 9.5). After the base layer was poured, time was allowed for repair and then plates were overlayed either with VRB agar (Speck et al. 1975) or VRB-2 agar that contained twice the usual levels of inhibitors (Hartman et al. 1975). The resuscitation procedure increases yields; for example, Reber and Marshall (1982) obtained 20% greater productivity with resuscitation when acidified half-and-half was assayed for content of viable coliforms.

Various modifications of the VRB resuscitation-overlay procedure have been used. The procedure described in *Standard Methods* (APHA 1985b) was formulated after an exchange of ideas between Bibek Ray and the authors of the chapter on coliforms so that an optimum procedure could be prescribed for dairy products and the procedure would coincide with that prescribed for other foods. The base layer consists of 8 to 10 mL of standard methods

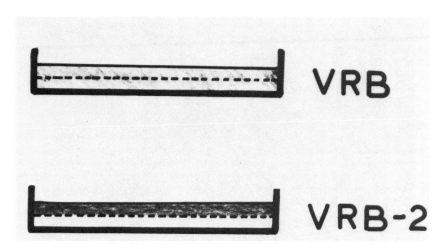

FIG. 9.5 Conventional VRB-agar procedure in which VRB agar is used for both the base layer and overlay (top). VRB-2 procedure involving resuscitation in a base layer of nonselective medium followed by an overlay of single-strength or double-strengh VRB agar (bottom). (See text.)

agar or tryptic soy agar. Plates are incubated at room temperature for 2 hr, and then an overlay of 8 to 10 mL of single-strength VRB agar is added. Increased recoveries of coliforms can be expected for several reasons. First, there is a resuscitation step. Second, only the overlay contains inhibitors, so the final concentrations of inhibitors in the modified VRB procedure are only half those used in the normal VRB/VRB procedure. Selectivity and formation of typical colonies seem not to be affected by the lower concentration of bile and dyes, but yields are increased (C. J. Brown and P. A. Hartman, unpublished data 1978). The medium used for the base layer can also affect results. Standard methods agar contains glucose, which facilitates cell repair (Draughon and Nelson 1981) as well as growth of some lactose-negative bacteria (C. J. Brown and P. A. Hartman, unpublished data, 1978). Tryptic soy agar would be the preferred basal for most purposes.

A study was recently completed (S. G. Campbell and P. A. Hartman, unpublished data) on a "baggie" method for making total counts and coliform counts on samples that contain very low numbers of bacteria. Plastic Whirl-Pak bags of 42-oz (1.2 kg) capacity (B1027[A]WA, Nasco, Fort Atkinson, WI) were used as the plating containers. The bags cost about 13 cents each. For a coliform count, 100 mL of sample were mixed with 100 mL of either double-strength VRB agar or with 50 mL each of double-strength VRB and trypticase soy agars. The bag was closed, sample and agar were mixed, the

FIG. 9.6   Bag-plate containing 100 mL of VRB agar and 100 mL of sample.

bag was rolled down to the agar level and fastened, and the bag was placed flat on a table top until the agar had solidified (Fig. 9.6). The bags were placed in an incubator in stacks three or four deep, and the ends unclasped and opened for better aeration and to facilitate evaporation of water of syneresis. After incubation, a modified Quebec counting box was used to aid in colony enumeration. Average percentage yields on 12 samples analyzed by using five methods are shown in Table 9.7. The conventional MPN method (APHA 1985b, 1985c) resulted in the highest average counts and the

Table 9.7.   Mean Percentage Yields of MPN, VRB, and Bag Methods on 12 Samples

Method	% Yield
MPN (lauryl tryptose broth)	100
VRB over VRB	25
VRB over trypticase soy agar	52
Bag with double-strength VRB	59
Bag with 50% 2X VRB: 50% 2X TSA	81

(Campbell and Hartman, unpublished data)

conventional VRB agar method the lowest mean counts. Counts made by using the VRB overlay on a TSA agar basal were twice as high as those on VRB/VRB agar. Two baggie methods yielded even higher counts; the mixture of VRB and TSA agars resulted in counts 19% lower than the MPN counts, but this difference was not statistically significant at the 5% level. All other methods yielded coliform counts that were significantly lower than those obtained using the MPN method. We conclude that this baggie method is a satisfactory alternative to membrane filtration for low-count samples. The bags are less expensive than filters, but because of the large volume of agar needed, the cost of a "baggie" assay is about the same as a membrane-filter assay.

Enhanced recovery of injured *E. coli* without the use of a resuscitation step has been obtained by adding 3,3'-thiodipropionic acid to VRB agar to prevent accumulation of H_2O_2, which is detrimental to injured cells (McDonald et al. 1983).

A new dry-medium-film (Petrifilm VRB) for coliform analysis was recently tested by Nelson et al. (1984). The Petrifilm VRB consists of a bottom foam circle containing dry VRB nutrients and a top film containing a dehydrated gelling agent and a tetrazolium dye (Nelson et al. 1984). Tests are made by adding 1 mL of sample to the foam circle and spreading the sample by exerting pressure on the covering top film. Upon incubation, coliforms growing in the gel reduce the tetrazolium to produce red colonies; gas bubbles can be observed near aerogenic colonies. Counts obtained by using the Petrifilm VRB were simlar to those obtained by using VRB agar or a MPN technique (Nelson et al. 1984).

Feng and Hartman (1982; Alvarez 1984; Van Wart and Moberg 1984) added MUG to the VRB-agar overlay and could detect *E. coli* among a mixture of coliforms growing in the agar. MUG may be added to MacConkey agar also (Trepeta and Edberg 1984b) for the same purpose, to reduce the number of confirmatory tests needed to identify colonies of *E. coli* in mixtures.

Several investigators have combined VRB-agar plating with elevated-temperature incubation. Klein and Fung (1976) plated water samples in VRB agar and incubated the plates without resuscitation at 44.5°C. They reported that the procedure was as reliable as MPN and MF methods to detect fecal coliforms; however, Stiles and Ng (1980) obtained higher fecal coliform counts from hamburger when a 2-hr resuscitation in nutrient agar was used before overlaying with VRB agar. Powers and Latt (1979) used a base layer of trypticase soy agar and a 2-hr resuscitation period to recover *E. coli* injured by freezing. Oblinger et al. (1982) compared 45°C with 7, 20, and 35°C for incubation of VRB plates (without resuscitation). Mean counts of food samples incubated at 45°C were less than half of those obtained at 20 and 35°C. Incubation at 45°C was somewhat selective for *E. coli*, but many bacteria belonging to other genera also grew at that temperature.

Because VRB agar is inhibitory to coliforms, especially injured cells, an improved plating medium is needed. Wright (1984) developed an enriched lauryl sulfate-aniline blue (ELSAB) agar that gave higher counts of coliforms and *E. coli* than VRB, MacConkey, or deoxycholate agars, which all contain bile. Fecal, water, and food samples were examined. Colonies of *E. coli* were readily differentiated from other coliforms on ELSAB agar. A similar type of medium, containing brom thymol blue as the indicator, was described earlier (Francis et al. 1974; Phirke 1976); results could be obtained within 8 hr. LeChevallier et al. (1983a, 1984) devised a membrane-filter medium, m-T7 (membrane filter-tergitol 7) agar, for improved recovery of coliforms with the MF method. An entirely new concept for *E. coli* determinations was proposed by Damaré et al. (1984). They devised a peptone-tergitol-glucuronide (PTG) agar that contained MUG but no carbohydrate. Because 4-methylumbelliferone (the fluorescent product of MUG hydrolysis) fluoresces more brightly at alkaline pH values than at an acid pH, low levels (50 μg/mL) of MUG could be used, and discrimination of MUG-hydrolyzing colonies was improved. PTG agar was not inhibitory to *E. coli* injured by heat and only slightly inhibitory to cells injured by freezing (Table 9.8). Recoveries of *E. coli* from meats were as high or higher than those obtained by using a standard 5-tube MPN procedure (APHA 1985c). Media such as these should be used to replace VRB agar for the direct-plating of food samples and, possibly, water.

ENTEROBACTERIACEAE

Henriksen (1955) suggested that acid and gas production from mannitol should be used in coliform tests because many coliforms that may be significant ecologically ferment lactose slowly if at all. Mossel (1957) agreed

Table 9.8. Percentage Recoveries (Relative to Trypticase Soy Agar) of *E. coli* Injured by Heating or Freezing and Examined by Using Different Media

Medium	Heated	Frozen
Anderson and Baird-Parker	92	70
Violet red bile agar	40	12
Peptone-tergitol-glucuronide agar	100	70

(*From Damaré et al. 1984*)

with this concept and proposed the addition of 1% *d*-mannitol to VRB agar to increase the detection of *Enterobacteriaceae*. Later, he recommended the addition of glucose instead of mannitol to MacConkey agar (Mossel 1962a) or VRB agar (VRBG agar—Mossel 1962b; Mossel et al. 1979; APHA 1984).

Mercuri and Cox (1979) compared VRB and VRBG agars for the analysis of poultry and meat products. About 34% of VRB isolates and only 20% of VRBG isolates were fecal coliforms or *E. coli*. Oblinger et al. (1982) obtained average percentage values for *E. coli* from foods of 10 to 11% on VRB agar and 3 to 8% on VRBG agar (Table 9.9). Mercuri and Cox (1979; see also Stadhouders et al. 1982) concluded that the use of *Enterobacteriaceae* counts for raw foods could be counterproductive because the *Enterobacteriaceae* count would include too many noncoliforms. There are, however, many situations for which an *Enterobacteriaceae* count would be useful (Van Schothorst and Oosterom 1984).

The sample type and temperature of incubation can influence results of *Enterobacteriaceae* counts by affecting the spectrum of coliforms recovered (Hartman and Hartman 1976; Mossel et al. 1979; Oblinger et al. 1982). There is general agreement that incubation at temperatures below 35°C results in greater recoveries of coliforms if the incubation period is sufficient. The increased recoveries are caused by the growth of bacteria with low optimal growth temperatures that may be significant in the spoilage of foods when refrigerated but may or may not be of public health significance. Farmer et al. (1985; see also Bouvet et al. 1985 and Hickman-Brenner et al. 1985) published a comprehensive description of all new organisms that comprise the 22 genera, 69 species, and 29 biogroups or enteric groups of the

Table 9.9 Percentage Distributions of Bacteria Isolated from VRB and VRBG Agars Incubated at 35°C

Organism	Retail foods		Fresh meats		Processed meats	
	VRB	VRBG '	VRB	VRBG	VRB	VRBG
Aeromonas spp.	9	10	14	24	0	0
Citrobacter spp.	6	10	0	7	21	19
Enterobacter spp.	15	7	19	7	16	12
Erwinia herbicola	27	36	11	24	16	8
Escherichia coli	10	6	11	3	11	8
Hafnia alvei	4	4	9	10	0	0
Klebsiella pneumoniae	7	6	11	3	5	12
Serratia marcescens	18	22	17	21	32	42
Yersinia enterocolitica	3	0	6	0	0	0

(*Data from Oblinger et al. 1982*)

Enterobacteriaceae. Included are indole-negative *Escherichia* and indole-positive *Klebsiella* groups and other bacteria that might serve as indicator organisms as well as being opportunistic pathogens. Whether attempts should be made to recover as many of these bacteria as possible during the examination of water and foods would depend on the purpose of the assay.

A DNA-DNA hybridization test for *Enterobacteriaceae* was recently described (Palva 1983). This assay might have utility in food analysis for the rapid determination of the presence of significant numbers of *Enterobacteriaceae* in bacterial mixtures or in confirming that isolates are indeed *Enterobacteriaceae*.

TOTAL GRAM-NEGATIVE BACTERIA

Gram-negative bacteria are more sensitive than many gram-positive bacteria to heat. Therefore, the presence of gram-negative bacteria in a thermally processed food signifies inadequate heating or postheating contamination (Mossel 1962b, 1982b; APHA 1984). By enumerating all gram-negative bacteria, not just those of enteric origin, the assay should be more sensitive.

Early literature on methods to selectively determine numbers of gram-negatives in food and other materials was reviewed by Mossel et al. (1977), Cyzeska et al. (1981), and Petzel (1984). A crystal violet-tetrazolium (CVT) agar has been recommended (APHA 1984) for the determination of psychotrophic microorganisms. CVT agar is not satisfactory for the estimation of total gram-negatives because crystal violet is inhibitory to some gram negatives (Mossel 1962b) and does not inhibit all gram-positive bacteria (Mossel et al. 1977; Cyzeska et al. 1981).

Two selective media for obtaining maximum yields of gram-negatives were described recently. Peptone-bile-amphotericin-cycloheximide (PBAC) agar was developed by Cyzeska et al. (1981). PBAC agar recovered 55 to 71% more gram-negatives from hamburger than when the VRB agar-overlay method was used; 95% of the isolates from PBAC agar were gram-negative, whereas only 70% of colonies selected from plate count agar were gram-negative. Thus, performance of PBAC agar was very good.

Cyzeska et al. (1981) did not report on percentages of gram-negatives that were not recovered on PBAC agar. We started a project to determine this and to attempt to improve PBAC agar; however, our efforts were directed toward developing an entirely new medium when the results of another research project indicated that low levels of the antibiotic monensin were inhibitory to all gram-positives tested but not to gram-negatives. A new medium (Table 9.10), plate count-monensin-KC1 (PMK) agar was developed (Petzel and Hartman 1985). When a variety of food and environmental samples was examined with PMK agar, 96% were gram negative, compared with 68% of colonies from plate count agar. PMK agar was more selective than CVT and PBAC agars against gram-positive bacteria. MUG could be added to PMK agar to obtain estimates of *E. coli* if the samples did not contain flavobacteria and other nonenterics that hydrolyze MUG. The formulation of PMK agar (Table 9.10) specifies the addition of monensin aseptically to sterilized basal medium. That procedure was used during the research (Petzel and Hartman 1985). Monensin is a relatively stable antibiotic and it may be possible to sterilize all ingredients together; in this case, the initial monensin concentration should be about 60 mg/L, rather than 35 mg/L.

Both PBAC and PMK agars can be recommended for the determination of total gram-negatives in foods. Slightly different flora are recovered on the two media (Petzel 1984; Petzel and Hartman 1985), so one medium may be preferred over the other for a specific purpose.

ENTEROCOCCI (FECAL STREPTOCOCCI)

The enterococci consist of the streptococcal species *faecalis*, *faecium* (including *durans*), *bovis*, *equinus*, and *avium* (APHA 1984). The taxonomy of these bacteria is in a state of flux (Knight et al. 1984; Farrow and Collins 1985), and these bacteria may soon possess new names. Recent emphasis placed on the relationships of these bacteria to each other and on their ecology (Hoadley and Dutka 1977; Skinner and Quesnel 1978; Mundt 1982) should lead to a better understanding of these bacteria and improved media and methods. The enterococci hold promise of being the most useful of all indicator organisms, and they presently are underutilized as pollution indicators. They are

Table 9.10.   Composition of PMK Agar

Plate count agar	23.5	g/L
KCl (omit for water samples)	7.5	g/L
Monensin (see text)	35.0	mg/L
MUG (optional; see text)	75.0	mg/L

(From Petzel and Hartman 1985)

relatively resistant to heat, salts, freezing, and other environmental insults that would kill most other indicator organisms (Skinner and Quesnel 1978; APHA 1984), so they are useful for certain purposes, such as an index of the sanitary quality of butter (APHA 1985b). Their presence in some foods should, however, be interpreted with caution (Mundt 1982; Stadhouders et al. 1982).

Almost 100 media have been described for the enumeration of the enterococci (Hartman et al. 1966; Barnes 1976; Mossel et al. 1982b). Only those described in the APHA manuals (1984, 1985b,c), recent improvements to those media, and selected new media and methods that hold promise for water and food analyses will be discussed here.

As shown in Table 9.11, all the media presently recommended for food and water analyses (APHA 1984, 1985b,c), except GTC agar, originated in the decades 1950 to 1970 and contain sodium azide as the primary selective ingredient. Azide-containing media have several disadvantages (Hartman et al. 1966; Skinner and Quesnel 1978; Beaudoin and Litsky 1981), including inability to promote growth of injured cells, selectivity against *S. bovis*, *S. equinus*, and *S. avium*, and a lengthy (48-hr) incubation time. GTC agar requires only 24 hr of incubation for colony development and recovers a wider variety of enterococci; however, the false-positive rate is high on this medium with some types of environmental samples (Donnelly and Hartman 1978). Alvarez (1982) reported that counts from seafoods on KF and GTC agars were equivalent and that both media yielded relatively high percentages of enterococci. Althaus et al. (1982) demonstrated that GTC agar permitted

Table 9.11. Media Recommended for Entercocci

Medium	Purpose	% Azide	Year	Reference
KF agar	food	0.40	1961	APHA 1984
GTC agar	food	none	1978	APHA 1984
Citrate azide agar	butter	0.01	1953	APHA 1985b
Azide dextrose broth	water	0.02	1950	APHA 1985c
KF	water	0.04	1961	APHA 1985c
PSE (esculin-azide)	water	0.025	1970	APHA 1985c

growth of more enterococcal isolates than KF agar or five other media tested, but some *Bacillus* spp. grew on GTC agar and produced false-positive esculin reactions.

Better media than all those shown in Table 9.11 are now available. Some of these rely on the use of fluorogenic substrates for specific colony detection and species recognition. Facklam et al. (1982) observed that, of a wide variety of streptococci examined, only group A streptococci (bile-esculin negative) and enterococci (bile-esculin positive) hydrolyzed L-pyroglutamic acid-β-naphthylamide (PYR); nonenterococcal group D streptococci were PYR-negative. Their results were confirmed by Hussain et al. (1984). Littel and Hartman (1983) examined a large series of β-naphthylamide and 4-methylumbelliferyl substrates (see also Slifkin and Gil 1983). The 4-methylumbelliferyl substrates resulted in greater fluorescence and were less toxic to the bacteria than the β-naphthylamides. A modification of GTC agar (Donnelly and Hartman 1978; APHA 1984) was proposed (Littel and Hartman 1983). They modified GTC agar (Table 9.12) by substituting galactose for the glucose in GTC agar; this increased specificity of the medium without decreasing productivity. A colorimetric starch substrate was added to detect amylase-positive colonies. And 4-methylumbelliferyl-α-D-galactoside (α-D-MUGAL) was added to detect enzyme activity. The new medium was named fGTC agar (Littel and Hartman 1983). Fecal streptococci could be differentiated into three phenotypic groups directly on the isolation plate: (1) amylase+ fluorescence+ (*S. bovis* from sewage; many bovine strains were amylase−), (2) amylase− fluorescence+ (*S. faecium,* including *S. durans* and *S. casseliflavus,* and (3) amylase− fluorescence− (*S. faecalis, S. equinus, S. avium, S. mitis,* and *S. salivarius.* No amylase+ fluorescence− cultures were encountered.

Use of a more sensitive colorimetric amylase detection system in place of dyed starch (Trepeta and Edberg 1984a) might result in improved detection

Table 9.12.   Ingredients of fGTC Agar

Trypticase soy agar	40.0	g/L
Galactose	1.0	g/L
KH$_2$PO$_4$	5.0	g/L
NaHCO$_3$	2.0	g/L
Thallous acetate	0.5	g/L
Gentamicin sulfate	2.5	mg/L
Tween 80	0.75	mL/L
Amylose azure	2.0	g/L
4-MUGAL[a]	100.0	mg/L

[a]4-methylumbelliferyl-α-D-galactoside.
(*From Littel and Hartman 1983*)

of starch-hydrolyzing *S. bovis* strains. A similar type of colorimetric test for β-glucosidase (esculinase) was also described recently (Edberg et al. 1985) and may have utility in formulating improved media.

A MF medium specific for *S. bovis* has been described (Oragui and Mara 1983); it might be modified for use as a plating medium to detect pollution from farm animals. All these new media hold promise for food analysis, as well as determining point-source pollution of water. It would be useful to have a single medium and method to determine point-source pollution, rather than relying on conventional FC/FS (fecal coliform/fecal streptococcus) ratios which rely on two determinations, each of which possesses a rather wide margin of error.

Several media have been proposed for the isolation of total streptococcal populations. Mossel et al. (1977; see also Skinner and Quesnel 1978) reviewed the literature and recommended a phenyl ethanol agar for gram-positives, including streptococci. Other media selective for only streptococci have been proposed; a new colistin-oxolinic acid-blood agar (Petts 1984) recovered all streptococci tested. This medium has not been used for water or food analyses, but modifications of it might be satisfactory.

Investigators interested in confirming and identifying enterococci (APHA 1984) should become familiar with latest developments on opitimal media for the production of group D antigen (Douglas et al. 1984) and precautions to take if using rapid latex-agglutination identification kits (Shlaes et al. 1984; Vanzo and Washington 1984, and references therein).

OTHER ORGANISMS

Bacteriophages

Bacteriophages, especially coliphages, have been suggested as indicators of pollution and virus survival in water and wastewater (Berg 1978; Melnick 1984). A number of methods have been suggested to assay coliphages; some take only six hours and are relatively easy to perform (Wentsel et al. 1982).

Purdy et al. (1985) described a method for the simultaneous concentration and determination of phages from water. Samples were treated with 1% v/v chloroform (a hazardous procedure) to kill indigenous bacteria, prefiltered to remove suspended solids, filtered, and aerated to remove the chloroform. About 3×10^7 host cells were placed on the filter by filtration, and the filter was incubated overnight. Plaques were counted after the membrane was treated with a tetrazolium compound to accentuate the background lawn. Kennedy et al. (1984) determined that chloroform treatment was detrimental to some coliphages and that its use could be avoided by producing the lawns on a selective medium; EC medium was best. The host strain used for phage detection is important (Kennedy et al. 1984; Stetler 1984). Since F pili are not synthesized in *E. coli* below 30°C, Primrose et al. (1982) suggested that all the male-specific phages in a sample that has been held at temperatures below 30°C must have originated in the intestine of warm-blooded animals. Therefore, male-specific phages should be a direct index of the extent of fecal pollution. If only a few phages are present in a large volume of sample, their numbers may be amplified by adding a host strain and incubating the mixture to permit phage multiplication before plating for plaque determinations (Hoch and László 1966).

A report on the incidence and numbers of coliphages in selected foods was published recently (Kennedy et al. 1984); an indicator *E. coli* carrying an *F*-factor was used as the host. Their results (Table 9.13) demonstrated that coliphage numbers in foods can be readily determined in a 16-hr test and that coliphages may offer a rapid method for indicating fecal contamination of foods.

Two observations made in our laboratory have a bearing on the potential efficacy of coliphage tests. First, the selection of diluent is important if one is used (W. R. Schwan and C. W. Kaspar, unpublished data). Second, we observed (W. R. Schwan and K. P. Raisch, unpublished data) that coliphages adsorb to a variety of gram-negative bacteria, not just *E. coli*. Some pseudomonads, for example, will remove from phage suspensions more coliphages than *E. coli* does. The union is nonproductive, however, and no lysis of the "host" occurs. These results indicate that the types and numbers of indigenous bacteria in samples may reduce the numbers of coliphages detected. This would be more of a problem when assaying liquids where phage and "hosts" are in suspension than when both were present in meat or another solid food (Trevors et al. 1984).

Table 9.13. Fecal Coliform, Coliform, and Coliphage Counts on Selected Foods

Food	No.	Coliforms	Fecal Coliforms	Coliphage
Chicken	9	4.33 ± 1.21	2.92 ± 0.68	3.99 ± 0.37
Pork sausage	9	2.00 ± 1.36	0.80 ± 0.86	2.58 ± 0.65
Roast corned beef	3	3.02 ± 1.25	1.13 ± 0.99	NR[a]
Roasted turkey breast	3	3.48 ± 0.69	2.55 ± 1.67	1.43 ± 1.37

[a]None recovered.
(*Data from Kennedy et al. 1984*)

Bifidobacteria

The value of bifidobacteria as indicator organisms has been limited because of significant extrafecal sources, poor survival in the external environment, and multiplication outside of the host (Berg 1978). Mara and Oragui (1983) recently reported, however, that sorbitol-fermenting strains were isolated only from samples of human feces (Table 9.14), and this species-specific characteristic might be of value for some applications.

Bacteroides

Bacteroides spp. are gram-negative bacteria that are present in human intestinal material in numbers over 100 times greater than those of *E. coli*. Furthermore, *Bacteroides* spp. are nutritionally fastidious, obligate anaerobes. Ordinarily they do not multiply outside the intestine. Media for their propagation have been developed (Allsop and Stickler 1984; Moench et al. 1984; Fiksdal et al. 1985). The use of *Bacteroides* spp. as an indicator of fecal pollution (Table 9.14), especially from humans (Allsop and Stickler 1985), might have application in food microbiology. Developments in analytical methodologies for both *Bifidobacterium* and *Bacteroides* spp. should be followed with interest. Creative food microbiologists might enter the arena to develop tests for these potential indicator organisms.

Rhodococcus coprophilus

Whereas *Bacteroides* spp. are characteristic of human wastes, *Rhodococcus coprophilus* is associated with animal excreta (Mara and Oragui 1981). The organism is an actinomycete (Mara and Oragui 1981). It is a very hardy organism

Table 9.14. Significant Properties of Three Potential Indicator Organisms

Potential indicator	Property	Reference
Bifidobacterium sp.	Sorbitol +; human source	Mara and Oragi (1983)
Bacterioides spp.	Human source; do not multiply outside host	Allsop and Stickler (1985)
Rhodococcus coprophilus	Animal source; very resistant	Oragui and Mara (1983) Mara and Oragui (1981)

(Oragui and Mara 1983). An adequate selective culture medium exists (Mara and Oragui 1981). *Rhodococcus coprophilus* has potential as an indicator specific for fecal pollution caused by farm-animal wastes (Table 9.14), so it has unique possibilities in food microbiology as an indicator organism. Also, a *R. coprophilus/Bacteroides* ratio or *R. coprophilus*/sorbitol-fermenting *Bifidobacterium* ratio might provide more meaningful results than the fecal coliform/fecal streptococcus ratio that has conventionally been used to determine point-source pollution of surface waters or to investigate sources of contamination of foods.

Other Microbial Indicator Organisms

Other microorganisms have been proposed as indicator organisms (Hoadley and Dutka 1977; Mossel 1982a; Petzel 1984), but there has been little activity in recent years to develop methods to determine their presence and numbers in water and foods.

REFERENCES

ABBISS, J. S. and BLOOD, R. M. 1982. The detection of *Escherichia coli* in foods. In *Isolation and Identification Methods for Food Poisoning Organisms*. Corry, J. E. L., Roberts, D., and Skinner, F. A. (Ed.). Academic Press, New York, NY.

ABBISS, J. S., WILSON, J. M., BLOOD, R. M., and JARVIS, B. 1981. A comparison of minerals modified glutamate medium with other media for the enumeration of coliforms in delicatessen foods. *J. Appl. Bacteriol.* 51: 121–127.

ABSHIRE, R. L. and GUTHRIE, R. K. 1973. Fluorescent antibody as a method for the detection of fecal pollution: *Escherichia coli* as indicator organisms. *Can. J. Microbiol.* 19: 201–206.

ALLSOP, K. and STICKLER, D. J. 1984. The enumeration of *Bacillus fragilis* group organisms from sewage and natural waters. *J. Appl. Bacteriol.* 56: 15–24.

ALLSOP, K. and STICKLER, D. J. 1985. An assessment of *Bacteroides fragilis* group organisms as indicators of human faecal pollution. *J. Appl. Bacteriol.* 58: 95–99.

ALTHAUS, H., DOTT, W., HAVEMEISTER, G., MÜLLER, H. E., and SACRÉ, C. 1982. Faecal streptococci as indicator organisms of drinking water. *Zentralbl. Bakteriol., Abt. I, Orig.* A252: 154–165.

ALVAREZ, R. J. 1982. Evaluation of various commercially available media for the recovery of enterococci from seafoods. Abstract 184. 42nd Annual Meeting Inst. of Food Technologists.

ALVAREZ, R. J. 1984. Use of fluorogenic assays for the enumeration of *Escherichia coli* from selected seafoods. *J. Food Sci.* 49: 1186–1187, 1232.

ANDERSON, J. G., MEADOWS, P. S., MULLINS, B. W., and PATEL, K. 1980. Gas production by *Escherichia coli* in selective lactose fermentation media. *FEMS Microbiol. Lett.* 8: 17–21.

ANDERSON, J. M. and BAIRD-PARKER, A. C. 1975. A rapid and direct plate method for enumerating *Escherichia coli* biotype I in food. *J. Appl. Bacteriol.* 39: 111–117.

ANDREW, M. H. E. and RUSSELL, A. D. (Ed.). 1984. *The Survival of Injured Microorganisms.* Academic Press, New York, NY.

ANDREWS, W. H., DURAN, A. P., McCLURE, F. D., and GENTILE, D. E. 1979. Use of two rapid A-1 methods for the recovery of fecal coliforms and *Escherichia coli* from selected food types. *J. Food Sci.* 44: 289–291.

ANDREWS, W. H. and PRESNELL, M. W. 1972. Rapid recovery of *Escherichia coli* from estuarine water. *Appl. Microbiol.* 23: 521–523.

ANDREWS, W. H. WILSON, C. R., POELMA, P. L., BULLOCK, L. K., McCLURE, F. D., and GENTILE, D. E. 1981. Interlaboratory evaluation of the AOAC method and the A-1 procedure for recovery of fecal coliforms from foods. *J. Assoc. Off. Anal. Chem.* 64: 1116–1121.

APHA. 1984. *Compendium of Methods for the Microbiological Examination of Foods.* 2nd ed. American Public Health Association, Washington, DC.

APHA. 1985a. *Laboratory Procedures for the Examination of Seawater and Shellfish.* 5th ed. American Public Health Association, Washington, DC.

APHA. 1985b. *Standard Methods for the Examination of Dairy Products.* 15th ed. American Public Health Association, Washington, DC.

APHA. 1985c. *Standard Methods for the Examination of Water and Wastewater.* 16th ed. American Public Health Association, Washington, DC.

ARMSTRONG, J. L., CALOMIRIS, J. J., and SEIDLER, R. J. 1982. Selection of antibiotic-resistant standard plate count bacteria during water treatment. *Appl. Environ. Microbiol.* 44: 308–316.

ARMSTRONG, J. L., SHIGENO, D. S., CALOMIRIS, J. J., and SEIDLER, R. J. 1981. Antibiotic-resistant bacteria in drinking water. *Appl. Environ. Microbiol.* 42: 277–283.

AUSTIN, B., HUSSONG, D., WEINER, R. M., and COLWELL, R. R. 1981. Numerical taxonomy analysis of bacteria isolated from the completed most probable numbers test for coliform bacilli. *J. Appl. Bacteriol.* 51: 101–112.

BARNES, E. M. 1976. Methods for the isolation of faecal streptococci. *Lab. Practice* 1976: 145–147.

BEAUDOIN, E. C. and LITSKY, W. 1981. Fecal streptococci. In *Membrane Filtration: Applications, Techniques, and Problems*. Dutka, B. J. (Ed.). Marcel Dekker, Inc., New York, NY.

BERG, G. (Ed.). 1978. *Indicators of Viruses in Water and Food*. Ann Arbor Science Publishers, Ann Arbor, MI.

BINDSCHEDLER, O., De MAN, J. C., and CURIAT, G. 1981. Comparative study of several culture media to determine coliforms and *E. coli* in dairy and cocoa products. *Zentralbl. Bakteriol.* Abt. II 136: 146–151.

BORDNER, R. H. 1983. Microbiology: methodology and quality assurance. *J. Water Pollut. Control Fed.* 55: 881–890.

BOUVET, O. M. M., GRIMONT, P. A. D., RICHARD, C., ALDOVA, E., HAUSNER, O., and GABRHELOVA, M. 1985. *Budvicia aquatica* gen. nov., sp. nov.: a hydrogen sulfide-producing member of the *Enterobacteriaceae*. *Int. J. System. Bacteriol.* 35: 60–64.

BUESCHKENS, D. H. and STILES, M. E. 1984. *Escherichia coli* variants for gas and indole production at elevated incubation temperatures. *Appl. Environ. Microbiol.* 48: 601–605.

BURAS, N. and KOTT, Y. 1972. A new approach in *E. coli* identification. In *Advances in Water Pollution Research*. Jenkins, S. H. (Ed.). Pergamon Press, Elmsford, NY.

BUSTA, F. F. 1976. Practical implications of injured microorganisms in food. *J. Milk Food Technol.* 39: 138–145.

CAPLENAS, N. R. and KANAREK, M. S. 1984. Thermotolerant non-fecal source *Klebsiella pneumoniae:* validity of the fecal coliform test in recreational waters. *Am. J. Publ. Health* 74: 1273–1275.

CHASLUS-DANCLA, E. and LAFONT, J.-P. 1985. IncH plasmids in *Escherichia coli* strains isolated from broiler chicken carcasses. *Appl. Environ. Microbiol.* 49: 1016–1018.

CLARK, J. A. 1968. A presence-absence (P-A) test providing sensitive and inexpensive detection of coliforms, fecal coliforms, and fecal streptococci in municipal drinking water supplies. *Can. J. Microbiol.* 14: 13–18.

CLARK, J. A. 1980. The influence of increasing numbers of nonindicator organisms by the membrane filter and presence-absence tests. *Can. J. Microbiol.* 26: 827–832.

CLEMESHA, W. W. 1912. A criticism of Dr. A. C. Houston's report on the biological characteristics of *B. coli* isolated from (1) raw, (2) stored river water, and (3) stored and filtered water. *J. Hyg.* 12: 463–478.

COOK, D. W. and PABST, G. S., Jr. 1984. Recommended modification of dilution procedure used for bacteriological examination of shellfish. *J. Assoc. Off. Anal. Chem.* 67: 197–198.

CRICHTON, P. B., IP, S. M., and OLD, D. C. 1981. Hemagglutinin typing as an aid in identification of biochemically atypical *Escherichia coli* strains. *J. Clin. Microbiol.* 14: 599–603.

CUNDELL, A. M. 1981. Rapid counting methods for coliform bacteria. *Adv. Appl. Microbiol.* 27: 169–181.

CYZESKA, F. J., SEITER, J. A., MARKS, S. N., and JAY, J. M. 1981. Culture medium for selective isolation and enumeration of Gram-negative bacteria from ground meats. *Appl. Environ. Microbiol.* 42: 303–307.

DAMARÉ, J. M., CAMPBELL, D. F., and JOHNSTON, R. W. 1984. An improved β-glucuronidase plating medium for *E. coli.* Abstract 234. 44th Annual Meeting, Inst. of Food Technologists.

De MAN, J. C. 1975. The probability of most probable numbers. *European J. Microbiol.* 1: 67–78.

De MAN, J. C. 1983. MPN tables, corrected. *Europ. J. Appl. Microbiol. Biotechnol.* 17: 301–305.

DEXTER, F. 1981. Modification of the standard most-probable-number procedure for fecal coliform bacteria in seawater and shellfish. *Appl. Environ. Microbiol.* 42: 184–185.

DOMEK, M. J., LeCHEVALLIER, M. W., CAMERON, S. C., and McFETERS, G. A. 1984. Evidence for the role of copper in the injury process of coliform bacteria in drinking water. *Appl. Environ. Microbiol.* 48: 289–293.

DONNELLY, L. S. and HARTMAN, P. A. 1978. Gentamicin-based medium for the isolation of group D streptococci and application of the medium to water analysis. *Appl. Environ. Microbiol.* 35: 576–581.

DOUGLAS, J., DHILLON, J., and SMITH, S. E. 1984. The general utility of a glycerophosphate-Tris buffered medium. *J. Appl. Bacteriol.* 56: 321–326.

DRAUGHON, F. A. and NELSON, P. J. 1981. Comparison of modified direct-plating procedures for the recovery of injured *Escherichia coli. J. Food Sci.* 46: 1188–1191.

DUTKA, B. J. 1973. Coliforms are an inadequate index of water quality. *J. Environ. Health* 36: 39–46.

DYCK, M. G. and QUINLEY, R. 1984. Speciation of coliform bacteria found in Kansas public water supply systems. Paper presented at the Am. Water Works Assoc. 1984 Water Qual. Technol. Conf., Denver, CO.

EDBERG, S. C., TREPETA, R. W., KONTNICK, C. M., and TORRES, A. R. 1985. Measurement of active β-D-glucosidase (esculinase) in the presence of sodium desoxycholate. *J. Clin. Microbiol.* 21: 363–365.

EIJKMAN, C. 1913. Die Gärungsprobe bei 46° als Hilfsmittel bei der Trinkwasseruntersuchung. *Centralbl. Bakteriol. Abt. I, Orig.* 37: 742–752.

ESCHERICH, T. 1885. Die Darmbacterien des Neugebornen und Säuglings. *Fortschr. Med.* 3: 515–522.

EVANS, T. M., LeCHEVALLIER, M. W., WAARVICK, C. E., and SEIDLER, R. J. 1981a. Coliform species recovered from untreated surface water and drinking water by the membrane filter, standard, and modified most-probable-number techniques. *Appl. Environ. Microbiol.* 41: 657–663.

EVANS, T. M., SEIDLER, R. J., and LeCHEVALLIER, M. W. 1981b. Impact of verification media and resuscitation on accuracy of the membrane filter total coliform enumeration technique. *Appl. Environ. Microbiol.* 41: 1144–1151.

EVANS, T. M., WAARVICK, C. W., SEIDLER, R. J., and LeCHEVALLIER, M. W. 1981c. Failure of the most-probable-number technique to detect coliforms in drinking water and raw water supplies. *Appl. Environ. Microbiol.* 41: 130–138.

FACKLAM, R. R., THACKER, L. G., FOX, B., and ERIQUEZ, L. 1982. Presumptive identification of streptococci with a new test system. *J. Clin. Microbiol.* 15: 987–990.

FARMER, J. J. III, DAVIS, B. R., HICKMAN-BRENNER, F. W., McWHORTER, A., HUNTLEY-CARTER, G. P., ASBURY, M. A., RIDDLE, C., WATHEN-GRADY, H. G., ELIAS, C., FANNING, G. R., STIEGERWALT, A. G., O'HARA, C. M., MORRIS, G. K., SMITH, P. B., and BRENNER, D. J. 1985. Biochemical identification of new species and biogroups of *Enterobacteriaceae* isolated from clinical specimens. *J. Clin. Microbiol.* 21: 46–76.

FARROW, J. A. E. and COLLINS, M. D. 1985. *Enterococcus hirae*, a new species than includes amino acid assay strain NCDO 1258 and strains causing growth depression in young chickens. *Int. J. Syst. Bacteriol.* 35: 73–75.

FENG, P. C. S. and HARTMAN, P. A. 1982. Fluorogenic assays for immediate confirmation of *Escherichia coli*. *Appl. Environ. Microbiol.* 43: 1320–1329.

FIKSDAL, L., MAKI, J. S., LaCROIX, S. J., and STALEY, J. T. 1985. Survival and detection of *Bacteroides* spp., prospective indicator bacteria. *Appl. Environ. Microbiol.* 49: 148–150.

FRANCIS, D. W., PEELER, J. T., and TWEDT, R. M. 1974. Rapid method for detection and enumeration of fecal coliforms in fresh chicken. *Appl. Microbiol.* 27: 1127–1130.

FUNG, D. Y. C. and KRAFT, A. A. 1969. Rapid evaluation of viable cell counts by using the Microtiter system and MPN techniques. *J. Milk Food Technol.* 32: 408–409.

FUNG, D. Y. C. and MILLER, R. D. 1972. Miniaturized techniques for IMViC tests. *J. Milk Food Technol.* 35: 328–329.

GADELLE, D., RAIBAUD, P., and SACQUET, E. 1985. β-Glucuronidase activities of intestinal bacteria determined both in vitro and in vivo in gnotobiotic rats. *Appl. Environ. Microbiol.* 49: 682–685.

GELDREICH, E. E. 1966. *Sanitary Significance of Fecal Coliforms in the Environment.* Water Pollution Control Publ. WP-20-3. Federal Water Pollution Control Administration, Washington, DC.

GELDREICH, E. E. 1983. Microbiology of water. *J. Water Pollution Control Fed.* 55: 869–881.

GELDREICH, E. E., ALLEN, M. J., and TAYLOR, R. H. 1978. Interferences to coliform detection in potable water supplies. In *Evaluation of the Microbiology Standards for Drinking Water.* Hendricks, C. W. (Ed.). U. S. Environmental Protection Agency, Washington, DC.

GOEPFERT, J. M. 1976. The aerobic plate count, coliform and *Escherichia coli* content of raw ground beef at the retail level. *J. Milk Food Technol.* 39: 175–178.

GOSHKO, M. A., PIPES, W. O., and CHRISTIAN, R. R. 1984. Possible confusion between *Enterobacter agglomerans* and *Escherichia coli. Pharm. Technol.* 8(2): 32, 34, 36, 38–39.

HANSEN, W. and YOURASSOWSKY, E. 1984. Detection of β-glucuronidase in lactose fermenting members of the family *Enterobacteriaceae* and its presence in bacterial urine culture. *J. Clin. Microbiol.* 20: 1177–1179.

HARTEL, P. C. and HAGEDORN, C. 1983. Microtechnique for isolating fecal coliforms from soil. *Appl. Environ. Microbiol.* 46: 518–520.

HARTMAN, P. A. 1979. Modification of conventional methods for recovery of injured coliforms and salmonellae. *J. Food Prot.* 42: 356–361.

HARTMAN, P. A., FENG, P. C. S., and MINNICH, S. A. 1982. Expanding horizons of miniaturized methods in food and water microbiology. In *Rapid Methods and Automation in Microbiology.* Tilton, R. C. (Ed.) American Society for Microbiology, Washington, DC.

HARTMAN, P. A. and HARTMAN, P. S. 1976. Coliform analysis at 30 C. *J. Milk Food Technol.* 39: 763–767.

HARTMAN, P. A., HARTMAN, P. S., and LANZ, W. W. 1975. Violet red bile 2 agar for stressed coliforms. *Appl. Microbiol.* 29: 537–539, 865.

HARTMAN, P. A., REINBOLD, G. W., and SARASWAT, D. S. 1966. Media and methods for isolation and enumeration of the enterococci. *Adv. Appl. Microbiol.* 8: 253–289.

HASTBACK, W. G. 1981. Short incubation of presumptive media for detection of fecal coliforms in shellfish. *Appl. Environ. Microbiol.* 42: 1125–1127.

HENRIKSEN, S. D. 1955. A study of the causes of discordant results of the presumptive and completed coliform tests on Norwegian waters. *Acta Pathol. Microbiol. Scand.* 36: 87–95.

HICKMAN-BRENNER, F. W., VOHRA, M. P., HUNTLEY-CARTER, G. P., FANNING, G. R., LOWERY, V. A. III, BRENNER, D. J. and FARMER, J. J. III. 1985. *Leminorella*, a new genus of *Enterobacteriaceae*: identification of *Leminorella grimontii* sp. nov. and *Leminorella richardii* sp. nov. found in clinical specimens. *J. Clin. Microbiol.* 21: 234–239.

HINTON, M., LINTON, A. H., and HEDGES, A. J. 1985. The ecology of *Escherichia coli* in calves reared as dairy-cow replacements. *J. Appl. Bacteriol.* 58: 131–138.

HIRAISHI, A. and HORIE, S. 1982. Species composition and growth-temperature characteristics of coliforms in relation to their sources. *J. Gen. Appl. Microbiol.* 28: 139–154.

HOADLEY, A. W. and DUTKA, B. J. (Ed.). 1977. *Bacterial Indicators/Health Hazards Associated with Water*. American Society for Testing and Materials, Philadelphia, PA.

HOCH, V. and LÁSZLÓ, V. 1966. Einführung einer empfindlichen schnell diagnostischen methode in die lebensmittelbakteriologie. *Zentralbl. Bakteriol., Abt. I, Orig.* 200: 394–397.

HOLBROOK, R. and ANDERSON, J. M. 1982. The rapid enumeration of *Escherichia coli* in foods by using a direct plating method. In *Isolation and Identification Methods for Food Poisoning Organisms*. Corry, J. E. L., Roberts, D., and Skinner, F. A. (Ed.). Academic Press, New York, NY.

HOLMBERG, S. D., OSTERHOLM, M. T., SENGER, K. A., and COHEN, M. L. 1984. Drug-resistant *Salmonella* from animals fed antimicrobials. *N. Engl. J. Med.* 311: 617–622.

HUNT, D. A., LUCAS, J. P., McCLURE, F. D., SPRINGER, J., and NEWELL, R. 1981. Comparison of modified A-1 method with standard EC test for recovery of fecal coliform bacteria for shellfish. *J. Assoc. Off. Anal. Chem.* 64: 607–610.

HURST, A. and NASIM, A. (Ed.). 1984. *Repairable Lesions in Microorganisms*. Academic Press, New York, NY.

HUSSAIN, Z., LANNIGAN, R., and STOAKES, L. 1984. A new approach for presumptive identification of clinically important streptococci. *Zentralbl. Bakteriol.* A258: 74–79.

HUSSONG, D., COLWELL, R. R., and WEINER, R. M. 1980. Rate of occurrence of false-positive results from total coliform most-probable-number analysis of shellfish and estuaries. *Appl. Environ. Microbiol.* 40: 981–983.

HUSSONG, D., DAMARÉ, J. M., WEINER, R. M., and COLWELL, R. R. 1981. Bacteria associated with false-positive most-probable-number coliform test results for shellfish and estuaries. *Appl. Environ. Microbiol.* 41: 35–45.

JILLY, B. J., SCHRECKENBERGER, P. C., and LeBEAU, L. J. 1984. Rapid glutamate decarboxylase test for identification of *Bacteroides* and *Clostridium* spp. *J. Clin. Microbiol.* 19: 592–593.

JOINT COMMITTEE. 1980. Single tube confirmatory tests for *Escherichia coli. J. Hyg.* 85: 51–57.

JOINT COMMITTEE. 1981. A comparison of confirmatory media for coliform organisms and *Escherichia coli* in water. *J. Hyg.* 87: 369–375.

KENNEDY, J. E., Jr., OBLINGER, J. L., and BITTON, G. 1984. Recovery of coliphages from chicken, pork sausage and delicatessen meats. *J. Food Prot.* 47: 623–626.

KILGEN, M., COLE, M., HACKNEY, C., and WARD, D. 1985. Evaluation of rapid methods for the seasonal enumeration of *E. coli* in oysters. Abstract Q38. Annual Meeting of the Am. Soc. Microbiol. 1985, 264.

KILIAN, M. and BÜLOW, P. 1976. Rapid diagnosis of *Enterobacteriaceae.* I. Detection of bacterial glycosidases. *Acta Pathol. Microbiol. Scand.* B84: 245–251.

KLEIN, H. and FUNG, D. Y. C. 1976. Identification and quantification of fecal coliforms using violet red bile agar at elevated temperature. *J. Milk Food Technol.* 39: 768–770.

KNIGHT, R. G., SHLAES, D. M., and MESSINEO, L. 1984. Deoxyribonucleic acid relatedness among major human enterococci. *Int. J. Syst. Bacteriol.* 34: 327–331.

KOBURGER, J. A. and MILLER, M. L. 1985. Evaluation of a fluorogenic MPN procedure for determining *Escherichia coli* in oysters. *J. Food Prot.* 48: 244–245.

KREGTEN, E. van, WESTERDAAL, N. A. C. and, WILLERS, J. M. N. 1984. New, simple medium for selective recovery of *Klebsiella pneumoniae* and *Klebsiella oxytoca* from human feces. *J. Clin. Microbiol.* 20: 936–941.

KRUMPERMAN, P. H. 1983. Multiple antibiotic resistance indexing of *Escherichia coli* to identify high-risk sources of fecal contamination of food. *Appl. Environ. Microbiol.* 46: 165–170.

LANGLOIS, B. E., CROMWELL, G. L., STAHLY, T. S., DAWSON, K. A., and HAYS, V. 1983. Antibiotic resistance of fecal coliforms after long-term withdrawal of therapeutic and subtherapeutic antibiotic use in a swine herd. *Appl. Environ. Microbiol.* 46: 1433–1434.

LeCHEVALLIER, M. W., CAMERON, S. C., and McFETERS, G. A. 1983a. New medium for improved recovery of coliform bacteria from drinking water. *Appl. Environ. Microbiol.* 45: 484–492.

LeCHEVALLIER, M. W., CAMERON, S. C., and McFETERS, G. A. 1983b. Comparison of verification procedures for the membrane filter total coliform technique. *Appl. Environ. Microbiol.* 45: 1126–1128, 1963.

LeCHEVALLIER, M. W., JAKANSKI, P. E., CAMPER, A. K., and McFETERS, G. A. 1984. Evaluation of m-T7 agar as a fecal coliform medium. *Appl. Environ. Microbiol.* 48: 371–375.

LEVIN, G. V., HARRISON, V. R., HESS, W. C., and GURNEY, H. C. 1956. A radioisotope technique for the rapid detection of coliform organisms. *Am. J. Publ. Health* 46: 1405–1414.

LEVINE, M. 1961. Facts and fancies of bacterial indices in standards for water and foods. *Food Technol.* 15: 29–38.

LEVVY, G. A. and MARSH, C. A. 1959. Preparation and properties of β-glucuronidase. *Adv. Carbohydr. Chem.* 14: 381–428.

LEVVY, G. A. and MARSH, C. A. 1960. β-Glucuronidase. In *The Enzymes.* 2nd ed., Volume 4. Boyer, P. D., Lardy H., and Myrback, K. (Ed.). Academic Press, New York, NY.

LILLARD, H. S. and THOMSON, J. E. 1983. Comparison of sampling methods for *Escherichica coli* and total aerobic counts on broiler carcasses. *J. Food Prot.* 46: 781–782.

LITTEL, K. J. and HARTMAN, P. A. 1983. Fluorogenic selective and differential medium for isolation of fecal streptococci. *Appl. Environ. Microbiol.* 45: 622–627.

LUPO, L., STRICKLAND, E., DUFOUR, A., and CABELLI, V. 1977. The effect of oxidase positive bacteria on total coliform density estimates. *Health Lab. Sci.* 14: 117–121.

MACCANI, J. E. 1979. Aerobically incubated medium for decarboxylase testing of *Enterobacteriaceae* by replica-plating methods. *J. Clin. Microbiol.* 10: 940–942.

MACKEY, B. M., DERRICK, C. M., and THOMAS, J. A. 1980. The recovery of sublethally injured *Escherichia coli* from frozen meat. *J. Appl. Bacteriol.* 48: 315–324.

MARA, D. D. and ORAGUI, J. I. 1981. Occurrence of *Rhodococcus coprophilus* and associated actinomycetes in feces, sewage, and freshwater. *Appl. Environ. Microbiol.* 42: 1037–1042.

MARA, D. D. and ORAGUI, J. I. 1983. Sorbitol-fermenting bifidobacteria as specific indicators of human faecal pollution. *J. Appl. Bacteriol.* 55: 349–357.

MARSHALL, B., TACHIBANA, C., and LEVY, S. B. 1983. Frequency of tetracycline resistance determinant classes among lactose-fermenting coliforms. *Antimicrob. Agents Chemother.* 24: 835–840.

MAUL, A. and BLOCK, J. C. 1983. Microplate fecal coliform method to monitor stream water pollution. *Appl. Environ. Microbiol.* 46: 1032–1037.

McDONALD, L. C., HACKNEY, C. R., and RAY, B. 1983. Enhanced recovery of injured *Escherichia coli* by compounds that degrade hydrogen peroxide or block its formation. *Appl. Environ. Microbiol.* 45: 360–365.

McFETERS, G. A., CAMERON, S. C., and LeCHEVALLIER, M. W. 1982. Influence of diluents, media, and membrane filters on the detection of injured waterborne coliform bacteria. *Appl. Environ. Microbiol.* 43: 97–103.

McFETERS, G. A. and CAMPER, A. K. 1983. Enumeration of indicator bacteria exposed to chlorine. *Adv. Appl. Microbiol.* 29: 177–193.

MEADOWS, P. S., ANDERSON, J. G., PATEL, K., and MULLINS, B. W. 1980. Variability in gas production by *Escherichia coli* in enrichment media and its relationship to pH. *Appl. Environ. Microbiol.* 40: 309–312.

MEANS, E. G. and OLSON, B. H. 1981. Coliform inhibition by bacteriocin-like substances in drinking water distribution systems. *Appl. Environ. Microbiol.* 42: 506–512.

MELNICK, J. L. (Ed.). 1984. *Enteric Viruses in Water.* S. Karger AG, Basel, Switzerland.

MERCURI, A. J. and COX, N. A. 1979. Coliforms and *Enterobacteriaceae* isolated from selected foods. *J. Food Prot.* 42: 712–714.

METCALF, H. 1905. Organisms on the surface of grain, with special reference to *Bacillus coli. Science* 22: 439–441.

METCALF, T. G. 1978. Indicators for viruses in natural waters. In *Water Pollution Microbiology.* Vol. 2. Mitchell, R. (Ed.). John Wiley and Sons, New York, NY.

MOENCH, T. T., JOHNSTONE, D. L., and STALEY, J. T. 1984. Rapid immunological methods for the detection of intestinal *Bacteroides* spp. as indicators of fecal contamination. Paper presented at the 1984 Water Qual. Technol. Conf., Am. Water Works Assoc., Denver, CO.

MORAN, J. W. and WITTER, L. D. 1976. An automated rapid test for *Escherichia coli* in milk. *J. Food Sci.* 41: 165–167.

MOSSEL, D. A. A. 1957. The presumptive enumeration of lactose negative as well as lactose positive *Enterobacteriaceae* in foods. *Appl. Microbiol.* 5: 379–381.

MOSSEL, D. A. A. 1962a. Use of a modified MacConkey agar medium for the selective growth and enumeration of *Enterobacteriaceae*. *J. Bacteriol.* 84: 381.

MOSSEL, D. A. A. 1962b. The significance of Gram-negative rod-shaped bacteria in foods. In *Biological and Microbiological Aspects of Foods*. Leitch, J. M. (Ed.). Gordon and Breach Science Publishers, New York, NY.

MOSSEL, D. A. A. 1967. Ecological principles and methodological aspects of the examination of foods and feeds for indicator microorganisms. *J. Assoc. Off. Anal. Chem.* 50: 91–104.

MOSSEL, D. A. A. 1978. Index and indicator organisms—A current assessment of their usefulness and significance. *Food Technol. Aust.* 30: 212–219.

MOSSEL, D. A. A. 1982a. *Microbiology of Foods. The Ecological Essentials of Assurance and Assessment of Safety and Quality*. 3rd ed. University of Utrecht, Utrecht, The Netherlands.

MOSSEL, D. A. A. 1982b. Marker (index and indicator) organisms in food and drinking water. Semantics, ecology, taxonomy and enumeration. *Antonie Leeuwenhoek J. Microbiol.* 48: 609–611 (and reviews by others on 612–644).

MOSSEL, D. A. A., EELDERINK, I., KOOPSMANS, M., and VAN ROSSEM, F. 1979. Influence of carbon source, bile salts and incubation temperature on recovery of *Enterobacteriaceae* from foods using MacConkey-type agars. *J. Food Prot.* 42: 470–475.

MOSSEL, D. A. A., VAN DOORNE, H., EELDERINK, I., and DE VOR, H. 1977. The selective enumeration of Gram positive and Gram negative bacteria in foods, water and medicinal and cosmetic preparations. *Pharmaceut. Week.* 112: 41–48.

MOTES, M. L., Jr., McPHEARSON, R. M., Jr., and DePAOLA, A., Jr. 1984. Comparison of three international methods with APHA method for enumeration of *Escherichia coli* in estuarine waters and shellfish. *J. Food Prot.* 47: 557–561.

MUNDT, J. O. 1982. The ecology of the streptococci. *Microbial Ecol.* 8: 355–369.

NELSON, C. L., FOX, T. L., and BUSTA, F. F. 1984. Evaluation of dry medium film (Petrifilm VRB) for coliform enumeration. *J. Food Prot.* 47: 520–525.

OBLINGER, J. L., KENNEDY, J. E., Jr., and LANGSTON, D. M. 1982. Microflora recovered from foods on violet red bile agar with and without glucose and incubated at different temperatures. *J. Food Prot.* 45: 948–952.

OLSON, B. H. 1978. Enhanced accuracy of coliform testing in seawater by a modification of the most-probable-number method. *Appl. Environ. Microbiol.* 36: 438–444.

ORAGUI, J. I. and MARA, D. D. 1983. Investigation of the survival characteristics of *Rhodococcus coprophilus* and certain fecal indicator bacteria. *Appl. Environ. Microbiol.* 46: 356–360.

PALVA, A. M. 1983. *ompA* gene in the detection of *Escherichia coli* and other *Enterobacteriacae* by nucleic acid sandwich hybridization. *J. Clin. Microbiol* 18: 92–100.

PERLMAN, D. (Ed.). 1978. *Adv. Appl. Microbiol.* 23: 195–285.

PETTS, D. N. 1984. Colistin-oxolinic acid-blood agar: a new selective medium for streptococci. *J. Clin. Microbiol.* 19: 4–7.

PETZEL, J. P. 1984. A monensin-based medium for the determination of total Gram-negatives and *Escherichia coli*. M. S. thesis, Parks Library, Iowa State University, Ames, IA.

PETZEL, J. P. and HARTMAN, P. A. 1985. Monensin-based medium for determination of total Gram-negative bacteria and *Escherichia coli*. *Appl. Environ. Microbiol.* 49: 925–933.

PHIRKE, P. M. 1976. Rapid agar pour-plate technique for detection and enumeration of faecal coliforms in sewage. *Indian J. Environ. Health* 18: 183–190.

PIPES, W. O. (Ed.). 1978. *Bacterial Indicators of Pollution.* CRC press, Inc., Boca Raton, FL.

PIPES, W. O., MUELLER, K. M., and MINNIGH, H. A. 1986. Comparison of coliform detection methods for water samples with low coliform densities. *Appl. Environ. Microbiol.* 50: in press.

POWERS, E. M. and LATT, T. G. 1979. Rapid enumeration and identification of stressed fecal coliforms. *J. Food Prot.* 42: 342–345.

PRESCOTT, S. C. 1902. On the apparent identity of the cultural reactions of *B. coli communis* and certain lactic bacteria. *Science* 15: 363.

PRESNELL, M. W. and ANDREWS, W. H. 1976. Use of the membrane filter and a filter aid for concentrating and enumerating indicator bacteria and *Salmonella* from estuarine waters. *Water Res.* 10: 549–554.

PRIMROSE, S. B., SEELEY, N. D., LOGAN, K. B., and NICOLSON, J. W. 1982. Methods for studying aquatic bacteriophage ecology. *Appl. Environ. Microbiol.* 43: 694–701.

PURDY, R. N., DANCER, B. N., DAY, M. J., and STICKLER, D. J. 1985. A note on a membrane filter method for the concentration and enumeration of bacteriophages from water. *J. Appl. Bacteriol.* 58: 231–233.

RAY, B. 1979. Methods to detect stressed microorganisms. *J. Food Prot.* 42: 346–355.

RAY, B. and SPECK, M. L. 1973. Freeze-injury in bacteria. *CRC Crit. Rev. Clin. Lab. Sci.* 4: 161–213.

RAYMAN, M. K. and ARIS, B. 1981. The Anderson-Baird-Parker direct plating method versus the most probable number procedure for enumeration of *Escherichia coli* in meats. *Can. J. Microbiol.* 27: 147–149.

REASONER, D. J. 1983. Microbiology of potable water and ground water. *J. Water Pollut. Control Fed.* 55: 891–895.

REBER, C. L. and MARSHALL, R. T. 1982. Comparison of VRB and VRB-2 agars for recovery of stressed coliforms from stored acidified half-and-half. *J. Food Prot.* 45: 584–585.

RIPPEY, S. R. and CHANDLER, L. A. 1985. A rapid, fluorometric method for the enumeration of *E. coli* in molluscan shellfish. Abstract N20. Annual Meeting of the Am. Soc. Microbiol. 1985, 220.

ROBISON, B. J. 1984. Evaluation of a fluorogenic assay for the detection of *Escherichia coli* in foods. *Appl. Environ. Microbiol.* 48: 285–288.

SCHARDINGER. 1892. Ueber das Vorkommen Gahrüng erregender Spaltpilze im Trinkwasser und ihre Bedeutung für die hygienische Beurtheilung desselben. *Wien. Klin. Wochschr.* 5: 403–405. (Cited by Mossel 1967).

SHARPE, A. N., RAYMAN, M. K., BURGENER, D. M., CONLEY, D., LOIT, A., MILLING, M., PETERKIN, P. I., PURVIS, V., and MALCOLM S. 1983. Collaborative study of the MPN, Anderson-Baird-Parker direct plating, and hydrophobic grid-membrane filter methods for the enumeration of *Escherichia coli* biotype I in foods. *Can. J. Microbiol.* 29: 1247–1252.

SHERRILL, J. M. 1985. Human colinic flora and its role in the metabolism of xenobiotics. Abstract I71. Annual Meeting of the Am. Soc. Microbiol. 1985, 158.

SHLAES, D. M., TOOSI, Z., and PATEL, A. 1984. Comparison of latex agglutination and immunofluorescence for direct Lancefield grouping of streptococci from blood cultures. *J. Clin. Microbiol.* 20: 195–198.

SILLIKER, J. H., GABIS, D. A., and MAY, A. 1979. ICMSF methods studies. XI. Collaborative/comparative studies on determination of coliforms using the most probable number procedure. *J. Food Prot.* 42: 638–644.

SKINNER, F. A. and QUESNEL, L. B. (Ed.). 1978. *Streptococci.* Academic Press, New York, NY.

SLIFKIN, M. and GIL, G. M. 1983. Rapid biochemical tests for the identification of groups A, B, C, F, and G streptococci from throat cultures. *J. Clin. Microbiol.* 18: 29–32.

SMITH, J. L. and ROCKLIFF, S. 1982. Rapid single-tube confirmatory test for *Escherichia coli. J. Hyg.* 89: 149–154.

SPECK, M. L., RAY, B., and READ, R. B., Jr. 1975. Repair and enumeration of injured coliforms by a plating procedure. *Appl. Environ. Microbiol.* 29: 549–550.

SPLITTSTOESSER, D. F., TOMPKIN, R. B., REINBOLD, G. W., MATCHES, J. R., and ABEYTA, C. 1983. Indicator organisms: a current look at their usefulness. *Food Technol.* 37(6): 105–117.

STADHOUDERS, J., HUP, G., and HASSIG, F. 1982. The conceptions index and indicator organisms discussed on the basis of the bacteriology of spray-dried milk powder. *Neth. Milk Dairy J.* 36: 231–260.

STANDRIDGE, J. H. and DELFINO, J. J. 1981. A-1 medium: alternative technique for fecal coliform organism enumeration in chlorinated wastewaters. *Appl. Environ. Microbiol.* 42: 918–920.

STANDRIDGE, J. H. and DELFINO, J. J. 1982. Underestimation of total-coliform counts by the membrane filter verification procedure. *Appl. Environ. Microbiol.* 44: 1001–1003.

STANDRIDGE, J. H. and DELFINO, J. J. 1983. Effect of ambient temperature storage on potable water coliform population estimations. *Appl. Environ. Microbiol.* 46: 1113–1117.

STETLER, R. E. 1984. Coliphages as indicators of enteroviruses. *Appl. Environ. Microbiol.* 48: 668–670.

STILES, M. E. and NG, L.-K. 1980. Estimation of *Escherichia coli* in raw ground beef. *Appl. Environ. Microbiol.* 40: 346–351.

TREPETA, R. W. and EDBERG, S. C. 1984a. Measurement of microbial alpha-amylases with p-nitrophenyl glycosides as the substrate complex. *J. Clin. Microbiol.* 19: 60–62.

TREPETA, R. W. and EDBERG, S. C. 1984b. Methylumbelliferyl-β-D-glucuronide-based medium for rapid isolation and identification of *Escherichia coli. J. Clin. Microbiol.* 19: 172–174.

TREVORS, K. E., HOLLEY, R. A., and KEMPTON, A. G. 1984. Effect of bacteriophage on the activity of lactic acid starter cultures used in the production of fermented sausage. *J. Food Sci.* 49: 650–651, 653.

TRINEL, P. A., HANOUNE, N., and LeCLERC, H. 1980. Automation of water bacteriological analysis: running test of an experimental prototype. *Appl. Environ. Microbiol.* 39: 976–982.

VAN SCHOTHORST, M. 1976. Resuscitation of injured bacteria in foods. In *Inhibition and Inactivation of Vegetative Microbes*. Skinner, F. A., and Hugo W. B. (Ed.). Academic Press, New York, NY.

VAN SCHOTHORST, M. and OOSTEROM, J. 1984. *Enterobacteriaceae* as indicators of good manufacturing practices in rendering plants. *Antonie Leeuwenhoek J. Microbiol.* 50: 1–6.

VAN WART, M. and MOBERG, L. J. 1984. Evaluation of a novel fluorogenic-based method for detection of *Escherichia coli*. Abstract P12. Annual Meeting of the Am. Soc. Microbiol. 1984, 201.

VANZO, S. J. and WASHINGTON, J. A., Jr. 1984. Evaluation of a rapid latex agglutination test for identification of group D streptococci. *J. Clin. Microbiol.* 20: 575–576.

VARGA, F. J., JENNINGS, B. A., and DiPERSO, J. R. 1985. Evaluation of a rapid identification method for *Escherichia coli*. Abstract C63. Annual Meeting of the Am. Soc. Microbiol. 1985, 310.

VARGA, S. and DOUCET, A. 1984. Quantitative estimation of fecal coliforms in fresh and frozen fishery products by APHA and modified A-1 procedures. *J. Food Prot.* 47: 602–603.

WARREN, L. S., BENOIT, R. E., and JESSEE, J. A. 1978. Rapid enumeration of fecal coliforms in water by a colorimetric β-galactosidase assay. *Appl. Environ. Microbiol.* 35: 136–141.

WEISS, J. E. and HUNTER, C. A. 1939. Simplified bacteriological examination of water. *J. Amer. Water Works Assoc.* 31: 707–713.

WEISS, K. F., CHOPRA, N., STOTLAND, P., REIDEL, G. W., and MALCOLM, S. 1983. Recovery of fecal coliforms and of *Escherichia coli* at 44.5, 45.0 and 45.5°C. *J. Food Prot.* 46: 172–177.

WENTSEL, R. S., O'NEILL, P. E., and KITCHENS, J. F. 1982. Evaluation of coliphage detection as a rapid indicator of water quality. *Appl. Environ. Microbiol.* 43: 430–434.

WONG, S. H., CULLIMORE, D. R., and BRUCE, D. L. 1985. Selective medium for the isolation and enumeration of *Klebsiella* spp. *Appl. Environ. Microbiol.* 49: 1022–1024.

WRIGHT, R. C. 1984. A new selective and differential agar medium for *Escherichia coli* and coliform organisms. *J. Appl. Bacteriol.* 56: 381–388.

YOOVIDHYA, T. and FLEET, G. H. 1981. An evaluation of the A-1 most probable number and the Anderson and Baird-Parker plate count methods for enumerating *Escherichia coli* in the Sydney rock oyster, *Crassotrea commercialis*. *J. Appl. Bacteriol.* 50: 519–528.

10

Microbial Spoilage Indicators and Metabolites

James M. Jáy

Wayne State University
Detroit, Michigan

INTRODUCTION

Although universal definitions of food microbial spoilage do not exist, all perishable foods reach a state of undesirability when held long enough under conditions that permit the growth of microorganisms. The lack of general agreement on the early signs of spoilage for the many classes and categories of foods makes all the more difficult the task of identifying spoilage indicators. In spite of this, attempts have been made since the turn of the century to develop tests to assess the overall microbial quality of foods from the standpoint of both safety and product quality. While there are few universally accepted spoilage indicators and metabolites, many of those proposed and used, and some that are being studied, are discussed in this chapter. A thorough review of chemical indicators of food quality was made in 1968 by Fields et al. which should be consulted for more detailed information up to that time. A more recent discussion of indicators of meat spoilage is that of Gill (1983).

Criteria

The criteria that a spoilage indicator or microbial metabolite should meet have been considered by Fields et al. (1968), and when combined with those suggested by other authors, the following list results:

1. The compound must be present at low levels or absent in sound foods.
2. With increased spoilage, there must be an increase in the amount of the indicator.
3. The compound should make it possible to differentiate low-quality raw materials from poor processing conditions.
4. The indicator should be produced by the dominant spoilage flora.
5. The indicator must be as reliable as organoleptic criteria, and should indicate stages of spoilage which cannot be established definitely by organoleptic testing.
6. To be useful for seafood and ground meats, the test for the compound must be rapid and the analysis must be simple.
7. The indicator should never yield a false positive test, and for this reason a companion test is desirable.

To these criteria may be added the following:

8. If the indicator is a microbial metabolite, its production should not be strain dependant, and it should be produced under all conditions that support the growth of producing organisms.
9. It should do more than indicate what is obvious; it should offer some predictive value relative to shelf life.
10. Ideally, the spoilage indicator should be responsive to certain food-borne pathogens in order that a food is not declared unspoiled and yet be unsafe for consumption.

With the criteria noted, viable counts come closer to being spoilage indicators than metabolic byproducts.

VIABLE COUNTS AS INDICATORS OF SPOILAGE

The determination of the "total" microbial flora of a food product is the most commonly used means of determining overall microbial quality. It is for this reason that so much attention has been and continues to be devoted to faster, simpler, and more reliable ways of determining the total viable count of foods. The use of impedimetry, luminometry, microcalorimetry, radiometry, dye reductions, and other related methods for food products is based upon the value of viable numbers in assessing food spoilage.

The overall significance of microbial numbers in a food is depicted in Fig. 10.1. Foods are free of any signs of microbial spoilage with aerobic plate counts (APC) of $< 10^4$/g. The same is true of most foods that contain between 10^4 and 10^5 viable bacteria/g. Raw and pasteurized milk may show some signs of off-flavors with viable numbers in this range. With counts between 10^5 and 10^6/g, some products are in states of spoilage incipiency (e.g., dark-firm-dry meats) while counts of 10^7 to 10^8 generally denote off-odors and/ or off-flavors. Except for the lactic acid bacteria, most foods that contain 10^8 bacteria/g may be presumed to be in some state of detectable spoilage, with definite structural changes in products having occurred when the APC attains 10^9/g or higher. The validity of microbial numbers as indicators of food spoilage has resulted in many studies on rapid methods for determining microbial numbers as noted above. The methods noted respond to viable cells, and their utility decreases if a food product has been treated so as to reduce the viable counts. Luminometry is less affected by the latter assuming that microbial ATP has not been dissipated. One method that responds to both viable and nonviable bacteria is the *Limulus* amoebocyte lysate (LAL) assay for gram-negative bacteria.

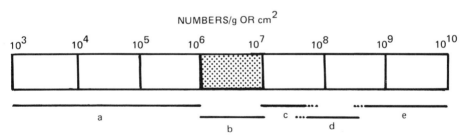

Fig. 10.1 Significance of total viable microbial numbers in food products relative to their use as indicators of spoilage. (a) Microbial spoilage generally not recognized with the possible exception of raw milk, which may sour in the 10^5–10^6 range. (b) Some food products show incipiency in this range. Vacuum-packaged meats often display objectionable odors and may be spoiled. (c) Off-odors generally associated with aerobically stored meats and some vegetables. (d) Most (all?) food products display obvious signs of spoilage. Slime is common on aerobically stored meats. (e) Definite structural changes in product occur in this range.

RAPID DETERMINATION OF GRAM-NEGATIVE BACTERIA

The most sensitive method known for measuring endotoxins or lipopolysaccharides (LPS) is the *Limulus* amoebocyte lysate (LAL) method. Its utility as an indicator of bacterial spoilage is based upon the fact that all gram-negative bacteria contain LPS, and the LAL reagent reacts with the LPS from both viable and nonviable cells. The method is most useful for foods that are spoiled by gram-negative bacteria, and essentially not useful for vacuum-packaged meats or other foods that undergo spoilage generally by gram-positive bacteria or fungi. On the assumption that the ratio of gram-negative to gram-positive bacteria is fairly constant for given categories of foods, rapid estimates of total viable bacterial numbers can be made by use of experimentally determined ratio values (Jay, 1981). It is conceivable that fungi can be represented in a similar manner although the numbers of yeasts in fresh ground beef have been found to be highly variable making for difficulty in relating their numbers to LAL-determined gram-negative bacteria (Jay and Margitic 1981).

The LAL test can be carried out in several ways. Perhaps the most widely used is the gelation tube method in which aliquots of food homogenates are added to 0.1 mL of LAL reagent in pyrogen-free tubes. Following mixing and incubation in a water bath at 37°C for 1 hr, LPS-containing samples cause the reagent to form a clot (gel) such that it remains intact when tubes are inverted. Because the reaction of endotoxin with the LAL reagent results in cloudiness or turbidity, endotoxin endpoints may be measured in this manner by use of spectrophotometry. When this method is employed, incubation is usually carried out for 30 min. Yet another way to employ the LAL reagent is by coupling it to a synthetic chromogenic substrate such that when reacted with endotoxin, the chromogen is released and measured by spectrophotometry. The quantity of chromogen released is proportional to the quantity of endotoxin present. Employing a chromogenic substrate, the detection of endotoxins has been automated making it possible to detect as little as 0.3 pg (Tsuji et al. 1984). Regardless of the way in which the LAL reagent is employed, the method is rapid, simple, reproducible, and very sensitive.

The LAL test has been applied to several categories of foods to assess overall hygienic quality or spoilage, and some of these are summarized in Table 10.1. European investigators have tended to stress the utility of LAL as a rapid test of hygienic quality of both raw and pasteurized milk. Since endotoxins are heat stable, they can be detected in pasteurized milk and thus one can determine the overall quality of the raw milk employed based upon content of gram-negative bacteria. The utility of LAL for aerobically stored

Table 10.1. Synopses of Some Applications of LAL for Determining Sanitary Quality or Spoilage of Various Foods

Products	Application	Synopsis of findings	References
Aerobically stored ground meats	Quality/spoilage	Significant correlations found between LAL-determined LPS and viable gram-negative counts for ground beef and pork	Jay (1977); Jay et al. (1979); Terplan et al. (1981)
Vacuum-packaged cooked turkey	Spoilage	Linear correlation found between LPS and *Enterobacteriaceae*; test was sensitive to < 100 cells, thus, more sensitive than Catalasemeter	Dodds et al. (1983)
Turkey carcass surfaces	Surface assessment	LAL values correlated with gram-negative viable counts	Terplan et al. (1981)
Lean fish	Spoilage	As test of spoilage, LPS correlated higher ($p < 0.001$) with total volatile bases	Sullivan et al. (1983)
Raw/pasteurized milk	Hygienic quality	Found suitable as test of hygienic quality (coliform detection) on 53 raw and 39 pasteurized milk samples	Terplan et al. (1975)
Milk and dairy products	Hygienic quality	Effective in assessing hygienic quality by measuring the total accumulated LPS. Fresh milk found to contain on average < 1 ng LPS/mL	Hansen et al. (1982); Jaksch et al. (1982); Zaadhof and Terplan (1981)
Cane and beet sugar	Pyrogens	Assessed the quality of sugar for use in parenteral fields. Swedish beet sugar contained < 1 ng/g while some imported sugars contained up to 100 mg/g of endotoxins or LPS	Haskå and Nystrand (1979)

fresh meats, poultry, and seafoods stems from the fact that such products undergo spoilage by gram-negative bacteria almost exclusively. Since the flora of vacuum-packaged meats is shifted to one dominated by lactic acid bacteria, LAL can be of value in determining that such products do not contain large numbers of gram-negative bacteria.

TESTS OF HYDRATION CAPACITY FOR MEATS

The microbial spoilage of meats, poultry, and seafoods can be assessed by use of one of several techniques that measure the hydration (water holding) capacity of these products. The method most often employed is the extract-release volume (ERV) test (Jay 1964). The test is conducted by homogenizing 25g of meat with 100 mL of pH 5.8 buffer for 2 min, followed by pouring the homogenate into a filter-funnel equipped with Whatman No. 1 paper, and collecting the extract that passes through the paper in 15 min. Beef, pork, and related meats of excellent microbial quality release 30–40 mL of extract in 15 min while the same meats following frank spoilage at refrigerator temperatures release no extract under the same conditions. A generalized curve depicting the response is noted in Fig. 10.2. The decrease in ERV (increase in water-holding capacity) is more or less linear, and the method allows for some prediction of shelf life. Sensory panel studies have indicated that ground beef with ERV below 25 may be presumed to be in a state of spoilage with APC of ca. $10^{8.5}$ (Kontou et al. 1966). The ERV test responds essentially the same to all red meats and to bony fish and shrimp, with the latter producing progressively lower volumes (Shelef and Jay 1971).

In addition to the ERV method, the filter-paper press method for determining water-holding capacity of meats and shrimp has been shown to respond to microbial spoilage and this method can be performed in 1 min (Jay 1965; Shelef and Jay 1971). Measurements of meat swelling and viscosity have been used to assess meat microbial spoilage (Shelef and Jay 1969a) but these methods are more time consuming and yet not any more effective than ERV.

The precise mechanism of the hydration tests as spoilage indicators is unclear. It appears that they are a response to changes in the primary structure of proteins. These changes lead to the unfolding of the protein molecules so they can bind more free water. It has been shown that the amino sugar complexes that accompany the growth of gram-negative spoilage bacteria have a positive effect on ERV (Shelef and Jay 1969b). For the increased hydration to occur, it is necessary to have the spoilage flora develop in the product since equal numbers of washed cells added to fresh meats do

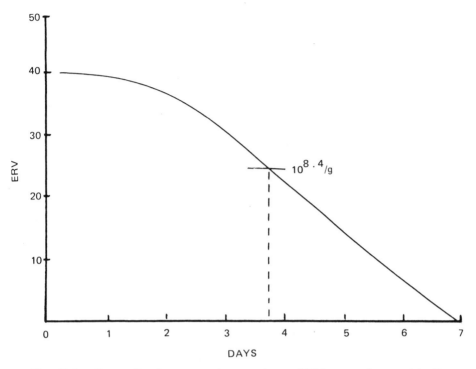

Fig. 10.2   Generalized extract release volume (ERV) curve for aerobically stored fresh ground beef held at 5–7°C for 7 days. In this example the meat was spoiled at an ERV of 25 and aerobic plate count of $10^{8.4}$/g.

not increase hydration capacity. The hydration tests are not directly applicable to vacuum-packaged meats, or to meats that do not undergo the normal spoilage that occurs in low-temperature, aerobically stored meats, but their use has been made to assess whether large numbers of gram-negative spoilage bacteria are present. With vacuum-packaged beef, ERV has been shown to decrease only slightly with storage time and thus confirmed that the lactic-acid bacteria were predominant (Sutherland et al. 1975). While pH increase accounts for some part of the hydration increase, it does not entirely explain the phenomenon (Shelef 1974).

    Overall, the hydration methods (ERV in particular) provide a rough measure of the growth and activity of gram-negative spoilage bacteria in low-temperature spoiled meats. They reflect the degree to which the spoilage flora has proliferated in meats since large numbers of washed cells do not affect hydration, and because of the linear-type response, they offer some predictive value regarding shelf-life of meats.

MICROBIAL METABOLITES

Numerous attempts have been made over the past 80 years to associate given metabolites with the microbial spoilage of given foods. In this way the metabolites could be used as spoilage predictors. Numerous methods for detecting spoilage in fresh meats have been proposed (see Jay 1986). The rationale for these methods is that as microorganisms grow in a food product, they utilize nutrients and produce metabolic byproducts. There is an inherent assumption that not only can spoilage be determined by the presence of the given metabolite(s) but that the quantity of same is directly referable to the degree of spoilage. While this assumption is reasonable, the ideal metabolite that can be used for spoilage assessment has eluded detection with a few possible exceptions.

The reasons for difficulty in assessing spoilage by measurement of metabolites include:

1. Given metabolites tend to be specific to certain organisms, and when these organisms are not present, or are present in high numbers, the metabolite provides incorrect spoilage information.

2. Most metabolites arise from specific product substrates but the absence of the given substrate or its presence in low quantities does not preclude spoilage.

3. Some metabolites are gaseous and consequently escape into the environment before and even during assessment.

4. The metabolic pathways and rates for some spoilage organisms are temperature and pH sensitive.

5. Although certain metabolites are produced in culture media, they may not be produced or produced at different levels when food substrates are used.

6. The accurate detection and measurement of some metabolites requires complicated procedures, equipment, and time.

7. Many metabolites reflect what is already obvious, i.e., that the product is, indeed, spoiled.

A list of some metabolites that have been studied and proposed as spoilage predictors is presented in Table 10.2 and synopses of some of the more promising are presented below.

Table 10.2. Some Metabolites Proposed/Studied/Employed as Microbial Spoilage Indicators for a Variety of Foods

Food	Metabolite(s)
Canned vegetables	Lactic acid
Frozen juice concentrate	Diacetyl
Ripened cheeses	(*see* Scombroid fish)
Oysters and clams	Lactic acid
Butter and cream	Volatile fatty acids
Apple juice	Ethanol
Aerobically stored ground meats and poultry	Mercaptans, H_2S, di- and trimethylamines, free amino acids, catalase, creatinine, hypoxanthine, ethanol, amino sugar complexes, nucleotides, titratable alkalinity, carbonyl residues (thiobarbituric acid values), ammonia
Vacuum-packed meats	Acetoin, acetic acid, isobutyric acid, lactic acid, isovaleric acid, diacetyl, diamines
Scombroid and related fish	Histamine, cadaverine, putrescine, spermine, spermindine
Other fish	Trimethylamine, total volatile substances, H_2S, tyrosine value, di- and trimethylsulfides, acetone, ethanol, acetoin (diacetyl), acetaldehyde, indole, diamines
Shrimp	Lactic acid, amino-N, total volatile substances, trimethylamine, hypoxanthine

Lactic Acid

Although it has been suggested as a spoilage indicator for molluscan shellfish and vacuum-packaged meats, lactic acid appears to be most useful as a means of determining spoilage in canned vegetables subject to flat-sour spoilage. A rapid method for detection of lactic acid in canned foods was presented by Ackland et al. (1981). In this method, a food sample is acidified with HCl, mixed with diethyl ether, shaken for 10 min, and centrifuged to separate the liquid phases. About 20 μL of the ether phase are spotted onto a silica-gel plate along with controls, and development is allowed to proceed until the solvent front has traveled 12 cm. Following drying and development, lactic and other organic acids appear as dark-blue spots. Results can be obtained within 2 hr. With this method, Ackland et al. examined 200 cans of potatoes and 1,000 cans of mashed vegetable products from lots containing swollen cans. Five of the 200 potato, and 21 of the 1,000 mashed vegetables were shown to be spoiled by leakage, and all contained lactic acid by the thin-layer chromatography method. The next most frequently found organic acid was formic which appeared in 9 of the 21 cans of vegetables. The lactic acid assay is a good alternative to the destructive testing of canned foods that may be spoiled by flat-sour bacteria. For ground meats, lactic acid concentration is more predictive of vacuum-packaged or anaerobically stored products than those stored aerobically (Nassos et al. 1985). The problem with this compound for meats is that it can be readily utilized by some members of the normal flora.

Diacetyl

Diacetyl is often a component of the volatile compounds of vacuum-packaged meats. Its production in meat is due to the activity of certain lactic acid bacteria. However, use of diacetyl as a sole predictor of spoilage in such products is unlikely because of its substrate dependance. Diacetyl is the single best predictor of product quality in frozen juice concentrates where at levels of 0.8 ppm it imparts a buttermilk aroma. The method employed by Murdock (1967) is a modification of the Voges-Proskauer method which employs alpha-naphthol with readings at 530 nm. When properly set up and run, diacetyl can be differentiated from acetoin, and results can be obtained within 30 min (Murdock 1968). According to the latter author, diacetyl in orange juice concentrate of 0.5 ppm represents a danger point, while the concentrate is undesirable if the concentration is 0.8 ppm or higher.

Alcohols

A variety of alcohols (methyl, ethyl, 3-methylbutyl, phenylethyl, isopropyl, propyl, etc.) have been identified among the volatile constituents of spoiled meats and fish. Holaday (1939) was apparently the first to associate a specific alcohol (ethanol) with the spoilage of fish. The potential value of ethanol as an indicator of canned fish quality was confirmed by Hillig (1958). In more recent studies with canned salmon, ethanol at levels up to 24 ppm was not associated with "offness" while from 25 to 74 ppm, some "offness" was evident, and at 75 ppm and above distinct "offness" was evident (Hollingworth and Throm 1982). In another study, ethanol at levels of 100 to 200 ppm occurred in spoiled canned salmon while volatile acids and volatile reducing substances (see below) were present at values of 50 to 100 and ca. 50 ppm, respectively (Crosgrove 1978). The latter author used a gas chromatographic method which produced results in less than 2 hr. The utility of ethanol as an index of canned tuna was shown by Lerke and Huck (1977).

In a more recent study, 244 bacterial fish spoilage isolates were tested for their capacity to produce ethanol, propanol, and isopropanol, and all were found to produce ethanol, 241 produced isopropanol, and 227 produced propanol (Ahamed and Matches, 1983). Of the three alcohols, ethanol was produced in highest quantities in a fish tissue extract at 5°C with average levels of 170 to 314 ppm for the various genera including gram-positives and gram-negatives. Average quantities of isopropanol ranged from 45 to 113 ppm while average propanol levels ranged from 13 to 30 ppm. Ethanol production was favored by aeration and it was produced from simple sugars or amino acids as substrates. The alcohols were determined by gas chromatography.

Regarding other alcohols, Chen et al. (1974) found that phenylethyl alcohol (along with phenol) was the major high-boiling volatile compound produced during refrigerator storage of haddock fillets. The phenylethanol was produced from L-phenylalanine and ethanol, and none of ten *Acinetobacter* and only one of nine *Moraxella* spp. produced the compound (Chen and Levin 1974).

From findings to date, ethanol appears to deserve more research as a spoilage indicator, especially for fishery products.

Catalase

Because of its production by most of the nonlactic acid bacteria, this enzyme has been employed as a rapid measure of numbers of aerobic bacteria in foods. A disc-flotation method using a Catalasemeter was employed by Dodds et al. (1983) to assess the load of catalase-positive bacteria (*Enterobacteriaceae*) in turkey rolls. When the log catalase-positive bacteria were plotted against the amount of catalase produced, the regression was significant at the 1% level, and results could be obtained in 300 seconds or less when the numbers of catalase-positive bacteria were $10^4/g$ or higher. The method was not reliable at numbers $<10^4/g$. This method is potentially useful for monitoring vacuum-packaged meats to determine if significant numbers of catalase-positive bacteria are present. While the same can be done with LAL or ERV, catalase measurement would reflect the numbers of catalase-positive, gram-positive bacteria present as well as the gram negatives.

Trimethylamine (TMA)

This amine is formed by the reduction of trimethylamine-N-oxide (TMAO) as shown:

$$H_3C$$
$$\diagdown$$
Trimethylamine-*N*-oxide →   N—CH$_3$
$$\diagup$$
$$H_3C$$
Trimethylamine

TMAO is present as a normal constituent of seafish. Little or no TMA is found in freshly caught fish, and its presence is presumed to be due solely to microbial activity, although some fish do contain muscle enzymes that reduce TMAO. In addition, some trace heavy metals (Fe, Co) are known to reduce TMAO to TMA in the absence of bacterial activity; some breakdown of TMAO occurs during freezer storage; some reduction occurs by irradiation; and some TMAO may be reduced to dimethylamine. Also, not all bacteria reduce TMAO to TMA with equal ease; its reduction is pH dependant; the content of TMAO in fish varies; and some organisms can utilize it as a terminal electron acceptor under anaerobic conditions. In spite of these exceptions, TMAO reduction continues to receive study and use as an indicator of seafish spoilage. Methods employed for the detection of TMA include its extraction from fish with toluene and KOH followed by reaction with picric acid, or its flushing from extracts and detection by use of alkaline permanganate solutions. The utility of TMAO reduction to TMA as a fish spoilage indicator has been discussed by Tarr (1954) and even more thoroughly by Fields et al. (1968).

Histamine, Diamines, and Polyamines

Histamine is produced from the amino acid histidine by the action of microbially produced histidine decarboxylase as noted.

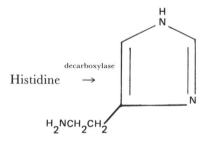

In addition to being a spoilage indicator, histamine is a toxic product, and histamine-associated or scombroid poisoning may result from its ingestion.

The seafoods that contain the largest quantity of histidine are the scombroid-type fish (tuna, bonita, mackerel, etc.), some nonscombroid fish (e.g., mahi-mahi), and some cheeses. While a large number of bacteria have been shown capable of producing histidine decarboxylase, the most active producers are *Proteus morganii*, *Klebsiella pneumoniae*, *Hafnia alvei*, and related gram negatives (Omura et al. 1978). As is true for many microbial metabolites, histamine production is temperature dependant. In one study the minimum temperature for production in a tuna fish infusion broth was 7°C for *K. pneumoniae*; 15°C for *P. morganii*; and 30°C for *H. alvei*, *Citrobacter freundii*, and *Escherichia coli* (Behling and Taylor 1982). The latter authors noted that the optimal conditions in general vary rather widely. Histamine has been employed as a quality index of canned tuna along with other amines. When histamine, putrescine, cadaverine, spermine, and spermidine were extracted and compared to other parameters of spoilage, they compared favorably with the organoleptic assessments of spoilage (Mietz and Karmus 1977).

Cadaverine and putrescine are the two most important diamines that have been evaluated as spoilage metabolites, and their production occurs in the manner depicted.

$$\text{Lysine} \quad \xrightarrow{\text{decarboxylase}} \quad \underset{\text{Cadaverine}}{\text{H}_2\text{N}(\text{CH}_2)_5\text{NH}_2}$$

$$\text{Ornithine or arginine} \quad \xrightarrow{\text{decarboxylase}} \quad \underset{\text{Putrescine}}{\text{H}_2\text{N}(\text{CH}_2)_4\text{NH}_2}$$

These compounds may be expected to occur in some quantity in all spoiled meats, fish, and poultry. More recently, their presence has been used to assess the quality of vacuum-packaged beef stored at 1°C for up to 8 weeks (Edwards et al. 1985). In this study, cadaverine increased more than putrescine for vacuum-packaged samples, which is the reverse of findings for aerobically stored samples (see below). Detectable levels were evident before maximum bacterial numbers were attained and before off-odors were evident; and the diamine concentration correlated better with total viable counts than with gram-negative bacteria. In sterile beef held for up to 8 weeks, there was no increase in concentration of these two diamines. The cadaverine levels attained over the incubation period were tenfold higher than the initial levels at total viable counts of $10^6/\text{cm}^2$ while there was little change in putrescine concentration at this level. Since the lactic-acid bacteria dominated the spoilage flora, the findings indicate that these organisms produce diamines in levels sufficient to be of value as spoilage indicators.

In contrast to vacuum-packaged meats, the production of these diamines in fresh meats is much more variable. In fresh beef, pork, and lamb, putrescine occurs at levels from 0.4 to 2.3 ppm; and cadaverine from 0.1 to 1.3 ppm (Nakamura et al. 1979; Edwards et al. 1983; Yamamoto et al. 1982). Putrescine is the major diamine produced by pseudomonads, and cadaverine by the *Enterobacteriaceae* (Slemr 1981). In one sample of naturally contaminated beef stored at 5°C for 4 days, putrescine increased from 1.2 to 26.1 ppm, cadaverine increased from 0.1 to only 0.6 ppm, while the APC increased from $10^{6.9}$ to $10^{9.57}$/g (Edwards et al. 1983). On the other hand, the two diamines increased almost equally in another sample of beef (see Table 10.3). Cadaverine is produced more by the *Enterobacteriaceae* than the pseudomonads, as noted above, and it can be seen from Table 10.3 that the *Enterobacteriaceae* were more predominant in the latter sample than in the former, apparently accounting for the higher concentration of cadaverine. The dependance of cadaverine production on the *Enterobacteriaceae* in aerobically stored meats renders it less valid as a quality index of products of this type. In ground beef, it is the only amine that correlates with coliforms (Sayem-El-Daher and Simard 1985). Edwards et al. (1983) found that significant changes in putrescine and cadaverine did not occur until the APC exceeded

Table 10.3. Development of Microbial Number and Diamine Concentrations on Naturally Contaminated Minced Beef Stored at 5°C

Sample[a]	Storage time (d)	Putrescine[b]	Cadaverine[b]	*Enterobacteri- aceae*	Aerobic plate count
		(μg/g)		($\log_{10}$no./g)	
E	0	1.2	0.1	3.81	6.29
	1	1.8	0.1	3.56	7.66
	2	4.2	0.5	4.57	8.49
	3	10.0	0.5	5.86	9.48
	4	26.1	0.6	7.54	9.97
F	0	2.3	1.3	6.18	7.49
	1	3.9	4.5	6.23	7.85
	2	12.4	17.9	6.69	8.73
	3	29.9	35.2	7.94	9.69
	4	59.2	40.8	9.00	9.91

[a]Samples E and F were obtained from two different retail outlets.
[b]Diamine values are the mean of two determinations.
(*From Edwards et al. 1983* Copyright © 1983, Blackwell Scientific Publications, Ltd.)

4.2×10^7/g when the meats were obviously spoiled, leading these investigators to question the utility of diamine assay as a predictor of spoilage or microbial quality for fresh, aerobically stored meats. In another study, no significant changes in the diamines or the polyamines (spermine and spermidine) occurred in fresh pork until the samples showed decomposition (Nakamura et al. 1979). In ground beef, total and psychotrophic counts correlated significantly with putrescine, 1,3-diaminopropane, tyramine, cadaverine, and spermidine (Sayem-El-Daher and Simard 1985). In contrast to Edwards et al. (1983), the latter authors suggested that putrescine is a potential count indicator for ground beef.

The diamines as spoilage indicators illustrate one of the many problems associated with metabolites in this regard—their production is organism dependant. Their combined use obviates this problem somewhat. Their use for vacuum-packaged meats seems more promising, however.

The determination of the di- and polyamines is best achieved by gasliquid chromatography and mass spectrometry as described by Yamamoto et al. (1982).

Total Volatile Substances

Originally developed to assess fish and seafood quality, several tests of volatile compounds are employed: Total volatile bases (TVB), total volatile acids (TVA), total volatile substances (TVS), and total volatile nitrogen (TVN). The volatile bases (TVB) include ammonia, dimethylamine, and trimethylamine (see above), while TVN includes TVB and other nitrogen compounds that are obtained by steam distillation of samples. TVS are those that can be aerated from a product and reduce alkaline permanganate solutions. Because of this reducing property, this method is sometimes designated volatile reducing substances (VRS), and a calorimetric method for VRS was developed by Farber and Lerke (1967). TVA include acetic, propionic, and related organic acids. TVN has been employed in Australia and Japan for shrimp with a maximum for acceptable quality being 30 mg TVN/100g along with a maximum of 5 mg trimethylamine nitrogen (TMN) of 5 mg/100g. Definite "offness" of shrimp has been noted when TVN is > 30 mg N/100g (Cobb and Vanderzant 1975). TVB values of ca. 45 mg TVB-N/100g of fish were found to correspond to ca. 10,000 ng of LPS by Sullivan et al. (1983), and to be reflective of lean fish of marginal quality.

The volatile substances tests have been employed rather widely for certain seafoods and red meats and the correlation of results with odor profiles is often found to be statistically significant. One of the advantages of these methods is their lack of dependance upon a single metabolite, although amino acids constitute the primary if not sole substrates. In general, they tend to confirm organoleptic assessments and do not provide enough information about spoilage incipiency.

Volatile Substances for Vacuum-Packaged Meats

The increasing practice of vacuum-packaging of meats has led to many studies on the microbiology of this technology, including studies on spoilage and indicators of spoilage. The most striking thing that occurs when meats are vacuum packaged, and stored in gas-impermeable films or in CO_2 atmospheres is the change in the spoilage flora from being predominantly or exclusively gram-negative to almost exclusively gram-positive. The gram-positive flora consist mainly of lactic acid bacteria and *Brochothrix thermosphacta* (see Table 10.4). Another significant difference between aerobically stored and vacuum-packaged meats is the restriction in the total number of bacteria that are attained upon spoilage, and the greater difficulty of determining when vacuum-packaged meats are spoiled. It may be noted from Table 10.4 that air-stored herring fillets had viable numbers of $10^{8.2}$ to $10^{8.7}$/g at the time of spoilage, while under CO_2 storage the numbers at spoilage were only $10^{6.5}$ to $10^{6.6}$/g (Molin and Stenstrom 1984). In vacuum-packaged beef held at 1°C for 8 weeks, the maximum numbers attained were ca. 10^7/cm^2 (Edwards et al. 1985). As noted previously, neither LAL nor ERV are useful in determining the spoilage of these products since gram-negative bacteria are generally absent. Since the products are characterized by high levels of volatile compounds, attempts to find spoilage indicators are being focused in this direction.

A large number of volatile compounds have been detected in spoiled vacuum-packaged meats, with the most frequently reported ones noted in

Table 10.4. Percent of Flora of Herring Fillets, at Time of Spoilage, Stored in Air and in 100% CO_2

		Air		CO_2	
Organisms	Initial	0°C	4°C	0°C	4°C
Gram negatives	95	98	100	0	0
Lactic acid bacteria	0	2.5[a]	0	100	97.5
Log APC/g	4.8	8.7	8.2	6.4	6.6

[a] *Brochothrix thermosphacta.*
(*From Molin and Stenstrom 1984*)

Table 10.5. In general, the volatiles are composed of a variety of sulfides, alcohols, carbonyls, amines, and organic acids. As noted above, the diamines have been studied for their potential as spoilage or quality indicators for vacuum-packaged meats with promising results. Among the other volatiles commonly found are diacetyl and acetoin (see above), and organic acids such as isobutyric, isovaleric, and acetic. These have been reported by several groups of investigators. One of the specific organisms that sometimes dominate the spoilage of vacuum-packaged meats is *B. thermosphacta*. Its end products have been shown by Dainty and Hibbard (1980) to be both substrate and pH dependant, with acetoin and acetate accounting for 80 to 90% of glucose metabolism at pH 7.0 and 7.5, but 100% at lower pH values. The organism was shown to produce acetic, isobutyric, and isovaleric acids both in meat and in APT broth at 1°C. Of the seven volatile compounds detected from spoiled vacuum-packaged sliced luncheon meat inoculated with *B. thermosphacta*, diacetyl and acetoin appeared to be of major sensory significance (Stanley et al. 1981). The others consisted of alcohols and a diol.

Finding spoilage indicators for vacuum-packaged meats is a relatively new challenge, and because spoilage in such products is strongly related to odors, the volatile constituent mixture appears to be the approach to take. A combination of carbonyls and organic acids appears to be promising.

SUMMARY

There is no universally agreed upon definition of microbial spoilage of food, and consequently, there is no universally agreed indicator of spoilage for most food products. Total viable microbial counts continue to be the most

Table 10.5. Some Volatile Compounds Produced by the Spoilage Flora of Meats, Poultry, and Seafoods

Dimethyl disulfide	Diacetyl
Dimethyl trisulfide	Acetoin
Hydrogen sulfide	Trimethylamine
Methyl mercaptan	Histamine
Methyl sulfide	Isobutyric acid
Ethanol	Isovaleric acid
Phenylethyl alcohol	N-Butyric acid
Methanol	Acetic acid
3-Methylbutanol	

widely used method for assessing quality attributes but there is no general agreement on the numbers that denote spoilage for given products. For those products that are spoiled by gram-negative bacteria, the *Limulus* test is the most rapid and accurate way to assess gram-negative bacteria, and because the test responds to both viable and nonviable cells, *Limulus* results provide some information on the history of a food product relative to its contamination by gram-negative bacteria. The hydration tests for fresh meat products provide rapid estimates of the degree to which gram-negative spoilage bacteria have proliferated in the products, and some predictive information is provided. One of the many problems associated with the use of microbial metabolites is the general lack of knowledge of the mechanisms by which most foods spoil, a problem which was noted some years ago (Jay 1972). The difficulty of employing a metabolite as spoilage indicator for meats has been addressed by Gill (1983) who noted that, " . . . it is not likely that a single, simple, unequivocal test could be devised to determine in all cases the spoilage status of meat before spoilage becomes evident to the senses." While this statement may seem a bit too prophetic, it does underscore the difficulty of using metabolites for complex substrates such as meats.

The metabolites that can be used with some degree of accuracy are lactic acid for certain canned foods; diacetyl for orange juice concentrates; ethanol for apple juice; and histamine for scombroid-type fish. Metabolites that show great promise as spoilage indicators are ethanol for fishery products; the diamines (cadaverine and putrescine) for fish and red meats; and the carbonyls (e.g., diacetyl) and organic acids for vacuum- or gas atmosphere-stored meats. More studies on the mechanisms by which foods spoil will facilitate the finding of usable indicators.

REFERENCES

ACKLAND, M. R., TREWHELLA, E. R., REEDER, J., and BEAN, F. G. 1981. The detection of microbial spoilage in canned foods using thin-layer chromatography. *J. Appl. Bacteriol.* 51: 277–281.

AHAMED, A. and MATCHES, J. R. 1983. Alcohol production by fish spoilage bacteria. *J. Food Protect.* 46: 1055–1069.

BEHLING, A. R. and TAYLOR, S. L. 1982. Bacterial histamine production as a function of temperature and time of incubation. *J. Food Sci.* 47: 1311–1314.

CHEN, T. C. and LEVIN, R. E. 1974. Taxonomic significance of phenethyl alcohol production by *Achromobacter* isolates from fishery sources. *Appl. Microbiol.* 28: 681–687.

CHEN, T. C., NAWAR, W. W., and LEVIN, R. E. 1974. Identification of major high-boiling volatile compounds produced during refrigerated storage of haddock fillets. *Appl. Microbiol.* 28: 679–680.

COBB, B. F., III, and VANDERZANT, C. 1975. Development of a chemical test for shrimp quality. *J. Food Sci.* 40: 121–124.

CROSGROVE, D. M. 1978. A rapid method for estimating ethanol in canned salmon. *J. Food Sci.* 43: 641 & 643.

DAINTY, R. H. and HIBBARD, C. M. 1980. Aerobic metabolism of *Brochothrix thermosphacta* growing on meat surfaces and in laboratory media. *J. Appl. Bacteriol.* 48: 387–396.

DODDS, K. L., HOLLEY, R. A., and KEMPTON, A. G. 1983. Evaluation of the catalase and *Limulus* amoebocyte lysate tests for rapid determination of the microbial quality of vacuum-packed cooked turkey. *Can. Inst. Food Sci. Technol. J.* 16: 167–172.

EDWARDS, R. A., DAINTY, R. H., and HIBBARD, C. M. 1983. The relationship of bacterial numbers and types to diamine concentration in fresh and aerobically stored beef, pork and lamb. *J. Food Technol.* 18: 777–788.

EDWARDS, R. A., DAINTY, R. H., and HIBBARD, C. M. 1985. Putrescine and cadaverine formation in vacuum packed beef. *J. Appl. Bacteriol.* 58: 13–19.

FARBER, L. and LERKE, P. 1967. Colorimetric determination of volatile reducing substances. *J. Food Sci.* 32: 616–617.

FIELDS, M. L., RICHMOND, B. S., and BALDWIN, R. E. 1968. Food quality as determined by metabolic by-products of microorganisms. *Adv. Food Res.* 16: 161–229.

GILL, C. O. 1983. Meat spoilage and evaluation of the potential storage life of fresh meat. *J. Food Protect.* 46: 444–452.

HANSEN, K., NIKKELSEN, T., and MOLLER-MADSEN, A. 1982. Use of the *Limulus* test to determine the hygienic status of milk products as characterized by levels of Gram-negative bacterial lipopolysaccharide present. *J. Dairy Res.* 49: 323–328.

HASKA, G. and NYSTRAND, R. 1979. Determination of endotoxins in sugar with the *Limulus* test. *Appl. Environ. Microbiol.* 38: 1078–1080.

HILLIG, F. 1958. Determination of alcohol in fish and egg products. *J. Assoc. Off. Agric. Chem.* 41: 776–781.

HOLADAY, D. A. 1939. The alcohols as a measure of spoilage in canned fish. *J. Assoc. Off. Agr. Chem.* 22: 418–420.

HOLLINGWORTH, T. A., JR. and THROM, H. R. 1982. Correlation of ethanol concentration with sensory classification of decomposition in canned salmon. *J. Food Sci.* 47: 1315–1317.

JAKSCH, P., ZAADHOF, K.-J., and TERPLAN, G. 1982. Zur Bewertung der hygienischen Qualität von Milchprodukten mit dem *Limulus*-Test. *Die Milkerei-Zeitung Welt der Milch* 36: 5–8.

JAY, J. M. 1964. Beef microbial quality determined by extract-release volume (ERV). *Food Technol.* 18: 1633–1636.

JAY, J. M. 1965. Relationship between water-holding capacity of meats and microbial quality. *Appl. Microbiol.* 13: 120–121.

JAY, J. M. 1972. Mechanism and detection of microbial spoilage in meats at low temperatures: A status report. *J. Milk Food Technol.* 35: 467–471.

JAY, J. M. 1977. The *Limulus* lysate endotoxin assay as a test of microbial quality of ground beef. *J. Appl. Bacteriol.* 43: 99–109.

JAY, J. M., MARGITIC, S., SHEREDA, A. L., and COVINGTON, H. V. 1979. Determining endotoxin content of ground beef by the *Limulus* amoebocyte lysate test as a rapid indicator of microbial quality. *Appl. Environ. Microbiol.* 38: 885–890.

JAY, J. M. 1981. Rapid estimation of microbial numbers in fresh ground beef by use of the *Limulus* test. *J. Food Protect.* 44: 275–278.

JAY, J. M. and MARGITIC, S. 1981. Incidence of yeasts in fresh ground beef and their ratios to bacteria. *J. Food Sci.* 46: 648–649.

JAY, J. M. 1986. *Modern Food Microbiology*, 3rd ed., Chap. 9. Van Nostrand Reinhold Co.: N.Y.

KONTOU, K. S., HUYCK, M. C., and JAY, J. M. 1966. Relationship between sensory test scores, bacterial numbers, and ERV on paired-raw and -cooked ground beef from freshness to spoilage. *Food Technol.* 20: 696–699.

LERKE, P. A. and HUCK, R. W. 1977. Objective determination of canned tuna quality: Identification of ethanol as a potentially useful index. *J. Food Sci.* 42: 755–758.

MIETZ, J. L. and KARMAS, E. 1977. Chemical quality index of canned tuna as determined by high-pressure liquid chromatography. *J. Food Sci.* 42: 155–158.

MOLIN, G. and STENSTROM, I. M. 1984. Effect of temperature on the microbial flora of herring fillets stored in air or carbon dioxide. *J. Appl. Bacteriol.* 56: 275–282.

MURDOCK, D. I. 1967. Methods employed by the citrus concentrate industry for detecting diacetyl and acetylmethylcarbinol. *Food Technol.* 21: 643–672.

MURDOCK, D. I. 1968. Diacetyl test as a quality control tool in processing frozen concentrated orange juice. *Food Technol.* 22: 90–94.

NAKAMURA, M., WADA, Y., SAWAYA, H., and KAWABATA, T. 1979. Polyamine content in fresh and processed pork. *J. Food Sci.* 44: 515–517 & 523.

NASSOS, P. S., KING, A. D. JR., and STAFFORD, A. E. 1985. Lactic acid concentration and microbial spoilage in anaerobically and aerobically stored ground beef. *J. Food Sci.* 50: 710–712, 715.

OMURA, Y., PRICE, R. J., and OLCOTT, H. S. 1978. Histamine-forming bacteria isolated from spoiled skipjack tuna and jack mackerel. *J. Food Sci.* 43: 1779–1781.

SAYEM-EL-DAHER, N. and SIMARD, R. E. 1985. Putrefactive amine changes in relation to microbial counts of ground beef during storage. *J. Food Protect.* 48: 54–58.

SHELEF, L. A. and JAY, J. M. 1969a. Relationship between meat swelling, viscosity, extract-release volume, and water-holding capacity in evaluating beef microbial quality. *J. Food Sci.* 34: 532–535.

SHELEF, L. A. and JAY, J. M. 1969b. Relationship between amino sugars and meat microbial quality. *Appl. Microbiol.* 17: 931–932.

SHELEF, L. A. and JAY, J. M. 1971. Hydration capacity as an index of shrimp microbial quality. *J. Food Sci.* 36: 994–997.

SHELEF, L. A. 1974. Hydration and pH of microbially spoiling beef. *J. Appl. Bacteriol.* 37: 531–536.

SLEMR, J. 1981. Biogene Amine als potentieller chemischer Qualitätsindikator für Fleisch. *Fleischwirtsch.* 61: 921–925.

STANLEY, G., SHAW, K. J., and EGAN, A. F. 1981. Volatile compounds associated with spoilage of vacuum-packaged sliced luncheon meat by *Brochothrix thermosphacta*. *Appl. Environ. Microbiol.* 41: 816–818.

SULLIVAN, J. D. JR., ELLIS, P. C., LEE, R. G., COMBS, W. S., JR., and WATSON, S. W. 1983. Comparison of the *Limulus* amoebocyte lysate test with plate counts and chemical analyses for assessment of the quality of lean fish. *Appl. Environ. Microbiol.* 45: 720–722.

SUTHERLAND, J. P., PATTERSON, J. T., and MURRARY, J. G. 1975. Changes in the microbiology of vacuum-packaged beef. *J. Appl. Bacteriol.* 39: 227–237.

TARR, H. L. A. 1954. Microbiological deterioration of fish post mortem, and its detection and control. *Bacteriol. Rev.* 18: 1–15.

TERPLAN, G., ZAADHOF, K.-J., and BUCHHOLZ-BERCHTOLD, S. 1975. Zum Nachweis von Endotoxinen gramnegativer Keime in Milch mit dem *Limulus*-Test. *Arch. Lebensmittelhyg.* 26: 217–221.

TERPLAN, G., BIERL, J., GROVE, H.-H., and K.-J. ZAADHOF. 1981. Zur Bewertung der Hygiene bei Gewinnung und Verarbeitung von Lebensmitteln mit dem Limulustest. *Arch. Lebensmittelhyg.* 32: 15–19.

TSUJI, K., MARTIN, P. A., and BUSSEY, D. M. 1984. Automation of chromogenic substrate *Limulus* amebocyte lysate assay method for endotoxin by robotic system. *Appl. Environ. Microbiol.* 48: 550–555.

YAMAMOTO, S., ITANO, H., KATAOKA, H., and MAKITA, M. 1982. Gas-liquid chromatographic method for analysis of di- and polyamines in foods. *J. Agric. Food Chem.* 30: 435–439.

ZAADHOF, K.-J. and TERPLAN, G. 1981. Der *Limulus*-Test—ein Verfahren zur Beurteilung der mikrobiologischen Qualität von Milch und Milchprodukten. *Deutsche Molkereinzeitung* 34: 1094–1098.

11

Newer Developments in Hybridoma Technology

Richard A. Goldsby

Amherst College
Amherst, Massachusetts

The manufacture of predefined specific antibodies by means of permanent tissue culture cell lines is of general interest. . . . We describe here
the derivation of a number of tissue culture cell lines which secrete anti-
sheep red blood cell (SRBC) antibodies. The cell lines are made by
fusion of a mouse myeloma and mouse spleen cells from an immunised
donor . . . the hybrid clones can be injected into BALB/c mice to produce
solid tumors and serum having anti-SRBC activity. Such cells can be
grown in vitro in massive cultures to provide specific antibody. Such
cultures could be valuable for medical and industrial use. (Kohler and
Milstein 1975)

The production and use of monoclonal antibodies has become a technology almost as widespread as the isolation and use of enzymes. Kohler's
and Milstein's visionary prediction that monoclonal antibodies would become
valuable tools for medicine and industry has been abundantly realized. In

the ten years since the publication of their now classic paper, we have seen the use of hybridoma technology to treat cancer, aid in the diagnoses of disease, and spawn a lively new industry. One of the striking features of this powerful technology is its accessibility. With a rather modest capital expenditure and the application of skilled and diligent cell culture techniques, almost any laboratory can produce useful monoclonal antibodies.

The basic elements of deriving and producing monoclonal antibodies have remained the same as those established by Kohler and Milstein a decade ago (see Hammerling et al. 1981; Kennett et al. 1980). First, one immunizes the system with the antigen of interest in order to predefine the specificity of the prospective hybridomas. Second, antibody producing cells from the immunized system are fused to a cell line which is permissive for immunoglobulin production. Third, the antibody products of hybridoma clones are screened to identify those antibodies possessing desired characteristics. Fourth, the desirable hybridomas are grown in mass culture and the supernatant harvested, or, more economically, as tumors whose antibody product appears in milligram concentrations in serum and *ascitic* fluids. Predictably, each of these steps has undergone technical evolution and we shall examine some of these advances in this review. We will also explore some ideas and technologies that were not anticipated, beginning with an inventory of the strategies of monoclonal antibody production to be examined:

1. Conventional

2. In vitro immunization

3. Electrofusion

4. Chimeric immunoglobulins

Each of these approaches to monoclonal antibody production is examined in turn.

CONVENTIONAL FUSION AND THE DESIGN OF SCREENING PROTOCOLS

The march of technology has increased the range and power of hybridoma methodology significantly. However, it is important to recognize that for the near future, the overwhelming majority of useful monoclonal antibodies will be made by the now classical method of PEG-assisted fusion of spleen cells from immunized donors with appropriate established cell lines. In large part one's success is obtaining hybridomas which secrete monoclonal antibodies possessing the desired characteristics of specificity, antibody class, and affinity will be critically dependent upon the intelligence and ingenuity invested in designing discriminating screening protocols. The cardinal rule of designing a screen is to make the screening procedure mirror, as nearly as possible, the actual situation in which one will use the antibody. This is important because different procedures demand antibodies with different properties. For example, assays based on complement dependent reactions such as cytoxicity or hemolysis will require monoclonal antibodies of the IgM class or only certain IgG subclasses (IgG_{2a} and IgG_{2b} in the mouse). Precipitation assays such as radial immunodiffusion or ouchterlony require a sufficiently multivalent interaction to build a latticework. The discrimination of closely related cell types, bacterial strains or viruses requires exquisite specificity. The ELISA or radioimmunoassay of compounds present in trace amounts (toxins, drugs, hormones) are dependent upon antibodies of high affinity and often high specificity as well. Here are some guidelines and procedural suggestions which point the way to engineering the appropriate monoclonal antibodies.

Antibody Class

First of all, the immunization schedule will be an important determinant of the broad general classes of monoclonal antibodies that will be obtained. In those cases where one wants antibodies of high avidity or high efficiency of complement fixation, say for cytotoxic assays, spleen cells should be harvested three days after priming and fused. Such a procedure tends to produce a high proportion of IgM class antibodies. On the other hand, if for reasons of ease of purification, handling, or tissue distribution, certain IgG classes are essential, two steps may be taken. First, the immunization schedule should allow an interval of four weeks between priming and boosting. Second, one should take the trouble to screen the library with a class specific reagent. For example, if [mouse] IgG_{2a} or IgG_{2b} antibodies are desired, suitably labeled protein A may be used as a screening reagent. One always has the option of screening the library with a class-specific, appropriately labeled anti-immunoglobulin.

Selection of Antibodies for Specificity

This is a straightforward exercise in which one constitutes a panel of antigens which includes the target antigen against which one seeks reactive monoclonal antibodies. The panel also should include one, or preferably, two or three related antigens and some antigens that bear no apparent relationship to the target antigen. The unrelated antigens will identify those monoclonal antibodies that are "sticky" and may bind the target antigen in a nonspecific and, therefore, not useful way. The related antigens, if carefully chosen, will reveal the extent to which a given target antigen-reactive monoclonal antibody can discriminate between it and closely related structures.

Monoclonal antibodies can be screened for high affinity in a variety of ways, two of the most straightforward are ligand blocking at low concentration and ligand capture at low concentration. These assays, all of which are conducted in microtiter plates, are schematized as follows:

Low Ligand Blocking

Step 1: (a) 2 hr incubation of 0.1 mL of hybridoma supernatant + 0.1 mL of ligand [10^{-5} to 10^{-7}M], (b) 2 hr incubation of 0.1 mL of hybridoma supernatant − 0.1 mL of ligand free solution

Step 2: ELISA or solid phase RIA of supernatants

Step 3: Comparison of ratio of [+] ligand/[−] ligand

Judgment criterion: Highest affinity monoclonal antibodies show smallest ratios.

Ligand Capture at Low Concentrations

Step 1: 16 hr incubation of 0.1 mL of hybridoma supernatant with 0.1 mL of radiolabeled ligand [low concentration + 1μg/mL]

Step 2: Addition of 0.1 mL sepharose to which anti-mouse Ig has been covalently attached

Step 3: Agitation for 30 minutes

Step 4: Three sequential washes of the beads

Step 5: Determine bead-associated radioactivity

Judgment criterion: Only high affinity antibodies will bind low concentrations of labeled antigen.

The thoughtful application of these considerations has allowed the construction and identification of conventionally prepared hybridomas which secrete monoclonal antibodies with useful constellations of desirable attributes. However, the application of recently developed, more advanced methodologies can overcome technical barriers inherent in the conventional approach. We turn now to an examination of the opportunities opened by these newer developments in hybridoma technology.

IN VITRO IMMUNIZATION

In vitro immunization provides a useful alternative to the traditional methods of in vivo immunization. It also offers some important additional advantages. Consider that (a) the immunization procedure requires only 5 to 7 days; (b) defined levels of antigen can be maintained throughout the immunization; (c) the procedure offers the option of utilizing regulatory lymphokines and monokines to attempt modulation of the response; (d) successful immunizations can be accomplished with extremely small antigen concentrations; (e) antigens which are toxic at the organismal level may be innocuous in cell culture; (f) it is possible to produce antibodies to "self" or to highly conserved antigens which are difficult to produce by conventional immunization because of tolerance. The following example provides an impressive demonstration of the power of the in vitro approach.

Luben and Mohler (1982) were interested in obtaining monoclonal antibodies to osteoclast activating factor (OAF), a T cell derived lymphokine which promotes bone resorption. A significant effort had to be expended to prepare the antigen in even microgram amounts. With few exceptions the conventional approach involving the multiple immunization of whole animals requires the expenditure of at least a few hundred micrograms of antigen. In an experiment that made a significant advance in the sensitivity and flexibility of the hybridoma technique, these workers demonstrated that naive BALB/c spleen cells could be immunized against human OAF in vitro. Strikingly, as shown in Table 11.1, significant numbers of hybridomas could be obtained from in vitro immunization with as little as 100 ng of antigen and some hybrids were obtained when only 10 ng were used.

Those who want to use the in vitro route to antibody producing hybridomas may want to purchase a kit (Hana Biologics, Inc., Berkeley, CA). Alternatively, those who wish to perform a do-it-yourself in vitro immunization may find the following protocol (adapted from Reading 1982; McHugh 1984) useful:

1.   Prepare mixed thymocyte culture conditioned medium (TCM) by sterilely removing the thymus glands from five young (4–8 weeks old) BALB/c mice and a similar number of C57/BL6 mice. The pooled glands are placed in HEPES-buffered (10 mM) Hank's balanced salt solution (HHBSS) and pressed through a stainless steel screen or ground between the frosted surfaces of glass slides. The thymocytes are counted and suspended at a concentration

Table 11.1   Production of Monoclonal
Antibodies to Osteoclast Activating Factor
(OAF) by in Vitro Immunization

Dose of OAF	No. of anti-OAF cultures/ total cultures	Maximum titer of anti-OAF activity
10 ug	23/48	1:10000
1	21/48	1:1000
0.1	14/48	1:100000
0.01	3/48	1:5000
0.0001	0/48	—

(*From Luben and Mohler 1982*)

of 5×10^6/mL in DMEN supplemented with 2 mM glutamine and 2% rabbit serum. Fifty milliliter aliquots of this suspension are cultured in 75 cm^2 flasks at 37°C for 48 hours. The cultures are then harvested by centrifugation and the supernatant, TCM, is filtered (0.2 μm), divided into 10 mL aliquots and stored at -80°C. Under these conditions TCM preparations retain their activity for at least six months and probabily indefinitely.

2.   Sterilely harvest the spleen from an unprimed BALB/c mouse and prepare a suspension of spleen cells as described above. Allow the clumps of tissue to settle for 30 seconds and harvest the spleen cell-containing supernatant.

3.   Adjust the volume of the suspension to 20 mL. Add 1–100 μg of soluble antigen to the flask of 10^7 irradiated (2500 rad) whole cells. A 10 mL vial of TCM is rapidly thawed at 37°C and added to the spleen cell suspension, mixed and the TCM supplemented suspension is transferred to a 75 cm^2 flask, flushed with 5% CO_2/95% air and placed on its culture face in a 37°C incubator. The flask is left undisturbed for five days and then harvested and fused to an appropriate established cell line.

4.   Note that the amounts of immunogen recommended are merely points of departure. In setting up an in vitro immunization, one should explore a variety of antigen concentrations in order to obtain optimal responses.

ELECTROFUSION

The exposure of cell membranes to pulsed electric fields of high intensity and short duration causes a reversible electrical breakdown in the membrane. The transient breakdown results in a brief (several seconds to a few minutes at 37°C) but dramatic increase in the permeability of the plasma membrane. This electric field induced increase in membrane permeability can be exploited to introduce particles, bring about the fusion of pairs or gorups of cells and even to transfect cells with DNA. A recent paper (Potter et al. 1984) describes the use of electroporation to introduce immunoglobulin genes into cells. A spectacular example of its use in cell fusion is provided by the use of electric field induced fusion to produce an interkingdom hybrid between a Friend virus induced erythroleukemic cell and petunia protoplasts. The fused cells displayed characteristics peculiar to each of the parental cells. Specifically, hybrid cells regenerated cell walls and were induced to synthesize hemoglobulin by treatment with dimethyl sulfoxide (Salhni, Zimmermann, Ward, and Cocking, unpublished; see Zimmermann and Vienken 1984). Perhaps the most striking application of the electrofusion technique to the production of hybridomas secreting monoclonal antibodies of a desired specificity is the highly selective procedure reported by Tsong and his colleagues (Lo et al. 1984).

This procedure, termed receptor-mediated electrically induced fusion, involves two essential elements. First, myeloma cells and antigen specific B cells are preferentially linked to each other by a biotin-antigen-immunoglobulin bridge. Second, the specifically associated B cell-myeloma complexes are efficiently fused by the application of an electric field. The preferential linkage is ingeniously engineered in the following manner. Biotin is attached to the surface of myeloma cells by reaction with N-hydroxysuccinimide linked biotin. The antigen of interest is cross-linked to avidin by means of 1,5-difluoro-2,4-dinitrobenzene. Addition of the avidin-antigen couple to a suspension of spleen cells from a mouse immunized with the antigen results in the specific binding of the couple to the subpopulation of B cells which bear surface immunoglobulin specific for that antigen. Now when biotinylated myeloma cells are added, there is preferential association with the B cells which have avidin attached via the bound antigen.

In an impressive demonstration of the potential of the technique these investigators derived monoclonal antibodies against angiotensin-converting-enzyme (ACE), against enkephalin convertase (a carboxypeptidase which forms enkephalin), and against bradykinin, a nine amino acid inflammatory peptide. In each case the antibodies were of high affinity ($+10^8$ and in some cases 10^{10}) and were raised by two injections of small (a few micrograms) amounts of antigens. An important feature of the hybridomas produced by this procuedure was that all of those recovered produced antibody of the desired specificity. Clearly, the use of the appropriate antigen-avidin conjugate can effectively restrict most of the fusions to biotinylated established cell lines and the small subset of B cells specific for the coupled antigen. It is of interest to see if this receptor mediated focussing technique, so usefully teamed with electrofusion by Tsong and colleagues, can be yoked with other fusion protocols to increase the specificity of fusion events and to increase the likelihood of obtaining high affinity antibodies.

CHIMERIC ANTIBODIES

Chimeric antibodies are the offspring of a fusion of recombinant DNA technology and hybridoma methodology. They are the protein products of chimeric genes, constructed by joining immunoglobulin V region genes from one species with genes from another species. The transfection of nonsecreting myeloma cell lines with appropriate expression vectors containing these recombinant genes results in the synthesis and secretion of the chimeric antibody.

There are three major reasons why chimeric antibodies are of great interest. First, mouse hybridomas secreting monoclonal antibodies of essentially any desired specificity exist or can be derived. Hence there is available a potential library of V region genes of enormous diversity. Second, the therapeutic administration of mouse monoclonal antibodies to humans or animals of veterinary interest raises problems of host hypersensitivity. Such reactions may be minimized if the C regions of the administered antibodies are host homologous. Also, most antibody-mediated defense mechanisms invoke such host-based effector mechanisms as transport, the complement system and phagocytosis. All of these involve the constant regions of the immunoglobulin molecule and are likely to operate more efficiently with homologous than with heterologous species constant regions. Third, chimeric molecules in which the antigen binding portion of an immunoglobulin is joined to some other functional protein moiety could find a variety of uses in diagnosis and therapy. For example, appropriate antibody binding sites linked to enzymes would be useful diagnostic reagents. Toxin-mediated tumor immunotherapy might be effected by the construction of chimeric molecules in which the binding site for tumor associated determinants is linked to cytotoxic polypeptides.

A number of groups have reported the construction of expression vectors which encode the production of chimeric antibodies. Boullanne et al. (1984) have produced TNP-specific antibodies which have mouse V regions and human mu constant regions. Phosphorylcholine-binding chimeric antibodies possess mouse heavy and light chain V regions and human kappa light chain C regions and human IgG_1 or IgG_2 heavy chain C regions. A novel antigen binding enzyme, an "immunase," in which the capacity to bind the hapten,

4-hydroxy-3-nitrophenacetyl (NP), is genetically conjugated to the *Staphylococcus aureus* nuclease gene, has been engineered and expressed by Neuberger et al. (1984). This anti-NP immunase retains 10% of the activity of the native *S. aureus* nuclease and the authors have demonstrated its use in an ELISA assay.

WHAT TO EXPECT

A review of these newer developments shows a clear evolutionary trend in the technology of antibody production. Serology began and remained for many years an art, albeit scientifically practiced, in which one performed certain procedures involving antigens, animals, and adjuvants and obtained all too finite quantities of antigen-reactive serums. In skilled hands these sera could be absorbed and standardized to produce still ill-defined, but extremely useful, polyclonal antisera of great analytical power. When one stripped away all the ingenious absorption protocols and elaborate immunochemical procedures of concentration and affinity purification, it was clear that investigators basically took what the animals gave and did the best they could. With the invention of monoclonal antibody technology by Kohler and Milstein, a dramatic change began. For the first time the investigator could introduce an important element of control over the definition of the antibodies obtained. Instead of a mixture of many antibodies, a single immunoglobulin of defined specificity was available without any program of absorption whatsoever. Furthermore, once a hybridoma producing a useful monoclonal antibody had been derived, its monoclonal antibody product could be obtained in unlimited amounts for the indefinite future. No longer was it required for some acceptable version of the wheel to be reinvented again and again. But as we have seen, the watershed year of 1975 was only the beginning, a point of departure.

Since its introduction, hybridoma technology has undergone a series of modifications, all of which provide the experimenter with ever greater control and an increasing freedom from the biological constraints inherent in conventional immunization procedures. In 1979, Parks and his colleagues demonstrated that the fluorescence-activated cell sorter could be used to select and clone hybridoma cells which had a desired antigen specificity. The method of receptor-mediated focussing of B cells with desirable antigen specificity on myeloma fusion partners described above makes preselection of fusion partners an approach that can be used even by laboratories of modest means. In vitro immunization frees one from animal immunization and many of the constraints imposed by tolerance while at the same time dramatically lowering the requirements for antigen. The demonstrations of the feasibility of chimeric antibody construction have made it clear that antibody combining sites are for hire. Thus V regions and C regions from diverse sources may be genetically conjugated to each other or even to other functional proteins to produce hybrid molecules yet unrealized by evolution. One must expect that things will go farther still. Certainly one will see the application of in vitro mutagenesis (Zoller and Smith 1983) to the deliberate tailoring of antibody combining sites. A fusion of hybridoma methodology and recombinant DNA technology has already begun to transform the antibody from the product of a specialized cell into a creation of the genetic engineer.

REFERENCES

BOULLANNE, G. L., HOZUMI, N., and SHULMAN, M. J. 1984. Production of functional chimaeric mouse/human antibody. *Nature* 312: 643.

HAMMERLING, G. J., HAMMERLING, U., and KEARNEY, J. F. (Ed.). 1981. *Monoclonal Antibodies and T Cell Hybridomas*. Elsevier/North Holland, Amsterdam.

KENNETT, R. H., McKEARN, T. J., and BECHTOL, K. (Ed.). 1980. *Monoclonal Antibodies*. Plenum Press, New York

KOHLER, G. and MILSTEIN, C. 1975. Continuous cultures of fused cells secreting antibody of predefined specificity. *Nature* 256: 495.

LO, M. M. S., TSONG, T. Y., CONRAD, M. K., STRITTMATTER, S. M., HESTER, L. D., and SNYDER, S. H. 1984. Monoclonal antibody production by receptor-mediated electrically induced cell fusion. *Nature* 310: 792.

LUBEN, R. A. and MOHLER, M. A. 1982. In vitro immunization as an adjunct to the production of hybridomas producing antibodies against the lymphokine osteoclast activating factor. *Mol. Immunol.* 17: 635.

McHUGH, Y. 1984. In vitro immunization for hybridomas production. In *Hybridoma Technology in Agricultural and Veterinary Research*. Stern, N. J. and Gamble, H. R. (Ed.), p. 216. Rowman and Allanheld, Totowa, NJ.

MORRISON, S. L., JOHNSON, J. M., HERZENBERG, L. A., and OI, V. T. 1984. Chimeric human antibody molecules: Mouse antigen-binding domains with human constant region domains. *Proc. Natl. Acad. Sci.* 81: 6851.

NEUBERGER, M. S., WILLIAMS, G. T., and FOX, R. O. 1984. Recombinant antibodies possessing novel effector functions. *Nature* 312: 604.

PARKS, D. R., BRYAN, V., OI, V. T., and HERZENBERG, L. A. 1979. Antigen-specific identification and cloning of hybridomas with a fluorescence-activated cell sorter. *Proc. Natl., Acad. Sci.* 76: 1962.

POTTER, H., WEIR, L., and LEDER, P. 1984. Enhancer-dependent expression of human kappa immunoglobulin genes introduced into mouse pre-B lymphocytes by electroporation. *Proc. Natl. Acad. Sci.* 81: 7161.

READING, C. L. 1982. Theory and methods for immunization in culture and monoclonal antibody production. *J. Immunol. Meth.* 53: 261.

ZIMMERMANN, U. and VIENKEN, J. 1984. Electrofusion of cells. In *Hybridoma Technology in Agricultural and Veterinary Research*. Stern, N.J. and Gamble, H. R. (Ed.), p. 173. Rowman and Allanheld, Totowa, NJ.

ZOLLER, M. J. and SMITH, M. 1983. Oligonucleotide directed mutagenesis of DNA fragments cloned into M13 vectors. In *Methods of Enzymology*, Vol. 100. Wu, R., Grossman, L., and Moldave, K. (Ed.), p. 468. Academic Press, New York.

12

Immunoassays for Detecting Foodborne Bacteria and Microbial Toxins

B. Swaminathan and Raymond L. Konger
Purdue University
West Lafayette, Indiana

INTRODUCTION

The reaction between an antigen and an antibody is a noncovalent reaction which depends primarily upon structurally complementary binding sites of the two molecules. An antigen may have from one to several thousand determinants; polyclonal antibodies are heterogeneous mixtures of antibodies directed against different individual epitopes on the antigen. Thus, antigen-antibody reactions assume a great deal of complexity.

Antigen-antibody reactions have been used for the identification and characterization of bacteria since the turn of the century. Even today, sero-agglutination with specific antisera is a major criterion for the compartmentalization of bacteria into genus, species, and types (Edwards and Ewing 1972); however, DNA-DNA hybridization techniques have become the most important tools of bacterial taxonomy during the past decade (Brenner 1983).

253

CO-AGGLUTINATION AND IMMUNOFLUORESCENCE

Co-agglutination is an agglutination-enhancement technique which is gaining popularity in diagnostic clinical microbiology. An antibody is used to sensitize nonviable cells of *Staphylococcus aureus* through the specific interaction between protein A of *S. aureus* and immunoglobulin G of the antiserum (Kronvall 1973). An alternative method is to coat latex microspheres with antibody (Essers and Radebold 1980). Suspect bacterial colonies from plating media are subjected to slide agglutination using the co-agglutination reagent. Edwards and Hilderbrand (1976) successfully used this technique to identify *Salmonella* and *Shigella* from primary isolation plates. Baker et al. (1985) found commercially available co-agglutination tests for *S. aureus* (Sero STAT; Scott Laboratories, Fiskeville, RI; Staphyloslide; BBL Microbiology Systems, Cockeysville, MD; Hemostaph; Remel, Lenexa, KS) to be more sensitive than conventional slide coagulase and tube coagulase tests for the rapid identification of *S. aureus*. However, co-agglutination tests are performed only after the isolation of pure cultures by pre-enrichment and/or selective enrichment followed by selective differential plating.

The immunofluorescence technique is the forerunner of immunoassays since it demonstrated the feasibility of labeling an antibody with a tracer without affecting the immunoreactivity of the antibody. Coons et al. (1942) reported on the use of a fluorescein labeled antibody for the detection of pneumococcal antigen in tissues. The immunofluorescence technique has been applied to the detection of salmonellae in foods by several investigators (Haglund et al. 1964; Swaminathan et al. 1978; Thomason 1981). In this method, bacteria from an enrichment culture are fixed to a microscope slide and treated with a fluorescein labeled anti-*Salmonella* antibody. After removing the excess antibody, the slide is observed under a fluorescent microscope for cells which have complexed with the antibody and are rendered fluorescent. The immunofluorescence technique was approved for the presumptive detection of salmonellae in foods and feeds (Anon 1975) but never enjoyed widespread use because of problems such as unacceptably high levels of cross-reactivity of the antibody, the subjectivity involved in the evaluation of test results, and the need for trained operators to perform the test.

RADIOIMMUNOASSAYS AND IMMUNORADIOMETRIC TECHNIQUES

Radioimmunoassay was developed about 25 years ago (Yalow and Berson 1959) and is an invaluable analytical tool for the estimation of antigens (or antibodies) in biological specimens and yields precise data in the nanogram to picogram range. The principle of the method is as follows: ligand from a test sample (Ag) competes with a constant amount of labeled (with radioisotope) ligand (Ag^*) for a limited number of binding sites on antibody molecules (Ab).

$$Ag^* + Ab \rightleftharpoons Ag^* - Ab$$
$$+$$
$$Ag$$
$$\Updownarrow$$
$$(Ag - Ab)$$

After equilibrium is attained, the bound label is separated from the free label by one of several methods: (a) immobilizing the antibody on an insoluble matrix such as Sepharose, (b) adsorption of antibody to a solid matrix (such as polystyrene), (c) precipitation of antigen-antibody complex by an antiserum prepared against the antibody, or (d) electrophoretic techniques (Kabat 1980). Some applications of radioimmunoassays to the detection of foodborne toxicants are shown in Table 12.1.

Radioimmunoassays, in spite of their great sensitivity, suffer from several drawbacks such as hazards associated with preparation, handling, and disposal of radioactive labels, chemical instability of many labels, and the requirement for expensive radioactivity measuring equipment. The food industry is particularly adverse to the idea of using radioisotopes in the vicinity of food processing operations.

Immunoradiometric techniques differ from radioimmunoassays in that radiolabeled antibodies are used in place of radiolabeled antigens (Hales and Woodhead 1980). The two-site immunoradiometric assay uses a specific antibody immobilized on a solid phase to selectively "capture" the antigen of interest. A second antibody (usually directed at a different epitope on the antigen) which is labeled with a radioactive tracer is used for the detection and quantitative estimation of the antigen.

ENZYME IMMUNOASSAYS

The enzyme immunoassay is a result of the aggressive search for alternatives to radiolabeling. Enzymes are attractive as labels in immunoassays because they provide an amplified response through their catalytic action in the conversion of a substrate to a product (Schuurs and Van Weeman 1977).

Table 12.1. Radioimmunoassay of Foodborne Toxicants

Toxin	Toxin type	Minimum detectable level (ng/mL)	Investigators
Staphylococcal enterotoxin	A	10.0	Collins et al. (1973)
Staphylococcal enterotoxin	B	1.0	Pober and Silverman (1977)
Staphylococcal enterotoxin	A,B,C	1.0	Orth (1977)
Staphylococcal enterotoxin	A,B,C,D,E	0.3	Miller et al. (1978)
C. perfringens enterotoxin	—	1.0	Stelma et al. (1983)
Aflatoxin	B_1	0.25	El-Nakib et al. (1981)
Aflatoxin	M_1	0.5	Pestka et al. (1981b)
T-2 toxin	—	10.0	Fontelo et al. (1983)
Zearalenone and Zearalanol	—	5.0	Thouvenot and Morfin (1983)

Enzyme immunoassays can be divided into two fundamentally different categories: homogeneous enzyme immunoassays and heterogeneous enzyme immunoassays.

Homogeneous Enzyme Immunoassay

The homogeneous enzyme immunoassay or enzyme multiplied immunoassay (EMIT) was developed at the Syva Research Institute, Palo Alto, CA (Rubinstein et al. 1972). This elegant and powerful immunochemical technique utilizes the steric inhibition of an enzyme by an antibody when a hapten is attached to the enzyme near its active site. In this system, the enzyme activity is regulated by the amount of antibody available for binding to the enzyme-bound hapten. The reactions are as follows where H is the unknown, *Ab* is the antibody, *Ei* is the enzyme in inhibited state, and Ea is active enzyme:

$$H + Ab - (H - Ei) \rightarrow Ab - H + H - Ea$$
$$H - Ea + \text{Substrate} \rightarrow \text{product}$$

The EMIT assay has been used primarily for the assay of small molecules such as drugs and hormones in serum and urine (Gibbons et al. 1980). However, at least two reports have been published on the application of EMIT to large molecules. Morita and Woodburn (1978) reported on the development of an EMIT assay for staphylococal enterotoxin B (SEB) using a β-amylase-SEB conjugate. They were able to detect SEB at levels as low as 5 ng/mL in extracts of mayonnaise, cornstarch, milk and wieners. Gibbons et al. (1980) developed an EMIT assay for proteins using a protein antigen-β-galactosidase conjugate, antibody directed against the protein, and a synthetic 40,000 kdal dextran linked o-nitrophenyl-β-galactoside substrate. It was possible to detect 25 ng/mL of human IgG in human serum (Gibbons et al. 1980).

Heterogeneous Enzyme Immunoassays

Heterogeneous enzyme-immunoassays (HET-EIA) require a separation step to remove reacted from unreacted enzyme-labeled material. This usually involves immobilization of a soluble antigen or antibody to an insoluble solid matrix in such a way that immunoreactivity of the anchored component is retained. This technique is also known as ELISA (Enzyme-Linked Immunosorbent Assay) (Engvall and Perlmann 1971).

HET-EIA can be divided into two major classes: competitive and noncompetitive. Both methods are used in the analysis of foods; some of the assay configurations are schematically represented in Fig. 12.1. In the competitive assay, antigen in the test sample competes with enzyme-labeled antigen for binding sites on specific antibody bound to a solid matrix. The binding of enzyme-linked antigen to immobilized antibody is decreased by the presence of antigen in the test sample. Therefore, the concentration of antigen in the test sample is inversely proportional to the concentration of product formed by enzyme action in the final reaction. A modification of this technique, the indirect competitive assay (indirect inhibition assay; Voller et al. 1979), is also frequently used in food analysis. In this method, antigen is immobilized to the solid phase rather than antibody. Competition is between test antigen and bound antigen for specific antibody. After an incubation period, antibody not bound to the immobilized antigen is washed off and an enzyme-linked anti-immunoglobulin, specific for the first antibody, is added. Again, concentration of test antigen is indicated by inhibition of enzyme product formation.

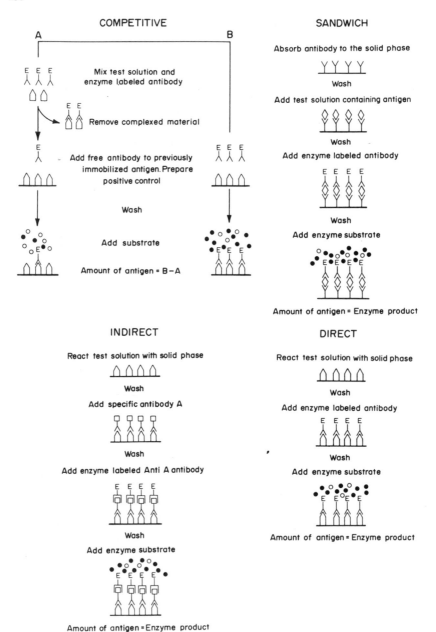

Fig. 12.1 Different configurations of heterogeneous enzyme immunoassays. (Reprinted from *Food Technology* with permission.)

The other assays shown in Fig. 12.1 are of the noncompetitive type. The "double antibody-sandwich" assay requires the antigen to have at least two binding sites for the antibody. One site is used for the capture of the antigen by immobilized antibody. The second site is for the binding of enzyme labeled antibody. In the direct assay, the antigen is reacted directly with enzyme labeled antibody while the indirect assay involves the reaction of antigen with unlabeled antibody followed by reaction with enzyme labeled protein A or antibody prepared against the first antibody.

Each type of enzyme immunoassay has its advantages and disadvantages. The competitive assay is rapid because it can be performed with one incubation and one washing step. However, purified antigen is required for the competitive assay, which poses a problem for most laboratories. Also, materials present in the food sample may interfere in the assay since the conjugate is reacted directly with the sample. Modifying enzymes such as proteases and noncompetitive enzyme inhibitors present in the test sample could substantially alter enzyme activity (Clark and Engvall 1980).

These interference problems are avoided in noncompetitive and indirect competitive assays where the test sample does not directly react with the enzyme-antibody conjugate. Additional advantages are the possibility of an amplification effect due to binding of several enzyme labeled antibody molecules to a polyvalent antigen molecule (or antibody in the case of indirect competitive assays) and the convenience of using a single conjugate to detect a variety of antigens in an indirect assay (Clark and Engvall 1980). The major disadvantage of noncompetitive and indirect competitive assays is the requirement for at least two incubations and several washings. Sandwich assays are reported to be less sensitive than other types of enzyme immunoassays (van Weeman and Schuurs, 1974); this could be particularly true for sandwich assays employing monoclonal antibodies since only one or very few types of antibody binding sites in the antigen molecule are being used. On the other hand, sandwich assays should be used when testing mixtures of proteins, such as food specimens, because of the competition among proteins for binding sites on the solid matrix. Another limitation of both the competitive and the indirect competitive assays is that antigen should be of relatively low molecular weight to prevent precipitation, agglutination, or steric hindrance of soluble reactants (Voller et al. 1979).

Mycotoxins are almost exclusively assayed by competitive HET-EIA (Chu 1984). Bacterial enterotoxins may be assayed by competitive and noncompetitive methods (Freed et al. 1982; Kuo and Silverman 1980), but noncompetitive methods are more commonly used. Noncompetitive methods are nearly always used for the detection of bacterial structural antigens because of problems associated with antigen purification.

Table 12.2. Application of Heterogeneous Enzyme Immunoassays (HET-EIA) to the Detection and Estimation of Foodborne Bacteria and Microbial Toxins

Contaminant	Type of HET-EIA	Matrix	Specific antibody	Conjugate	Sensitivity	Investigators
Staphylococcus aureus enterotoxin B	Direct	Nitrocellulose disc	Anti-SEB	Anti-SEB-protein A-HRPO	500 pg/colony	Peterkin and Sharpe (1984)
Staphylococcus aureus enterotoxins	Double antibody sandwich	Polystyrene balls	Anti-SE IgG	Anti-SE Ig-G-HRPO	$\leqslant$ 1 ng/g	Freed et al. (1982)
	Double antibody sandwich	Microtiter plate	Anti-SE IgG	Anti-SE IgG-HRPO	$\leqslant$ 1 ng/g	Freed et al. (1982)
	Double antibody sandwich	Microtiter plate	Anti-SE	Anti-SE-HRPO	0.5 g/100g	Notermans et al. (1983)
Clostridium perfringens type A toxin	Indirect	Nitrocellulose disc	Rabbit anti-toxin IgG	Anti-rabbit IgG-HRPO	0.6 ng/colony	Stelma et al. (1985)
Clostridium botulinum type G toxin	Double antibody sandwich	60 well polystyrene plates	Goat anti-type G toxin	Rabbit-anti-goat IgG-AK	less than 1 mouse intraperitoneal median lethal dose (LD_{50})	Lewis et al. (1981)
Escherichia coli heat-labile (LT) enterotoxin	Indirect	Nitrocellulose membrane	Rabbit anti-LT antiserum	Anti-LT serum-HRPO	1 ng/mm^2	Rhea and Shah (1985)
Ochratoxin A	Direct competitive	Microtissue plate	Rabbit anti-OA	OA-HRPO	25 pg/assay	Pestka et al. (1981a)

Analyte	Assay	Solid phase	Antibody	Conjugate	Sensitivity	Reference
T-2 Toxin	Indirect competitive	Microtiter plate	Monoclonal IgG₁	Rabbit anti-mouse IgG₁	50 ng/assay	Hunter et al. (1985)
	Indirect competitive	Microtiter plate	Rabbit anti-T-2-IgG-HRPO	Goat anti-rabbit IgG₁	0.2 ng/mL	Fan et al. (1984a)
	Direct competitive	Microtiter plate	Rabbit anti-T-2-IgG	T-2-HRPO	0.05 ng/mL	Gendloff et al. (1984)
	Direct competitive	Microtiter plate, Nylon beads	Rabbit anti-T-2-IgG	T-2-HRPO	0.1 ng/mL	Pestka and Chu (1984)
Salmonella typhimurium	Indirect	Cellulose acetate membrane filter	Rabbit antiflagellar monovalent	Antibody-HRPO	10⁵ cells/mL	Krysinski and Heimsch (1977)
Salmonella lipopolysaccharide	Inhibition by Salmonella lipopolysaccharide	Microtitration plate	Rabbit anti-Salmonella serum group A to G	Goat-antirabbit IgG-HRPO	—	Rigby (1984)
Aflatoxin B₁	Direct competitive	Microtiter plate, Terasaki microtissue plate, Nylon beads	Rabbit anti-AFB₁ IgG	AFB₁-HRPO	1.0 ng/mL	Pestka and Chu (1984)
	Direct competitive	Microtiter plate	Rabbit AFB₁ IgG	AFB₁-HRPO	25-2500 pg/assay	Pestka et al. (1980)
	Indirect competitive	Microtiter plate	Rabbit anti-AFB₁ IgG	Goat anti-rabbit IgG-HRPO	25 pg/assay	Fan and Chu (1984)

(Continued)

Table 12.2. (Continued)

Contaminant	Type of HET-EIA	Matrix	Specific antibody	Conjugate	Sensitivity	Investigators
Aflatoxin M_1	Direct competitive	Microtiter plate	Rabbit anti-BSA-AFM$_1$ IgG	AFM$_1$-HRPO	10–25 pg/mL	Hu et al. (1984)
	Direct competitive	Microtiter plate, Terasaki microtissue plate, Nylon beads	Rabbit anti-AFM$_1$ IgG	AFM$_1$-HRPO	0.05–0.1 ng/mL	Pestka and Chu (1984)
Aflatoxin Q_1	Direct competitive, Indirect competitive	Microtiter plate	Rabbit anti-AFQ$_{2a}$-IgG	AFQ$_{2a}$-HRPO	2 ng/mL	Fan et al. (1984b)
Salmonella spp.	Direct	Microtiter plate/ Centrifugation	Rabbit antiflagellar Polyvalent	Antibody-ALK. PHOS.	10^6 cells/mL	Minnich et al. (1982)
	Double antibody sandwich	Microtiter plate	Monoclonal (M467)	M467-HRPO	10^6 cells/mL	Robison et al. (1983)
	Competitive	Microtiter plate	Monocolonal (M467)	M467-ALK.PHOS	10^3–10^5 cells/mL	Smith and Jones (1983)

Direct	Microtitration plate	Spicer Edwards anti-serum pool	Protein A-β-galactosidase	10^6 cells/mL	Aleixo et al. (1984)
Double antibody sandwich	Polystyrene coated ferromagnetic beads	Monoclonal (M467)	M467-HRPO	10^5 cells/mL	Mattingly and Gehle (1984)
Double antibody sandwich	Polystyrene coated ferromagnetic beads	Monoclonal (M467)	M467-HRPO	—	Emswiler-Rose et al. (1984)
Double antibody	Polystyrene coated ferromagnetic beads	Monoclonal	Monoclonal-HRPO	—	Mattingly (1984)
Double antibody sandwich	Microtitration plate	Spicer Edwards antiserum pool	Antiserum-protein A-β-galactosidase	10^6–10^7 cells/mL	Anderson and Hartman
Double antibody sandwich	Microtiter plate	Monoclonal (M467)	M467-β-galactosidase	10^4 cells/mL	Swaminathan et al. (1985)

SE = Staphylococcal enterotoxin
OA = Ochratoxin A
AF = Aflatoxin
HRPO = Horseradish peroxidase
AK = Alkaline phosphatase

Within the last decade, numerous laboratories have investigated the use of HET-EIA for the detection and enumeration of the major bacterial agents of foodborne disease and their toxins (Table 12.2). *Salmonella* spp., *Clostridium botulinum* toxins (Notermans et al. 1982), *Clostridium perfringens* type *A* toxin, and staphylococcal enterotoxin *A* (SEA), *B* (SEB), *C* (SEC), *D* (SED), and *E* (SEE) (Freed et al. 1982) have all been assayed by HET-EIA with sensitivities comparable to or better than alternative methods currently in use.

Lewis et al. (1981) reported the use of a double antibody "sandwich" HET-EIA to detect *Clostridium botulinum* type *G* toxin. The level of detection of this assay was equivalent to levels obtained by mouse bioassays. Sandwich assays have also been described for the detection of staphylococcal enterotoxins (Freed et al. 1982; Notermans et al. 1983). In general, sensitivity of immunoassays for staphylococcal enterotoxins in foods range from 100 pg for SEC to less than 0.1 mg per g for SEA, SEB, SED, or SEE (Kuo and Silverman 1980). A direct HET-EIA for SEB (Peterkin and Sharpe 1984) and an indirect HET-EIA for *Clostridium perfringens* (Stelma et al. 1985) have been developed. These methods involve the blotting, or adsorption of the enterotoxin directly from colonies grown on a solid media on to nitrocellulose which serves as the solid phase in the enzyme immunoassay.

HET-EIA's have been extensively applied to the detection of salmonellae in foods. A major problem in the detection of *Salmonella* is that contaminated processed foods contain low numbers of *Salmonella*, as low as 1 cell per 25 g of food sample (Andrews 1985). Prolonged cultural procedures are required to revive and multiply the *Salmonella* to detectable levels. The first reported EIA for the detection of *Salmonella* (Krysinski and Heimsch 1977) was an indirect method utilizing an antiserum prepared against the flagella of *Salmonella typhimurium*. However, attempts to expand the above method to the detection of other serotypes were troubled by false positives due to crossreactivity of the polyclonal antisera with "O" antigens of other bacteria. Various attempts were made to purify the antisera to remove crossreactive components of polyclonal antisera (Minnich et al. 1982; Swaminathan et al. 1978) resulting in improvements. With the introduction of a mouse myeloma protein (M467) by Robison et al. (1983) and Smith and Jones (1983), the problem of crossreactivity was significantly reduced. The myeloma protein, M467, recognizes a common antigenic determinant present on many serotypes of *Salmonella*. However, a small number of *Salmonella* serotypes (5%) are not reactive with M467, including several of significant clinical importance. Current work with enzyme immunoassays have utilized "sandwich" HET-EIA using monoclonal antibody mixed with M467 to broaden the range of detection (Mattingly 1984).

The low molecular weight of mycotoxins and their availability in purified form allows use of competitive HET-EIA as a diagnostic tool for their detection and quantitative determination. Competitive HET-EIA have been developed for detection of aflatoxins, T-2 toxin, ochratoxin A (OA), and zearalenone, with sensitivities in the nanogram to picogram range. Most competitive HET-EIA used for mycotoxin detection are the direct, more rapid, and simple competitive type, although indirect competitive HET-EIA have also been adapted for the assay of mycotoxins.

Fan et al. (1984a, b) and Fan and Chu (1984) reported on the development of indirect competitive assays for detection of T-2 toxin, aflatoxin B_1, and aflatoxin Q_1, respectively, with sensitivities equal to those of direct assays but using 50–100 times less specific antibody per assay. This is important as antisera produced against mycotoxins are of universal low titer due to the poor immunogenic qualities of mycotoxins (low molecular weight, non-protein structure, and cytotoxicity; Chu 1984). Another recent approach utilizes an indirect assay and monoclonal antibodies against T-2 toxin (Hunter et al. 1985). Although sensitivites were somewhat lower than in other reported assays, unlimited availability of defined antibody is a positive feature. The development of two prepacked silica gel cartridges has greatly simplified the procedures for "clean-up" of test samples and has increased sensitivities of assays (Chu 1984; Hu et al. 1984; Fan et al. 1984b). The cartridges can be loaded, washed, and samples eluted with a simple hypodermic syringe (Chu 1984).

SELECTION OF ENZYMES FOR IMMUNOASSAYS

The catalytic properties of enzymes allow them to act as amplifiers of reactions. Many enzyme molecules can catalyze the formation of more than 10^5 product molecules per minute. However, an enzyme must meet several criteria to be considered useful for EIA. Some of the important criteria are: high molecular activity or catalytic center activity, stability during conjugation and under assay and storage conditions, solubility, availability of suitable and safe substrates, and commercial availability at reasonable prices. While there is no one enzyme which meets all the above criteria, a number of enzymes meet several of the above criteria and have been used in enzyme immunoassays. These are shown in Table 12.3.

Of these enzymes, peroxidase and alkaline phosphatase are most frequently used. Some of the substrates initially used for horseradish peroxidase were suspect carcinogens (e.g., 3-3'-diaminobenzidine); however, several alternate substrates (4-aminoantipyrine, ABTS) are now available. Where several preparations of a given enzyme are available, the preparation with highest specific activity must be selected for use. For example, the sensitivity

Table 12.3. Enzymes Used as Labels in Enzyme Immunoassays

Types of enzyme immunoassay	Enzyme	Source	Enzyme commission no.	Mol. wt. (K dal)	Subunits
HET-EIA	Acetylcholinesterase	*Electrophorus electricus*	3.1.1.7	259	12
	Alkaline phosphatase	Calf intestine	3.1.3.1	190	—
	β-Galactosidase	*Escherichia coli* *E. coli*	3.2.1.23	135 or 320	4 4
	Glucose 6-phosphate dehydrogenase	*Leuconostoc mesenteroides*	1.1.1.49	120	—
	Glucose oxidase	*Aspergillus niger*	1.1.3.4	186	—
	Penicillinase (β-Lactamase)	*Bacillus cereus*	3.5.2.6	32	—
	Peroxidase	Horseradish	1.11.1.7	40	—
	Luciferase	Firefly	—	—	—
	Exo-1,4-β-glucosidase (Glucoamylase)	*Coniophora cerebella*	3.2.1.3	48	—
	Carbonate dehydrolase (Carbonic anhydrase)	Hen erythrocytes	4.2.1.1.	28	—
	Catalase	*Micrococcus lysodekticus*	1.11.1.6	232	4
HOM-EIA	N-acetylmuramide glycano-hydrolase (Lysozyme)	Egg white	3.2.1.17	14	6
	Malate dehydrogenase	Pig heart	1.1.1.37	70	2
	Glucose-6-phosphate dehydrogenase	*L. mesenteroides*	1.1.1.49	190	—
	β-Amylase	Sweet potato	3.2.1.2	215	4
	β-Galactosidase	*E. coli*	3.2.1.23	135 or 320	4 4

of an enzyme immunoassay can be increased eightfold by using alkaline phosphatase with a specific activity of 45 U/mg instead of a preparation with an activity of 15 U/mg (Avrameas et al. 1978).

Coupling of Enzymes to Proteins

Several homobifunctional and heterobifunctional reagents have been used to conjugate enzymes to other proteins. Homobifunctional reagents (e.g., glutaraldehyde) offer simple means of conjugating enzymes to proteins; however, they generally yield heterogeneous mixtures of conjugates along with significant quantities of homoconjugates of enzymes and/or protein antibodies (O'Sullivan and Marks 1981). Recently introduced heterobifunctional reagents offer a means of controlling or preventing the formation of such homoconjugates.

The ideal conjugation method should be technically simple to use, yield a homogeneous conjugate, should not substantially affect the activity of either enzyme or antibody, minimize formation of enzyme-enzyme or antibody-antibody conjugates, provide a stable conjugate, and must be flexible and controllable so that the enzyme-antibody ratios can be optimized for each application (O'Sullivan and Marks 1981).

One step glutaraldehyde method. Glutaraldehyde is a homobifunctional dialdehyde which reacts with amino residues on protein to form a Schiff's base. However, the Schiff's base is unlikely to be the final reaction product in view of the stability of the cross-link. The reaction mechanism is:

$$E - NH_2 + CHO \cdot CH_2 \cdot CH_2 \cdot CH_2 \cdot CHO + NH_2 - Ab$$
$$\downarrow$$
$$E - N = CH \cdot CH_2 \cdot CH_2 \cdot CH_2 \cdot CH = N - Ab$$
$$\downarrow$$
$$\text{Further Complex Reactions}$$
$$\downarrow$$
$$\text{Conjugate}$$
$$E = \text{Enzyme} \qquad Ab = \text{Antibody}$$

This method has been used to prepare conjugates of peroxidase, alkaline phosphatase, glucose oxidase and glucoamylase (Wisdom 1976). Enzyme and antibody are simply mixed in the presence of glutaraldehyde (0.2%) to obtain the conjugate. The efficiency of coupling protein to peroxidase and alkaline phosphatase is poor, considerable inactivation of enzyme occurs, and the conjugates are highly polymerized (Wisdom 1976; O'Sullivan and Marks 1981).

Two-step glutaraldehyde procedure. This procedure is useful for peroxidase because one molecule of the enzyme normally reacts with only one aldehyde group of the cross-linker (Avrameas and Ternynck 1971). After removal of excess glutaraldehyde, the activated enzyme is allowed to react with the antibody. A conjugate of immunoglobulin G and peroxidase has a molecular weight of approximately 210 kdal indicating that it is composed of one molecule of antibody and one molecule of enzyme. The efficiency of the two-step procedure is poor but labels prepared by this method yield increased sensitivity in enzyme immunoassays when compared with labels prepared by one step procedures (O'Sullivan and Marks 1981).

Periodate oxidation. This method has been applied only to horseradish peroxidase, a glycoprotein, in which the carbohydrate component is not required for enzyme activity. The peroxidase is first treated with 1-fluoro-2,4-dinitrobenzene to block its free amino groups and prevent self-linking. The carbohydrate moieties are oxidized by periodate to yield aldehydes. The activated peroxidase is allowed to react with amino groups of a second protein (antibody) and the resulting Schiff's bases are reduced with sodium borohydride to provide stable cross-links. Nakane and Kawaoi (1974) reported that under optimal conditions 68% of the enzyme activity and 99% of immunoglobulin G were incorporated in the conjugate. However, other evaluations indicated much lower efficiency of conjugation. Peroxidase-antibody conjugates prepared by the periodate method yielded much steeper dose response curves in enzyme immunoassays than one step and two step glutaraldehyde procedures (Adams and Wisdom 1979).

Cross-Linking with $N,N'-o$-phenylenedimaleimide. $N,N'-o$-Phenylenedimaleimide is a homobifunctional maleimide which reacts rapidly and selectively with sulfhydryl groups under mild conditions (Kato et al. 1975). Sulfhydryl groups are first introduced into the antibody by reduction of dislufide bridges. The modified antibody is reacted with maleimide and the activated antibody, after the removal of excess maleimide, is finally reacted with β-D-galactosidase which contains free thiol groups. This method is reported to efficiently couple β-D-galactosidase to antibody with little or no loss of enzyme or antibody activity (O'Sullivan and Marks 1981); however, it is technically more demanding.

Cross-linking with m-maleimidobenzoyl-N-hydroxysuccinimide ester (MBS). MBS is a heterobifunctional reagent. Under mild conditions, the hydroxysuccinimide moiety of MBS reacts rapidly and selectively with amino groups whereas the maleimide reacts rapidly and selectively with thiol groups (Kitagawa et al. 1978). MBS has been used in a two-step procedure to couple β-galactosidase to antibody. In the first reaction, maleimide residues are introduced into the antibody by the reaction of the hydroxysuccinimide of

MBS with amino groups of antibody. Since the antibody does not contain free sulfhydryl groups, the reagent will not cross-link the antibody. After removal of excess reagent, the activated antibody is reacted with β-galactosidase. The procedure is simpler than the N-N'-o-phenylenedimaleimide method (O'Sullivan and Marks 1981).

Cross-linking with N-succinimidyl 3-(2-pyridyldithio) propionate.

Carlsson et al. (1978) introduced a heterobifunctional reagent, N-succinimidyl 3-(2-pyridyldithio) propionate (SPDP) for use in protein-protein conjugation. Peroxidase, alkaline phosphatase, and β-galactosidase have been conjugated to antibodies by the procedure. Since β-galactosidase possesses free sulfhydryl groups which are not required for enzyme activity, no derivatization of this enzyme is necessary (Aleixo and Swaminathan 1985).

FACTORS AFFECTING THE SENSITIVITY OF ENZYME IMMUNOASSAY

One of the major criticisms of enzyme immunoassays has been that its sensitivity does not approach that of radioimmunoassays (10^{-17} mol). Several factors influence sensitivity of an enzyme immunoassay and many of these factors can be optimized to yield increased sensitivity.

Immunoreactant Affinity

The strength with which an antibody binds to its antigen is denoted as affinity. Mathematically, the interaction at equilibrium between a monovalent antibody and an antigen with a single antigenic determinant (hapten) may be expressed as follows:

$$[Ab] + [Ag] \underset{kd}{\overset{ka}{\rightleftharpoons}} [Ab - Ag] \tag{1}$$

where $[Ab]$ represents the antibody, $[Ag]$ the antigen, and $[Ab\text{-}Ag]$ the antibody-antigen complex, and ka and kd represents the association and dissociation rate constants. Applying the Law of Mass Action to Eq. (1),

$$K = \frac{ka}{kd} = \frac{[Ab - Ag]}{[Ab][Ag]} \tag{2}$$

The $[Ab\text{-}Ag]$ complex is stabilized by forces such as hydrogen bonding, Van der Waals forces, London forces, and hydrophobic and Coloumbic interactions (Steward and Stensgaard 1983). Further mathematical manipulation of Eq. (2) leads to the following form of Langmuir Adsorption isotherm,

$$\frac{[Ab - Ag]}{[Ab]} = r = \frac{nK[Ab]}{1 + K[Ab]} \tag{3}$$

where r = moles of antigen bound per mole of antibody; $[Ab\text{-}Ag]$ = bound antigen concentration; $[Ab]$ = total antibody concentration; $[Ag]$ = free antigen concentration (at equilibrium); n = antibody valence; K = association equilibrium constant or affinity. A rearrangement of Eq. (3) leads to the Scratchard equation

$$\frac{r}{[Ag]} = nK - rK = -rK + nK \tag{4}$$

Therefore, a plot of $r/[Ag]$ vs. r allows the determination of antibody affinity (K) and antibody valence (n). An alternate equation for calculation of affinity is given below

$$\frac{1}{r} = \frac{1}{n} \times \frac{1}{Ag} \times \frac{1}{K} - \frac{1}{n}$$

Using this equation, a plot of $1/r$ vs. $1/(Ag)$ yields values for affinity and valence. Several methods are available for experimental determination of antibody affinity. These include equilibrium dialysis, fluorescence quenching and fluorescence polarization, ammonium sulfate precipitation, competitive radioimmunoassay, equilibrium molecular sieving, and electrophoresis (Steward and Stensgaard 1983). High affinity antibodies yield better sensitivities than low affinity antibodies in immunoassays (Butler et al. 1978; Lehotonen and Ferola 1982; Nimmo et al. 1984).

Method of Preparation of Enzyme-Antibody Conjugate

The method used for preparation of antibody-enzyme conjugates appears to have a significant influence on the sensitivity of enzyme immunoassays. Nygren (1982) reported that the periodate method (Nakane and Kawaoi 1974) is superior to a method utilizing SPDP. However, Yoshitake et al. (1982) observed a 10–100-fold increase in sensitivity in sandwich enzyme immunoassay with a peroxidase-antibody conjugate prepared using a maleimide compound when compared with conjugates prepared by the periodate method. A peroxidase-antibody conjugate prepared by the SPDP method was superior to one prepared by the two-step glutaraldehyde procedure when evaluated against various antigens in enzyme immunoassays (Nilsson et al. 1981). Experience in our laboratory indicates that SPDP conjugates of antibody with β-galactosidase or alkaline phosphatase yielded a 10–100-fold increase in sensitivity in enzyme immunoassays when compared with glutaraldehyde conjugates (Aleixo 1984; Aleixo and Swaminathan, unpublished data).

SUBSTRATES AND QUANTITATION OF FINAL REACTION PRODUCT

The substrates available for commonly used enzymes in enzyme immunoassays are shown in Table 12.4. The choice of a substrate for an enzyme immunoassay would depend upon the final configuration of the assay. In general, chromogenic immunoassays are most common at present although that situation is expected to change by 1990. Chromogenic substrates used to measure the activity of hydrolytic enzymes are more stable than those used for oxidoreductases such as peroxidase and glucose oxidase (Guesdon and Avrameas 1981). Among the substrates for peroxidase, ABTS is most commonly employed although o-phenylenediamine may yield greater sensitivity (Avrameas et al. 1978).

The use of a substrate which is converted to a highly fluorescent product after reaction with an enzyme would allow for the measurement of very low concentrations of substrate products and consequently low levels of enzyme-labeled antibody and antigens. Such systems are gaining increased acceptance with the introduction of fluorometric immunoassay readers and fluorogenic substrates for enzymes. Zaitsu and Ohkura (1980) found that by using 3-(p-hydroxyphenyl)propionic acid, peroxidase activity can be assayed down to a level of 7.8U. Yolken and Leister (1982) reported that the use of high-energy fluorescent substrates (4-methylumbelliferyl phosphate) led to 64-fold increase in sensitivity over colorigenic EIA for the measurement of *Haemophilus influenzae* polyribose phosphate with a substrate reaction time of 10 minutes. Shalev et al. (1980) attained a 16–39-fold increase in sensitivity by utilizing fluorogenic substrates. By optimizing various parameters of fluorescent immunoassay, they were able to detect 3–10 attog/mL (3–10 × 10^{-18}g)mL or 24,000 molecules of purified IgG. Swaminathan et al. (1985) reported a 10–100-fold increase in sensitivity in the detection of *Salmonella* by using a heterobifunctional agent for conjugation and a fluorescent enzyme immunoassay system.

Table 12.4 Substrates for Selected Enzymes Used in Enzyme
Immunoassays

Enzyme	Substrates
Alkaline phosphatase	p-nitrophenyl phosphate k-Phos-Eiken (disodium phenyl phosphate + 4-aminoantipyrene) 4-methyl umbelliferyl phosphate[F]
β-Galactosidase	o-nitrophenyl β-D-galactopyranoside 4-methyl umbelliferyl β-D-galactopyranoside[F]
Glucose-6-phosphate dehydrogenase	NAD + glucose-6-phosphate → NADH NADH measured with immobilized oxidoreductase and luciferase
Glucose oxidase	sodium, 3,5-dicholoro-2 hydroxybenzene sulfonate (DHSA), 4-aminoantipyrine glucose peroxidase o-dianisidine + horseradish peroxidase
Penicillinase	starch + penicillin G + iodine + potassium iodide
Peroxidase	3-3′ diaminobenzidine + H_2O_2 o-tolidine + H_2O_2 2-2′-azino-dl(3-ethyl-benzthiazolin)-6′-sulfonate (ABTS) + H_2O_2 3-(p-hydroxyphenyl)propionic acid (HPPA)[F]

F = fluorogenic substrate

OTHER DEVELOPMENTS AND PERSPECTIVES FOR THE FUTURE

Chemiluminescence precursors, i.e. luminol (3-aminophthalhydrazide), have been used as labels in immunoassays. However, such assays have low sensitivity because the photon yields of the labels are very low, on the order of

1% or less (Schall and Tenoso 1981). Bioluminescent immunoassays utilize enzyme-substrate combinations which produce light as one of the products. One procedure involves conjugating an antigen to firefly luciferase. The labeled antigen is used in a competitive binding assay with increasing amounts of free antigen and a constant amount of antibody. The sensitivity of this assay (10^{-15} mol) is comparable to that of radioimmunoassay (Wannlund and DeLuca 1983). The sensitivity of a bioluminescent immunoassay can be further enhanced to approximately 10 attomoles (10^{-17} moles) by linking the antigen to an enzyme such as glucose-6-phosphate dehydrogenase which has a high turnover number. The NADH produced is measured with bacterial luminescent enzymes (Wannlund and DeLuca 1983).

$$NADH + H^+ + FMN \rightarrow NAD^+ + FMNH_2$$
$$FMNH_2 + RCHO + O_2 \rightarrow RMN + RCOOH + h\nu + H_2O$$

Thermometric enzyme immunoassay (TEIA) is based on the principle that a measurable amount of heat is liberated when certain enzymes convert their substrates. An enzyme which meets this requirement is catalase (ΔH of reaction $= -30$ kcal/mol, turnover number $3.7 \times 10^7 sec^{-1}$). TEIA has been used to determine human serum albumin down to a concentration of 10^{-10}M (Mattiason et al. 1977).

The enzyme immunoassay will play an increasingly important role in detection of foodborne microorganisms and quantitative determination of microbial toxins in foods. The argument that enzyme immunoassays can never approach the sensitivity and precision of radioimmunoassays has already been disproven in some instances (Chu 1984; Pestka et al. 1981b). Improving the sensitivity of enzyme immunoassays is currently receiving a major research emphasis and we are already beginning to see the results of such attempts in techniques such as fluorescence enzyme immunoassay and biolumines-cence enzyme immunoassay. The exceptionally strong affinity ($K_d \sim 10^{-15}$M) between avidin and biotin (compared with a dissociation constant of 10^{-8}M) typical of antigen-antibody reactions) has been utilized to enhance the sensitivity of enzyme immunoassays (Guesdon et al. 1979). In an avidin-biotin mediated enzyme immunoassay, enzyme labeled avidin attaches to multiple sites on a biotin labeled antibody and greatly amplifies the signal. In spite of such improvements in signal detection to achieve greater sensitivity, the specificity of an enzyme immunoassay (or any other immunological method) is dependant on the quality and nature of the antibody used for the assay. Previous attempts to apply such techniques to detection of gram-negative bacterial pathogens were not successful because of cross-reactivity problems associated with polyclonal polvalent antisera. Monoclonal antibodies have greatly alleviated such cross-reactivity problems (Robison et al. 1983; Smith and Jones 1983; Mattingly and Gehle 1984; Mattingly 1984) and has made it possible to reliably detect *Salmonella* in foods. An immunoassay test for *Salmonella* detection is now commercially available (Litton Bionetics, Charleston, SC) and others will soon become available. Monoclonal antibodies against the enterotoxins of *S. aureus* have been developed (Meyer et al. 1984; Edwin et al. 1984) and enzyme immunoassays for staphylococcal enterotoxins employing these monoclonal antibodies will soon be developed. Many more assays for the detection of other clinically important foodborne pathogens (e.g., *Campylobacter jejuni* and *C. coli; Yersinia enterocolitica*), microbial toxins, and food quality and sanitation indicators (e.g., *Geotrichum candidum*) are expected to become available in the near future.

REFERENCES

ADAMS, T. H. and WISDOM, G. B. 1979. Peroxidase labelling of antibodies for use in enzyme immunoassay. *Biochem. Soc. Trans.* 7: 55–57.

ALEIXO, J. A. G. 1984. Enzyme immunoassays for the rapid detection of salmonellae in foods. Ph.D. dissertation, Purdue University, West Lafayette, IN.

ALEIXO, J. A. G., SWAMINATHAN, B., and MINNICH, S. A. 1984. Salmonella detection in foods and feeds in 27 hours by an enzyme immunoassay. *J. Microbiol. Methods* 2: 135–145.

ALEIXO, J. A. G. and SWAMINATHAN, B. 1985. The use of homo- and heterobifunctional reagents for the preparation of β-galactosidase-antibody conjugates. *Abstracts Ann. Meet. Am. Soc. Microbiol.* V15: 391.

ANDERSON, J. M. and HARTMAN, P. A. 1985. Direct immunoassay for detection of salmonellae in foods and feeds. *Appl. Environ. Microbiol.* 49: 1124–1127.

ANDREWS, W. H. 1985. A review of cultural methods and their relation to rapid methods for the detection of *Salmonella* in foods. *Food Technol.* 39(3): 77–82.

ANONYMOUS. 1975. Changes in methods. *J. Assoc. Offic. Anal. Chem.* 58: 417–419.

AVRAMEAS, S. and TERNYNCK, T. 1971. Peroxidase labeled antibody and Fab conjugates for enhanced intracellular penetration. *Immunochemistry* 8: 1175–1179.

AVRAMEAS, S., TERNYNCK, T., and GUESDON, J. L. 1978. Coupling of enzymes to antibodies and antigens. *Scand. J. Immunol.* (Suppl.) 7: 7–23.

BAKER, J. S., BORMANN, M. A., and BOUDREAU, D. H. 1985. Evaluation of various rapid agglutination methods for the identification of *Staphylococcus aureus. J. Clin. Microbiol.* 21: 726–729.

BRENNER, D. J. 1983. Impact of modern taxonomy on clinical microbiology. *ASM News* 49: 58–63.

BUTLER, J. E., FELDBUSH, T. L., McGIVERN, P. L., and STEWART, N. 1978. The enzyme-linked immunosorbent assay (ELISA): A measure of antibody concentration or affinity? *Immunochemistry* 15: 131–136.

CARLSSON, J., DREVIN, H., and AXEN, R. 1978. Protein thiolation and reversible protein-protein conjugation. *Biochem. J.* 173: 723–737.

CHU, F. S. 1984. Immunoassays for analysis of mycotoxins. *J. Food Prot.* 47: 562–569.

CLARK, B. R. and ENGVALL, E. 1980. Enzyme linked immunosorbent assay (ELISA): Theoretical and practical aspects. In *Enzyme Immunoassay.* Maggio, E. T. (Ed.). CRC Press, Boca Raton, FL.

COLLINS, W. S., JOHNSON, A. D., METZGER, J. F., and BENNETT, R. W. 1973. Rapid solid phase radioimmunoassay for staphylococcal enterotoxin A. *Appl. Environ. Microbiol.* 25: 774–777.

COONS, A. H., CREECH, H. J., JONES, R. N., and BERLINER, E. 1942. The demonstration of pneumococcal antigen in tissues by the use of fluorescent antibody. *J. Immunol.* 45: 159–170.

EDWARDS, P. R. and EWING, W. H. 1972. *Identification of Enterobacteriaceae.* 3rd ed. Burgess Publishing Company, Minneapolis, MN.

EDWARDS, E. A. and HILDERBRAND. 1976. Method for identifying *Salmonella* and *Shigella* directly from the primary isolation plate by coagglutination of protein A-containing staphylococci sensitized with specific antibody. *J. Clin. Microbiol.* 3: 339–343.

EDWIN, C., TATINI, S. R., STROBEL, R. S. and MAHESWARAN, S. K. 1984. Production of monoclonal antibodies to staphylococcal enterotoxin A. *Appl. Environ. Microbiol.* 48: 1171–1175.

EL-NAKIB, O., PESTKA, J. J., and CHU, F. S. 1981. Determination of aflatoxin B_1 in corn, wheat, and peanut butter by enzyme linked immunosorbent assay and solid phase radioimmunoassay. *J. Assoc. Off. Anal. Chem.* 64: 1077–1082.

EMSWILER-ROSE, B., GEHLE, W. D., JOHNSTON, R. W., OKREND, A., MORAN, A., and BENNETT, B. 1984. An enzyme immunoassay technique for detection of salmonellae in meat and poultry products. *J. Food Sci.* 49: 1018–1020.

ENGVALL, E. and PERLMANN, P. 1971. Enzyme-linked immunosorbent assay (ELISA). Quantitative assay of immunoglobulin G. *Immunochemistry* 8: 871–874.

ESSERS, L. and RADEBOLD, K. 1980. Rapid and reliable identificatio of *Staphylococcus aureus* by a latex agglutination test. *J. Clin. Microbiol.* 12: 641–643.

FAN, T. S. L. and CHU, F. S. 1984. Indirect enzyme-linked immunosorbent assay for detection of aflatoxin B_1 in corn and peanut butter. *J. Food Prot.* 47: 263–266.

FAN, T. S. L., ZHANG, G. S., and CHU, F. S. 1984(a). An indirect enzyme-linked immunosorbent assay for T-2 toxin in biological fluids. *J. Food Prot.* 47: 964–967.

FAN, T. S. L., ZHANG, G. S., and CHU, F. S. 1984(b). Production and characterization of antibody against aflatoxin Q_1. *Appl. Environ. Microbiol.* 47: 526–532.

FLOWERS, R. S. 1985. Comparison of rapid *Salmonella* screening methods and the conventional culture method. *Food Technol.* 39(3): 103–108.

FONTELO, P. A., BEHELER, J., BUNNER, D. L., and CHU, F. S. 1983. Detection of T-2 toxins by an improved radioimmunoassay. *Appl. Environ. Microbiol.* 45: 640–643.

FREED, R. C., EVENSON, M. L., REISER, R. F., and BERGDOLL, M. S. 1982. Enzyme-linked immunosorbent assay for detection of enterotoxins in foods. *Appl. Environ. Microbiol.* 44: 1349–1355.

GENDLOFF, E. H., PESTKA, J. J., SWANSON, S. P., and HART, L. P. 1984. Detection of T-2 toxin in *Fusarium sporotrichiodes* infected corn by enzyme-linked immunosorbent assay. *Appl. Environ. Microbiol.* 47: 1161–1163.

GUESDON, J-L. and AVRAMEAS, S. 1981. Solid phase enzyme immunoassays. *Appl. Biochem. Bioeng.* 3: 207–232

GUESDON, J-L., TERNYNCK, T., and AVRAMEAS, S. 1979. The use of avidin-biotin interaction in immunoenzymatic techniques. *J. Histochem. Chytochen.* 27: 1131–1139.

GIBBONS, I., SKOLD, C., ROWLEY, G. L., and NUMAN, E. F. 1980. Homogeneous enzyme immunoassay for protein employing -galactosidase. *Anal. Biochem.* 102: 167–170.

HAGLUND, J. R., AYRES, J. C., PATON, A. M., KRAFT, A. A., and QUINN, L. Y. 1964. Detection of salmonellae in eggs and egg products with fluorescent antibody. *Appl. Microbiol.* 12: 447–450.

HALES, C. N. and WOODHEAD, J. S. 1980. Labeled antibodies and their use in the immunoradiometric assays. In *Methods in Enzymology*, Vol. 70. Vurakis, H. V. and Langone, J. J. (Ed.). Academic Press, New York.

HU, W. J., CHIK, N. W., and CHU, F. S. 1984. A research note: ELISA of picogram quantities of aflatoxin M_1 in urine and milk. *J. Food Prot.* 47: 126–127.

HUNTER, JR., K. W., BRIMFIELD, A. A., MILLER, M., FINKELMAN, F. D., and CHU, F. S. 1985. Preparation and characterization of monoclonal antibodies to the tricothecene mycotoxin T-2. *Appl. Environ. Microbiol.* 49: 168–172.

KABAT, E. A. 1980. Basic principles of antigen-antibody reactions. In *Methods in Immunology*, Vol. 70. Van Vunakis, H. and Langone, J. J. (Ed.). Academic Press, New York.

KATO, K., MAMAGUCHI, Y., FUKUI, H., and ISHIFAWA, E. 1975. Enzyme linked immunoassay. II. A simple method for synthesis of the rabbit antibody-D-galactosidase complex and its general applicability. *J. Biochem.* 78: 423–425.

KITAGAWA, T., FUJITAKE, T., TANUYAMA, H., and TADAOMI, A. 1978. Enzyme immunoassay of viomycin. New cross-linking reagent for enzyme labeling and a preparation method for antiserum to viomycin. *J. Biochem.* 83: 1493–1501.

KRONVALL, G. 1973. A rapid slide-agglutination method for typing pneumococci by means of specific antibody absorbed to protein A-containing staphylococci. *J. Med. Microbiol.* 6: 187–190.

KRYSINSKI, E. P. and HEIMSCH, R. C. 1977. Use of enzyme labeled antibodies to detect *Salmonella* in foods. *Appl. Environ. Microbiol.* 33: 947–954.

KUO, J. K. S. and SILVERMAN, G. J. 1980. Application of enzyme-linked immunosorbent assay for detection of staphylococcal enterotoxin in food. *J. Food Prot.* 43: 404–407.

LEHOTONEN, O. P. and FEROLA, E. 1982. The effect of different antibody affinities on ELISA absorbance and titer. *J. Immunol. Methods* 54: 233–240.

LEWIS, JR., G. E., KULINSKI, S. S., REICHARD, D. W., and METZGER, J. F. 1981. Detection of *Clostridium botulinum* type G toxin by enzyme-linked immunosorbent assay. *Appl. Environ. Microbiol.* 42: 1018–1022.

MATTIASSON, B., BORREBAECK, C., SANFRIDSON, B., and MOSBACH, K. 1977. Thermometric enzyme linked immunosorbent assay. *Biochem. Biophys. Acta* 483: 221–227.

MATTINGLY, J. A. 1984. An enzyme immunoassay for the detection of all *Salmonella* using a combination of a myeloma protein and a hybridoma antibody. *J. Immunol. Methods* 73: 147–156.

MATTINGLY, J. A., and GEHLE, W. D. 1984. An improved enzyme immunoassay for the detection of *Salmonella*. *J. Food Sci.* 49: 807–809.

MEYER, R. F., MILLER, L., BENNETT, R. W., and MACMILLAN, J. D. 1984. Development of a monoclonal antibody capable of interacting with five serotypes of *Staphylococcus aureus* enterotoxin. *Appl. Environ. Microbiol.* 47: 283–287.

MILLER, B. A., REISER, R. F., and BERGDOLL, M. S. 1978. Detection of staphylococcal cells containing protein A as immunosorbent. *Appl. Environ. Microbiol.* 36: 421–426.

MINNICH, S. A., HARTMAN, P. A., and HEIMSCH, R. C. 1982. Enzyme immunoassay for detection of salmonellae in foods. *Appl. Environ. Microbiol.* 43: 877–883.

MORITA, T. N. and M. J. WOODBURN. 1978. Homogeneous enzyme immune assay for staphylococcal enterotoxin B. *Infect. Immun.* 21: 666–668.

NAKANE, P. K. and KAWOI, A. 1974. Peroxidase labeled antibody. A new method of conjugation. *J. Histochem. Cytochem.* 22: 1084–1091.

NILSSON, P., BERGQUIST, N. R., and GRUNDY, M. S. 1981. A technique for preparing defined conjugates of horseradish peroxidase and immunoglobulin. *J. Immunol. Methods* 41: 81–93.

NIMMO, G. R., LEW, A. M., STANLEY, C. M., and STEWARD, M. W. 1984. Influence of antibody affinity on the performance of different antibody assays. *J. Immunol. Methods* 72: 177–187.

NOTERMANS, S., HAGENAARO, A. M., and KOZAKI, S. 1982. The enzyme-linked immunosorbent assay (ELISA) for the detection and determination of *Clostridium botulinum* toxins A, B, and E. In *Methods in Immunology*. Vol. 84. Langore, J. J. and Vunakis, H. V. (Ed.). Academic Press, New York.

NOTERMANS, S., BOOT, R., TIPS, P. D., and DENOOIJ, M. P. 1983. Extraction of staphylococcal enterotoxins (SE) from minced meat and subsequent detection of SE with enzyme-linked immunosorbent assay (ELISA). *J. Food Prot.* 46: 238–241.

NYGREN, H. 1982. Conjugation of horseradish peroxidase to Fab fragments with different homobifunctional and heterobifunctional cross-linking reagents. *J. Histochem. Chytochem.* 30: 407–412.

ORTH, D. S. 1977. Statistical analysis and quality control in radioimmunoassays for staphylococcol entertoxins A, B, and C. *Appl. Environ. Microbiol.* 34: 710–714.

O'SULLIVAN, M. J. and MARKS, V. 1981. Methods for the preparation of enzyme-antibody conjugates for use in enzyme immunoassay. In *Methods in Enzymology*. Vol. 73. Langone, J. J. and Vunakis, H. V. (Ed.). Academic Press, New York.

PESTKA, J. J. and CHU, F. S. 1984. Enzyme-linked immunosorbent assay of mycotoxins using nylon bead and Terasaki plate solid phases. *J. Food Prot.* 47: 305–308.

PESTKA, J. J., GAUS, P. K., and CHU, F. S. 1980. Quantitation of aflatoxin B_1 and aflatoxin B_1 antibody by an enzyme-linked immunosorbent microassay. *Appl. Environ. Microbiol.* 40, 1027–1031.

PESTKA, J. J., STEINERT, B. W., and CHU, F. S. 1981(a). Enzyme-linked immunosorbent assay for detection of ochratoxin A. *Appl. Environ. Microbiol.* 4: 1472–1474.

PESTKA, J. J., LI, Y., HARDEN, W. O., and CHU, F. S. 1981(b). Comparison of radioimmunoassay and enzyme-linked immunosorbent assay for aflatoxin M_1 in milk. *J. Assoc. Off. Anal. Chem.* 64: 294–301.

PETERKIN, P. I., and SHARPE, A. N. 1984. Rapid enumeration of *Staphylococcus aureus* in foods by direct demonstration of enterotoxigenic colonies on membrane filters by enzyme immunoassay. *Appl. Environ. Microbiol.* 47: 1047–1053.

POBER, Z. and SILVERMAN, G. J. 1977. Modified radioimmunoassay for staphylococcal enterotoxin B in foods. *Appl. Environ. Microbiol.* 33: 620–625.

RHEA, U. S. and SHAH, D. B. 1985. Foodborne enterotoxigenic *Escherichia coli*: Detection and enumeration on nitrocellulose membrane by enzyme immunoassay. *Abstracts. Ann. Meet. Am. Soc. Microbiol.* 34: 256.

RIGBY, C. E. 1984. Enzyme-linked immunosorbent assay for detection of *Salmonella* lipopolysaccharide in poultry specimen. *Appl. Environ. Microbiol.* 47: 1327–1330.

ROBISON, B. J., PRETZMAN, C. I., and J. A. MATTINGLY. 1983. Enzyme immunoassay in which a myeloma protein is used for detection of salmonellae. *Appl. Environ. Microbiol.* 45: 1816–1821.

RUBENSTEIN, K. E., SCHNEIDER, R. S., and ULLMAN, E. F. 1972. "Homogeneous" enzyme immunoassay. A new immunochemical technique. *Biochem. Biophys. Res. Commun.* 47: 846–851.

SCHALL, JR., R. F., and TENOSO, H. J. 1981. Alternatives to radioimmunoassay: Labels and methods. *Clin. Chem.* 27: 1157–1164.

SHALEV, A., GREENBERG, A. H., and McALPINE, P. J. 1980. Detection of attograms of antigen by a high sensitivity enzyme-linked immunosorbent assay (HS-ELISA) using a fluorogenic substrate. *J. Immunol. Methods* 38: 125–139.

SCHUURS, A. H. W. M. and VAN WEEMAN, B. K. 1977. Enzyme immunoassay. *Clin. Chem. Acta* 81: 1–40.

SMITH, A. M. and JONES, C. 1983. Use of murine myeloma protein M467
for detecting *Salmonella* spp. in milk. *Appl. Environ. Microbiol.* 46: 826–831.

STELMA, JR., G. N., WIMSATT, J. C., KAUFFMAN, P. E., and
SHAH, D. B. 1983. Radioimmunoassay for *Clostridium perfringens* enterotoxin and its use in screening isolates implicated in food-poisoning outbreaks. *J. Food Prot.* 46: 1069–1973.

STELMA, JR., G. N., JOHNSON, C. H., and SHAH, D. B. 1985. Detection
of enterotoxin in colonies of *Clostridium perfringens* by solid phase enzyme-
linked immunosorbent assay. *J. Food Prot.* 48: 227–231.

STEWARD, M. W. and STENSGAARD, J. 1983. *Antibody Affinity: Ther-
modynamic Aspects and Biological Significance.* CRC Press, Boca Raton, FL.

SWAMINATHAN, B., AYRES, J. C., and WILLIAMS, J. E. 1978. Control
of non-specific staining in the fluorescent antibody technique for the detection of salmonellae in foods. *Appl. Environ. Microbiol.* 35: 911–919.

SWAMINATHAN, B., ALEIXO, J. A. G., and MINNICH, S. A. 1985.
Enzyme immunoassays for *Salmonella*: One day testing is now a reality.
Food Technol. 39(3): 83–89.

THOMASON, B. M. 1981. Current status of immunofluorescent methodology for salmonellae. *J. Food Prot.* 44: 381–384.

THOUVENOT, D. and MORFIN, R. F. 1983. Radioimmunoassay for zearalenone and zernalanol in human serum. *Appl. Environ. Microbiol.* 45: 16–
23.

VAN WEEMAN, B. K. and SCHUURS, A. H. W. M. 1974. Immunoassay
using antibody-enzyme conjugates. *FEBS Letters* 43: 215–218.

VOLLER, A., BIDWELL, D., and BARTLETT, A. 1979. The enzyme
linked immunosorbent assay (ELISA). Nuffield Laboratories of Comparative Medicine, The Zoological Society of London, London.

WANNLUND, J. and DELUCA, M. 1983. Bioluminescent immunoassays.
In *Methods in Enzymology*. Vol. 92 Colowick, S. P. and Kaplan, N. O. (Ed.).
Academic Press, New York.

WISDOM, B. 1976. Enzyme immunoassay. *Clin. Chem.* 22: 1243–1255.

YALOW, R. S. and BERSON, S. A. 1959. Assay of plasma insulin in human
subjects by immunological methods. *Nature* (London) 184: 1648–1649.

YOLKEN, R. H. and LEISTER, F. J. 1982. Comparison of fluorescent and
colorigenic substrates for enzyme immunoassays. *J. Clin. Microbiol.* 15:
757–760.

YOSHITAKE, S., IMAGAWA, M., ISHIKAWA, E., NIITSU, Y., URUSHIZAKI, I., NISHIURA, M., KANAZAWA, R., KURO-SAKI, H., TACHIBANA, S., NAKAZAWA, N., and OGAWA, H. 1982. Mild and efficient conjugation of rabbit Fab and horseradish peroxidase using a maleimide compound and its use in enzyme immunoassay. *J. Biochem* (Japan) 92: 1413–1424.

ZAITSU, K. and OHKURA, Y. 1980. New fluorogenic substrates for horse-radish peroxidase: Rapid and sensitive assays for hydrogen peroxide and the peroxidase. *Anal. Biochem.* 109: 109–113.

13

Detection of Foodborne Microorganisms by DNA Hybridization

Renee A. Fitts

Massachusetts Institute of Technology
Cambridge, Massachusetts

DNA probe technology is an exciting new approach to the detection of virtually any organism in foods, clinical samples, or the environment. An increasing amount of research is underway to demonstrate the potential uses of these probes, although field studies utilizing these techniques have only just begun. It is now possible to detect a wide variety of viral, bacterial, and protozoan pathogens in urine, stools, tissues, and sputum, using traditional radiolabeled probes and newer nonisotopic assay systems. Many of the examples we have for the use of DNA hybridization assays come from clinical applications, but we can extend this work to diagnostic problems in the food industry as well. This review is intended only as a basic introduction to the field and as a guide to those investigators who would like to design a hybridization assay for their own systems, but who are newcomers to the field. The reader is encouraged to refer to Fitts (in press) and Meinkoth and Wahl (1984) for a more technical discussion.

HYBRIDIZATION CONDITIONS

A hybridization assay typically begins with preparation of the test sample. In the traditional and most commonly used formats, a small volume of the test sample is applied to a solid support (Meinkoth and Wahl 1984; Southern 1975; Grunstein and Hogness 1975; Benton and Davis 1977). The test sample may be a pure solution of DNA, a mixture of whole bacteria or viruses in growth medium, or a more complex mixture which includes food particles or body exudates such as sputum or urine. The solid support is usually a nitrocellulose or nylon membrane. Once the sample has been applied, either by direct spotting onto the membrane support or by filtration through the membrane, it is necessary to make the DNA of the target organism available for interaction with the probe molecule. In the simplest format, this is done by treatment of the sample-loaded filters with a solution containing sodium hydroxide, which causes the bacteria to lyse and thereby release their DNA, and also denatures the DNA into single strands. In more detailed protocols, the filters are treated with proteinases, detergents, and phenol or chloroform, to remove debris from the filter that may either cause reduction of the signal in the assay or contribute to background noise.

When a solid support is used to hold the test sample DNA, it is necessary to attach the DNA to the support. Usually, this is done by baking filters in a vacuum oven, but it can also be done by exposure to heat lamps for a short time or by actual cross-linking of DNA to the filter support (Church and Gilbert 1984). At this point, these prepared filters are ready for a pre-hybridization step. Although some protocols omit this step, it can be very helpful in decreasing background noise. The components of the cocktail used for soaking filters in this step usually include Denhardt's solution (0.02% polyvinylpyrrolidone, 0.02% Ficoll, and 0.02% bovine serum albumen) and sodium chloride. Sodium phosphate and sodium citrate are sometimes added as well. Carrier DNA, such as salmon sperm or calf thymus DNA, and other agents, such as nonfat dry milk, often help to decrease background noise, presumably by binding to sites on the membrane that would otherwise non-specifically bind probe DNA. Sometimes background noise can be further reduced through the addition of detergents such as sodium dodecyl sulfate to the system.

In the hybridization step, the formulation of the cocktail in which the DNA hybridization will occur depends on the desired degree of stringency. The DNA probe, which is a single-stranded molecule, will seek out its complementary sequence in the DNA of the test sample and then base-pair with it to form a double-stranded structure. The degree to which mismatching of the bases in the helix is allowed is a measure of the stringency of the hybridization. To avoid cross-hybridization with sequences other than the desired target DNA, one wishes to demand as perfect a match between the probe sequence and the target DNA as is possible. Thus, the specificity of the hybridization can be determined by using very stringent conditions; this is achieved through the temperature and salt concentration of the hybridization solution. An excellent discussion of these parameters is provided by Meinkoth and Wahl (1984). One can also use formamide, a helix-destabilizing agent, to increase stringency. The rate of the reannealing of the probe sequence with target DNA can be increased by adjusting the temperature and components of the hybridization cocktail. For example, anionic dextran polymers such as dextran sulfate can be used to accelerate the rate of reannealing up to 100-fold. After the hybridization step, it is necessary to wash away any unhybridized probe DNA. As described above, the salt concentration and temperature of the washes can be adjusted for the desired degree of specificity of hybridization. Detection of hybrid molecules on the filter can be done by scintillation counting or autoradiography if the probe molecule has been labeled with a radionuclide.

PROBE SEQUENCES

There are a number of considerations in choosing an appropriate DNA sequence to serve as a probe. The first question addresses the nature of the target organism. Does one wish to detect a particular genus, species, or variety of organisms? The second question addresses the environment of the target organism. What other organisms are likely to be present that might be closely enough related to the target organism so as to cross-react with the probe?

The most straightforward example of probe sequence selection is in the identification of viral pathogens. The presence of hepatitis B virus in blood can be done using the entire hepatitis B viral genome (Berninger et al. 1982; Scotto et al. 1983). Larger viruses, such as cytomegalovirus, may have nucleotide sequence homology with other viruses or even host cell DNA; in these instances, it is necessary to dissect the viral genome into smaller segments to find an appropriate probe sequence (Spector et al. 1984; Gadler 1983; Chou and Merigan 1983). Each segment is used in hybridizations to other viruses and host cells to rule out those potential probes that cross-hybridize with other DNAs.

For bacteria and other pathogens which have genomes that may be several hundred or thousand times larger than that of viruses, it is necessary to look harder to find a good candidate for a probe sequence. When the target organism is known to have some trait or property not present in other organisms, the gene for that trait can be cloned and used as a probe. Examples are the use of toxin genes to detect enterotoxigenic *E. coli* (Moseley et al. 1980) or cloned virulence factor genes to detect *Y. enterocolitica* (Hill et al. 1983). These approaches can be used when one works to detect a particular variety of organism, i.e., virulent or toxigenic, in a background of related organisms that are otherwise innocuous.

When such traits are not directly obvious, it may be possible to find instead a plasmid that is characteristic of the target organism. This had been done by Totten and associates (Totten et al. 1983) to detect *N. gonorrhoeae* in men with urethritis, using the cryptic plasmid of the organism as a probe. A similar approach by Wirth and Pratt (1982) utilized organelle DNA found only in target *Leishmania* species.

When the organism of interest is sufficiently different from other bacteria or viruses, etc., in the environment, it may be possible to identify DNA fragments of that organism that empirically do not cross-hybridize with other DNAs. In other words, when no special trait or plasmid or other characteristic feature of the target organism is apparent, one can simply look at its chromosomal DNA to find those regions present in it that are not present in other bacteria without knowing beforehand what the function of that DNA is in the living cell. Grimont et al. (1985) used this method to find a DNA probe for *Legionella pneumophila*. In this report, the investigators prepared a restriction digest of *L. pneumophila* DNA on an agarose gel, then hybridized DNAs of other organisms to the digested *L. pneumophila* DNA. They noted that a particular size range of digested DNA fragments did not cross-hybridize to those other DNAs, and so used those fragments as their probe.

My associates and I approached the problem of *Salmonella* detection in a similar way. We, however, were interested in finding a probe that would detect all members of the *Salmonella* genus, as opposed to one particular species. We constructed a library of *Salmonella* DNA by cloning restriction fragments of chromosomal DNA, and then screened these clones one by one to identify those DNA sequences that did not cross-hybridize with other DNAs. These *Salmonella*-specific clones were then used as probes to survey a large collection of *Salmonella* isolates so as to determine which *Salmonella*-specific clones would hybridize to every *Salmonella* isolate. In this manner, we found several restriction fragments that could be used to detect members of the *Salmonella* genus (Fitts et al. 1983; Fitts 1985).

PROBE LABELING AND DETECTION SYSTEMS

Traditionally, probe molecules are labeled by incorporation of a radiolabeled nucleotide during a process termed "nick-translation" (Rigby et al. 1977). Beginning with a double-stranded probe DNA molecule, a DNAase is added, which nicks one or the other DNA strand at random sites. Then nucleoside triphosphates, one of which is radiolabeled, are provided, along with DNA polymerase. The polymerase begins synthesis at each nick, incorporating the nucleotides as it copies the DNA sequence. The resulting labeled double-stranded structure must be denatured into single strands before use as a probe in the hybridization assay.

When a radiolabeled probe is generated, detection of the hybrids formed in the hybridization assay is straightforward. Scintillation counting or auto-radiography can be done with the DNA-loaded filters. However, to some, nonisotopic labeling methods are preferable. The vitamin biotin is frequently used for this purpose (Langer et al. 1981; Singer and Ward 1982; Broker et al. 1978). Biotin is linked to a nucleotide and then the nucleotide is incor-porated into the probe DNA. Biotin serves as a "reporter molecule" after the hybridization step, when another compound, avidin, is added to the system. The avidin molecule binds to biotin very strongly. Usually an enzyme such as horseradish peroxidase or alkaline phosphotase is linked beforehand to the avidin reagent. At the end of these reactions, the probe molecule hybridized to target DNA can be detected via the biotin-avidin-enzyme aggregate by adding the substrate molecule for the enzyme, which when cleaved, yields a colored product.

Other possibilities for nonisotopic detection include use of haptens as reporter molecules. During nick-translation of probe sequences, Vincent et al. (1982) incorporated a nucleotide labeled with a dinitrophenol group. The dinitrophenol group is later detected by anti-dinitrophenol antibodies labeled with an enzyme.

Renz and Kurz (1984) have linked alkaline phosphostase and horseradish peroxidase directly to probe DNA, thereby eliminating several steps required in the biotin-avidin-enzyme system.

It is not always necessary to use a double-stranded probe molecule labeled by nick-translation. One can synthesize an oligonucleotide sequence *de novo* to serve as a probe and at the same time, incorporate an isotopically or nonisotopically labeled nucleotide during synthesis (Meinkoth and Wahl 1984). This procedure does require, though, that one know the exact nucleo-tide sequence of the probe molecules beforehand. Oligonucleotide probes are usually 14 to 20 bases in length and are single-stranded.

Another method to generate single-stranded probes utilizes probe DNA sequences cloned into single-stranded bacteriophage vectors (Hu and Mess-ing 1982). An oligonucleotide primer sequence is first hybridized to the recombinant bacteriophage molecule, then nucleotides and DNA polymerase are added to the system. DNA synthesis begins at the primer and copies a part of the recombinant molecule, but not the probe sequence. Reporter molecules can be incorporated during syntheses. These "primer-extended" probes can be used directly in hybridization because the probe sequence itself remains single-stranded in this only partly double-stranded molecule. One can depart completely from DNA probes and make RNA probes instead (Butler and Chamberlin 1982; Kassavetis et al. 1982). This method begins with a special cloning vector that carries the *S. typhimurium* bacteriophage SP6 promoter adjacent to the desired probe sequence. When the SP6 RNA polymerase is added, RNA synthesis begins at the promoter and makes an RNA copy of the probe. The DNA template is removed by DNAase treatment to leave a single-stranded RNA probe. This probe can be labeled isotopically or nonisotopically during synthesis, as in other systems. The RNA probe can be used in the same way as DNA probes in most assays (Church and Gilbert 1984; Zinn et al. 1982; Lynn et al. 1983).

OUTLOOK FOR THE FUTURE

DNA hydbridization technology has already clearly made an impact on how we think about diagnostic problems. These methods can be used to detect virtually any organism of interest in almost any setting. There are, of course, some situations in which DNA hybridization methods work better than in others, because of problems in sensitivity, sample composition, and competitive flora. However, DNA hybridization assays are still in their very earliest beginnings. As the applications of these assays continue, there is every reason to believe that what may appear to be present difficulties will be overcome by streamlined protocols and ever more sophisticated probes and detection reagents.

REFERENCES

BENTON, W. D. and DAVIS, R. W. 1977. Screening lambda gt recombinant clones by hybridization to single plaques *in situ. Science* 196: 180–181.

BERNINGER, M., HAMMER, M., HOYER, B., and GERIN, J. L. 1982. An assay for the detection of the DNA genomes of hepatitis B virus in serum. *J. Med. Virol.* 9: 57–68.

BROKER, T. R., ANGERER, L. M., YEN, P. H., HERSHEY, N. D., and DAVIDSON, N. 1978. Electron microscope visualization of tRNA genes with ferritin-avidin: biotin labels. *Nucleic Acids Res.* 5: 363–384.

BUTLER, E. T. and CHAMBERLIN, M. J. 1982. Bacteriophage SP6 specific RNA polymerase I. Isolation and characterization of the enzyme. *J. Biol. Chem.* 257: 5772–5778.

CHOU, S. and MERIGAN, T. C. 1983. Rapid detection and quantitation of human cytomegalovirus in urine through DNA hybridization. *New Engl. J. Med.* 380: 921–925.

CHURCH, G. M. and GILBERT, W. 1984. Genomic screening. *Proc. Natl. Acad. Sci. USA.* 81: 1991–1995.

FITTS, R., DIAMOND, M., HAMILTON, C., and NERI, M. 1983. A DNA: DNA hybridization assay for Salmonella spp. in foods. *Appl. Environ. Microbiol.* 46: 1146–1151.

FITTS, R. 1985. Development of a DNA hybridization test for the presence of Salmonella in foods. *Food Technol.* 39: 95–102.

FITTS, R. in press. DNA probes and hybridization assays. In *Topics in Food Microbiology, Vol. II: Methods.* Montville, T. J. (Ed.). CRC Press, Cleveland, OH

GADLER, H. 1983. Nucleic acid hybridization for measurement of effects of antiviral compounds on human cytomegalovirus DNA replication. *Antimicrob. Agents Chemother.* 24: 370–374.

GRIMONT, P. A. D., GRIMONT, F., DESPLACES, N., and TCHEN, P. 1985. DNA probe specific for *Legionella pneumophila*. *J. Clin. Micro.* 21: 431–437.

GRUNSTEIN, M. and HOGNESS, D. S. 1975. Colony hybridization: a method for the isolation of cloned DNAs that contain a specific gene. *Proc. Natl. Acad. Sci. USA.* 72: 3961–3965.

HILL, W. E., PAYNE, W. L., and AULISIO, C. C. G. 1983. Detection and enumeration of virulent *Yersinia enterocolitica* in food by colony hybridization. *Appl. Environ. Microbiol.* 46: 636–641.

HU, N-t. and MESSING, J. 1982. The making of strand-specific M13 probes. *Gene* 17: 271–277.

KASSAVETIS, G. A., BUTLER, E. T., ROULLAND, D., and CHAMBERLIN, M. J. 1982. Bacterophage SP6-specific RNA polymerase. II. Mapping of SP6 DNA and selective *in vitro* transcription. *J. Biol.. Chem.* 257: 5779–5788.

LANGER, P. R., WALDROP, A. A., and WARD, D. C. 1981. Enzymatic synthesis of biotin-labeled polynucleotides: novel nucleic acid affinity probes. *Proc. Natl. Acad. Sci. USA.* 78: 6633–6637.

LYNN, D. A., ANGERER, L. M., BRUSKIN, A. M., KLEIN, W. H., and ANGERER, R. C. 1983. Localization of a family of mRNAs in a single cell type and its precursors in sea urchin embryos. *Proc. Natl. Acad. Sci. USA.* 80: 2656–2660.

MEINKOTH, J. and WAHL, G. 1984. Hybridization of nucleic acid immobilized on solid supports. *Anal. Biochem.* 138: 267–284.

MOSELEY, S. L., HUQ, I., ALIM, A. R. M. A., SO, M., SAMADPOUR-MOTALEBI, M., and FALKOW, S. 1980. Detection of enterotoxigenic *Escherichia coli* by DNA hybridization. *J. Inf. Dis.* 142: 897–898.

RENZ, M. and KURZ, C. 1984. A colorimetric method for DNA hybridization. *Nucleic Acids Res.* 12: 3435–3444.

RIGBY, P. W. J., DIECKMAN, M., RHODES, C., and BERG, P. 1977. Labeling deoxyribonucleic acid to high specific activity *in vitro* by nick-translation with DNA polymerase I. *J. Mol. Biol.* 113: 237–252.

SCOTTO, J., HADCHOUEL, M., HENRY, C., ALVAREZ, F., YUART, J., TIOLLAIS, P., BERNARD, O., and BRECHOT, C. 1983. Hepatitis B virus DNA in children's liver diseases: detection by blot hybridizations in liver and serum. *Gut* 24: 618–624.

SINGER, R. H. and WARD, D. C. 1982. Actin gene expression visualized in chicken muscle tissue culture by using *in situ* hybridization with a biotinylated nucleotide analog. *Proc. Natl. Acad. Sci. USA.* 79: 7331–7335.

SOUTHERN, E. M. 1975. Detection of specific sequences among DNA fragments separated by gel electrophoresis. *J. Mol. Biol.* 98: 503–517.

SPECTOR, S. A., RUA, J. A., SPECTOR, D. H., and McMILLAN, R. 1984. Detection of human cytomegalovirus in clinical specimens by DNA-DNA hybridization. *J. Inf. Dis.* 150: 121–126.

TOTTEN, P. A., HOLMES, K. K., HANDSFIELD, H. H., KNAPP, P. L., PERINE, P. L., and FALKOW, S. 1983. DNA hybridization technique for the detection of *Neisseria gonorrhoeae* in men with urethritis. *J. Inf. Dis.* 148: 462–471.

VINCENT, C., TCHEN, P., COHEN-SOLAL, M., and KOURILSKY, P. 1982. Synthesis of 8-(2-4 dinitrophenyl 2-6 aminohexyl) amino-adenosine 5-triphosphate: biological properties and potential uses. *Nucleic Acids Res.* 10: 6787–6796.

WIRTH, D. F. and PRATT, D. M. 1982. Rapid identification of *Leishmania* species by specific hybridization of kinetoplast DNA in cutaneous lesions. *Proc. Natl. Acad. Sci. USA* 79: 6999–7003.

ZINN, K., DIMAIO, D., and MANIATIS, T. 1983. Identification of two distinct regulatory regions adjacent to the human β-interferon gene. *Cell* 34: 865–879.

14

Virulence Assessment
of Foodborne Microbes

Joseph M. Madden, Barbara A. McCardell,
and Douglas L. Archer
Food and Drug Administration
Washington, D.C.

Food poisoning in the United States is responsible for a major loss of economic resources (Sanders et al. 1984); it is second only to the common cold in causing time lost from work (Dingle et al. 1964). Foodborne illnesses may be divided into two distinct types: those caused by pure intoxications, and those dependent upon ingestion of the causative microbe followed by colonization and either invasion of the intestinal epithelium or production of enterotoxin(s). The former group is typified by such organisms as *Clostridium botulinum* and enterotoxic *Staphylococcus aureus* strains; ingestion of food containing the preformed toxin(s) of these organisms causes illness. The latter group includes the following microbes:

Aeromonas hydrophila   *Campylobacter coli/jejuni*

Bacillus cereus   *Escherichia coli*

Clostridium perfringens   *Klebsiella pneumoniae*

Plesiomonas shigelloides   *Vibrio mimicus*

Pseudomonas aeruginosa   *Vibrio parahaemolyticus*

Salmonella species   *Vibrio vulnificus*

Shigella species   *Yersinia enterocolitica*

Vibrio cholerae O1   *Yersinia pseudotuberculosis*

Vibrio cholerae non-O1

Detailed methods for routine identification of organisms and preformed toxins in foods have been published in the *Bacteriological Analytical Manual,* 6th edition, of the Food and Drug Administration (1984) and in the *Compendium of Methods for the Microbiological Examination of Foods* of the American Public Health Association (1984) and will not be discussed in this review.

The clinical microbiologist seldom has trouble identifying the etiological agent responsible for a patient's diarrhea since the microbe is usually present in large numbers within the diarrhetic stool submitted for examination. Unfortunately, however, the food microbiologist is faced with relatively few bacteria in most foods and food products. Because the simple speciation of isolates is insufficient to establish pathogenicity, the food microbiologist must demonstrate that isolated microbes are able to cause disease. To accomplish this, Koch's postulates must be fulfilled, i.e., a pure culture of the microbe is fed to a susceptible animal, the disease is thus produced in the animal, and the microbe is then isolated from it. This procedure poses many problems: Most laboratories do not have large-animal facilities, nor are their personnel trained in the surgical or other specialized techniques required to infect animals with suspected pathogens. It is precisely for these reasons (and for the development of vaccines) that microbial virulence factors are being studied. Simple yet definitive tests must be developed for use in all microbiology laboratories so that the pathogenicity of microbial food isolates can be determined.

Bacterial virulence (or pathogenicity) factors may be defined as all factors elaborated by a bacterial species that allow it to cause illness or infection. It is easiest to understand microbial virulence factors by examining exactly what a microbe must do to cause an enteric illness.

After it is ingested, a microbe must adhere to the host's intestinal lining, survive the acidity of the stomach (the gastric barrier), and be able to grow and reproduce. The enteric pathogen must then produce factors that will damage the host's tissues and, in some instances, allow it to invade the tissues or the blood stream. All this must be accomplished in the particular environment in which the microbe finds itself.

HOST DEFENSE MECHANISMS AND MICROBIAL STRATEGIES

The following defense mechanisms protect the healthy host from infection via the oral-gastric route:

Intestinal peristalsis	Immunoglobulin secreted
Mucous barrier	into intestine
Essential nutrient	Interferons
deprivation	
Stomach and intestinal pH	Intact intestinal cell surface
Lysozyme in secretions	Cell-mediated immunity

These defense mechanisms begin with the acidity encountered in the stomach, which rapidly kills some enteric pathogens (Nalin et al. 1978). The amount of free acid in the stomach is lower in individuals aged 1 to 4 years and declines again somewhat after age 55. This may account, in part, for the greater susceptibility of the extreme age groups to foodborne pathogens (Vanzant et al. 1932). An enteric pathogen must be able to attach itself to the mucosa of the intestine after surviving the acidity of the stomach. Intestinal peristalsis creates a hydrodynamic flow which prevents bacterial attachment, and a mucous barrier (glycocalyx) prevents the pathogen's direct access to the intestinal mucosa. To overcome these host defense mechanisms, microbes produce adhesions, substances which permit them to adhere directly to the glycocalyx, or enzymes (mucinases), which partially degrade the glycoproteins and thus allow direct access to the eucaryotic cells underlying the mucous layer (Prizont and Reed, 1980). The latter mechanism may apply only to nonmotile bacteria such as *Shigella* species; Freter et al. (1981a, b) demonstrated that these bacteria may gain entry to the intestinal epithelium by an active or a passive mechanism. The passive mechanism is identical to the passage of polystyrene particles through the mucous membrane to the epithelium. Motility, however, aids bacteria such as *V. cholerae* to penetrate the mucous gel when they are guided by chemotaxis to the epithelium (Freter et al. 1981a, b).

Although motility, adhesins, and chemotaxis may aid microbes to overcome the host's intestinal peristalsis and to penetrate the mucous layer, it is not absolutely necessary for pathogenic microbes to attach directly to the intestinal epithelium. Enterotoxic microbes such as heat-labile toxin (LT)-producing strains of *E. coli* bind strictly to the mucous layer and never reach

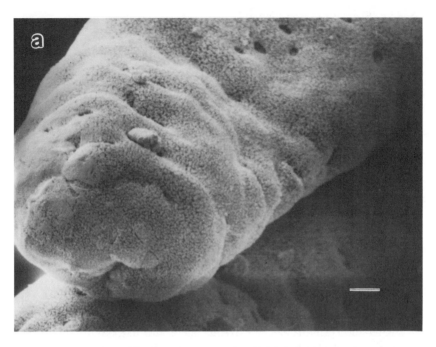

FIG. 14.1   Scanning electron micrographs of adult rabbit ileum 18 hr post-infection with: (a) sterile broth. Note normal appearance of microvillus; (b) *Vibrio cholerae*, biotype El Tor, serogroup Inaba, strain N16961. Typical microvillus observed after exposure to this cholera toxin-producing strain; (c) *V. cholerae*, strain JBK70, a genetically derived strain of N16961 from which the colera toxin gene has been deleted (Levine et al. 1983). Microvillus observed after exposure to strain JBK70. Note red and white blood cells, which signify an invasive process, and attachment of individual bacteria cells to microvillus. Neither observation is made in (b). Bar represents 1 μm unless otherwise indicated.

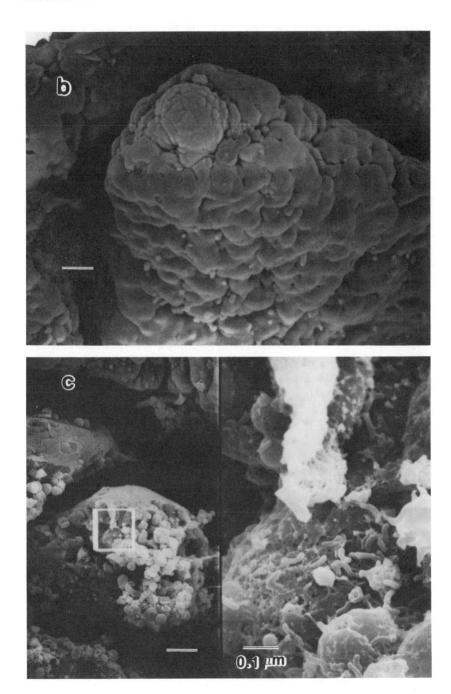

the intestinal epithelium (Jones and Rutter 1972), meanwhile achieving such high numbers that the effect of the enterotoxin on the intestinal epithelium is elicited by simple diffusion across the mucous layer. We have repeatedly observed that few cholera toxin (CT)-producing *V. cholerae* cells are bound to intestinal villi 18–24 hr after infection of ligated rabbit ileal loops. When intestinal samples are fixed in glutaraldehyde and critically point-dried in an atmosphere of carbon dioxide, and the dried tissue is coated with gold:palladium (60:40) and viewed in a scanning electron microscope, few attached bacterial cells can be seen (Fig. 14.1a and 14.1b). However, many cells of the same *V. cholerae* strain from which the CT gene had been deleted may be observed by the identical method 18–24 hr after infection (Fig. 14.1c). Interestingly, both the CT-producing strain and the derived negative strains, as viable cells, produce fluid accumulation in the ligated rabbit ileal loop model (Spira et al. 1983).

Other nonspecific defenses in the host's intestine include commensal microbial inhabitants, which occupy mucosal space needed for adherence by pathogens and compete for available nutrients (Freter 1980; Smith 1982; Freter et al. 1983). Pathogenic microbes must either have the various adhesins necessary for attachment to host intestinal epithelium at the time of ingestion or rapidly produce them before passage through the intestine. In their excellent review article on this subject, Freter and Jones (1983) explain that most bacterial adhesins use carbohydrates as receptors on mammalian cell membranes. Since many foodstuffs also contain both simple and complex sugars, glycoproteins, or glycolipids, a competitive inhibition between adhesin receptors on these foodstuffs will inhibit the adhesion of bacteria to the mouth and gastrointestinal tract. The competition for receptors is compounded if the host is a meat-eater, for most mammalian tissues contain chemically identical or similar membrane components. Pathogenic microbes attached to cells or to cell debris that is passing through the gastrointestinal tract would not be free to adhere to host receptors.

Immunologic host defenses in the gastrointestinal tract provide a formidable barrier to the invading microbe. Both cell-mediated immunity and humoral immunity function in the intestine (reviewed by Archer 1984). The principal humoral immune mechanism is secretory immunoglobulin A (sIgA). Because of its structure this specialized antibody remains associated with the glycocalyx and is protected from the action of normal digestive processes. The antimicrobial responses of sIgA are initiated locally in the gut and do not require the pathogen to have entered the systemic circulation. They prevent bacterial attachment to the epithelium, neutralize bacterial toxins, and act in concert with gut-associated lymphocytes in the antibody-dependent, cell-mediated killing of bacteria (Walker and Isselbacher 1977; Tagliabue et al. 1983). Should the invading organism penetrate the glyocalyx and invade the epithelium, mechanisms involving cell-mediated immunity (i.e.,

T-lymphocytes and macrophages) provide a second line of defense (reviewed in Collins and Carter 1974; LeFevre et al. 1979). Interferons, generally thought of as antiviral defenses, are often produced in response to bacterial invasion (Baron et al. 1982). All three characterized interferons (alpha, beta, and gamma) function in various ways to prevent successful bacterial invasion (Bukholm and Degre 1983; Bukholm et al. 1984; Izadkhah et al. 1980).

Before entry into the host's systemic circulation, an invading microbe must overcome a formidable array of immunologic responses (reviewed by Campbell 1976). Once in the host tissue, an invading microbe elicits a group of host responses collectively known as the acute-phase response (Dinarello 1984), which is principally activated by interleukin-1, a product of macrophages and monocytes in response to endotoxin. Interleukin-1 activates host-protective mechanisms that induce fever, cause infiltration of neutrophils to the invasion site(s), induce lymphokines to activate B and T lymphocytes, and release acute-phase proteins such as haptoglobulin, protease inhibitors, complement, and fibrinogen. A complete discussion of the acute-phase response and its components is presented by Dinarello (1984).

Adherence of pathogenic microbes to the gastrointestinal tract is only the beginning of the infectious process. As mentioned earlier, the pathogen must be able to compete with commensal microbes for available nutrients. If it survives the acidity of the stomach, it must then be able to withstand the pH of the host's intestine as well as bactericidal materials and phagocytes introduced into the lumen of the intestine. Pathogens evade these mechanisms by inhibiting phagocyte chemotaxis (Martin and Chaudhuri 1952) and the production of IgA proteases (Kornfeld and Plaut 1981). These are just a few of the ways that a pathogen may defeat host defenses. The interested reader is directed to several excellent review articles (Densen and Mandell 1980; Falconi et al. 1984; O'Grady and Smith 1981; Smith 1976, 1983).

Iron plays an interesting role in microbial virulence. It is required for the growth and reproduction of bacteria and regulates the production of toxins by at least two bacterial species: *Corynebacterium diphtheriae* (Uchida 1983) and *P. aeruginosa* (Iglewski and Sadoff 1979). Animals also require iron for their metabolic functions and have very good mechanisms for binding any iron found in such body fluids as mucin, mammalian milk, plasma (lactoferrin), and serum (transferrin). The pathogen must therefore possess some mechanism to bind the free iron encountered in the body fluids of the animal host and/or possess some means of releasing host-bound iron either by removing it from host chelators (transferrin or lactoferrin) or by invading host cells and using intracellular pools of iron within the cells. The iron-binding compounds produced by microbes generally have a molecular weight of less than 1,000 (Lankford 1973) and have been termed siderophores. From an enteric pathogen's point of view, lactoferrin is by far the most important iron chelator, for the pathogen must be able to grow and multiply in the intestinal tract to produce its enterotoxins or mount its invasive mechanisms. Finkelstein et al. (1983) present original data that demonstrate the inhibitory effects of lactoferrin on the number of cell divisions by various enteric pathogens. Together with the data of Spik et al. (1978), which demonstrated that ingested lactoferrins of human or bovine origin are not completely digested during their passage through the intestines of infants, these data strongly support the breast feeding of infants rather than reliance upon infant formula. Clinical studies (Rowland et al. 1980) have supported this by demonstrating that infants fed highly bacteriostatic milk (rich in lactoferrin, leukocytes, and antibody) had fewer episodes of bacterial-associated diarrhea than those fed milk with less bacteriostatic activity.

The in vitro studies of Finkelstein et al. (1983) show a correlation between the bacterial production of siderophores and the availability of iron in infected individuals. Data presented by Blake et al. (1980), concerning cases studied by the Centers for Disease Control between 1964 and 1977, demonstrated that individuals with liver damage, alcohol abuse problems, thalassemia major, diabetes, and/or hemachromatosis were highly susceptible to infection by the marine bacterium *V. vulnificus*, which may cause septicemia in individuals following the consumption of infected raw oysters. This epidemiological study was further supported by the work of Simpson and Oliver (1983), who showed a relationship between infection, the production of siderophores by this bacterium, and increased iron levels in infected individuals. Other enteric pathogens whose virulence is increased by the availability of iron include *C. perfringens, E. coli, Salmonella typhimurium, K. pneumoniae, Listeria monocytogenes* (Sussman 1974), *Y. enterocolitica* (Robins-Browne et al. 1979), and *C. jejuni* (Kazmi et al. 1984). Iron is only one of the factors in the host's intestine for which enteric pathogens must compete with the host and with commensal bacteria; other metal cations such as zinc (Sugarman 1983) are required as enzyme cofactors. It should also be remembered that the enteric pathogen must also compete for available nutrients.

The mechanisms by which microorganisms evade host defenses, both nonspecific and immunologic, were recently reviewed by Gotschlich (1983). An important aspect of evading host defenses, with potentially deleterious consequences to the host, is molecular mimicry, or the ability of an organism to mimic host tissue antigens. In his "cross-tolerance" hypothesis, Ebringer (1983) states that from the invading organism's viewpoint, partial but not complete antigenic mimicry would be ideal. A suboptimal immune response would be initiated and would ensure the survival of both host and pathogen; such a partial antigenic relationship may, however, lead to autoimmune disease in the host. A related antigenic variation may occur during the course of infection: A microorganism may alter its surface antigenic makeup and thus frustrate the host's immune responses. This antigenic variation was once attributed to the selection of a minor, antigenically different population of bacteria after the major population was eliminated by immunological mechanisms. Evidence now indicates that antigenic variation is a genetically preprogrammed event in bacteria, triggered by unknown aspects of the host response. The sequential switching-on of genes controlling surface antigenic makeup is now thought to occur in genera such as *Vibrio, Campylobacter,* and the thoroughly studied *Borrelia recurrentis.*

Bacteria facilitate invasion by producing a variety of enzymes, such as hemolysins (possibly involved in iron acquisition), proteases, lipases, neuraminidase, phospholipase C, collagenase, chondroitinase, and hyaluronidase. The functioning of these factors has been reviewed by Gotschlich (1983).

MODELS TO DETECT COLONIZATION

The surface of an enteric pathogen is extremely important in its establishment in the host's intestinal tract, for it is the surface that contains any adhesins, pili, siderophores, capsules, and flagellae. The mechanisms associated with the adherence of enterotoxigenic *E. coli* (ETEC) to animal cells have been well studied. In all cases, ETEC strains have adhered via fimbriae (also known as pili). Ørskov and Ørskov (1966) identified the first adhesion pili in ETECs in animal strains that caused diarrhea in neonatal piglets. These authors demonstrated that the antigen K88 was present only if the ETEC strains carried a plasmid encoding for that antigen. Smith and Linggood (1971) demonstrated that the gene encoding for enterotoxin production was also carried on the same plasmid. When the K88-encoding gene was deleted, the strains that had carried it failed to produce illness in piglets. In addition to the K88 antigen, the following antigens are required for the adherence of ETEC strains to animal cells and tissues: K99, associated with calf, lamb, and piglet pathogens (Moon et al. 1977; Ørskov et al. 1975); type 987 fimbriae, associated with porcine strains (Isaacson et al. 1977); and CFA/I, CFA/II, and E8775 antigens, associated with human ETEC pathogens (Evans and Evans 1978; Evans et al. 1975, 1978; Thomas et al. 1982). The presence of these colonization factors can be confirmed by a simple screening test, i.e., they cause hemagglutination of certain animal red blood cells in the presence of the carbohydrate mannose. Not all of the colonization factors have been identified (Levine et al. 1979; Lumish et al. 1980); some are not expressed in liquid media or in cultures grown at 18 to 22°C.

Because colonization factors have not yet been identified for most enteric pathogens, the colonization potential of a food isolate must be tested in an animal model. The species and age of the animal used and the methods for inoculation vary greatly. Some of the models for detecting the adherence and colonization potential of *V. cholerae* include intraintestinal inoculations of infant rabbits (Dutta and Habbu 1955), ingestion of vibrios by canines (Sack and Carpenter 1969), infant mouse inoculation (Ujiiye and Kobari 1970), guinea pig inoculation (Burrows et al. 1947), ingestion of vibrios by chinchillas (Blachman et al. 1974), and a recently proposed adult rabbit model known as RITARD (removable intestinal tie-adult rabbit model) (Spira et al. 1981). These whole animal models have the advantage of indicating the total pathogenic potential of a food isolate (i.e., its ability to establish itself in an animal's intestinal tract) and the production of other virulence factors that affect diarrhea. However, these models are mainly research tools and are inconvenient, if not impossible, to perform in a nonresearch laboratory. In addition, because whole animal model systems involve complex interactions between the bacteria and the intestinal epithelium, their usefulness is limited for isolating and studying the specific factors responsible for bacterial adhesion.

Jones et al. (1976) and Jones and Freter (1976) used rabbit brush borders to study the adhesion of *V. cholerae* to the intestinal epithelium of the adult rabbit. With this model, they demonstrated that the absence of motility, growth at a low temperature, and the presence of L-fucose or absence of divalent cations inhibit or reduce vibrio adhesion to the gut mucosa. The model devised by Thorne et al. (1979) for the adhesion of *E. coli* cells to human buccal cells is simple to establish and uses epithelial cells scraped from the mouth of human volunteers. The adherence of bacteria to erythrocytes or buccal cells demonstrates only some colonization factors that react after in vitro growth. In general, virulence is determined by more than one factor; growth in vitro may destroy one or more virulence factors and may even cause the expression of virulence factors in vitro but not in vivo (Smith 1958). It was recognized early in the history of bacteriology that the in vitro growth of bacteria may lead to nonpathogenicity and that in vivo passages of the resulting organisms may restore or increase pathogenicity. Despite the difficulties involved in the isolation and identification of true microbial virulence factors, a number of tissue culture, immunological, or simple animal models have been developed for routine use in food microbiology laboratories.

LABORATORY TESTS FOR VIRULENCE FACTORS

Heat-Labile Enterotoxins

One of the first virulence factors to be purified from an enteric pathogen was cholera toxin (CT), the enterotoxin produced by *V. cholerae*. Several assays were developed to detect CT once the purified toxin was isolated and demonstrated to induce a watery diarrhea when injected intragastrically into infant rabbits (Dutta and Habbu 1955). After an enterotoxin is purified, an antibody directed against it is produced and various tissue culture effects may be related directly to its presence. The CT antibody led to the discovery of the similarities between CT and the enterotoxins produced by *E. coli* (Clements and Finkelstein 1978; Holmgren et al. 1973b), *S. typhimurium* (Sandefur and Peterson 1977), and *C. fetus/jejuni* (Gubina et al. 1982; Ruiz-Palacios et al. 1983; McCardell et al. 1984).

Presently, two tissue culture models and a variety of immunological methods may routinely be applied to detect CT or cholera-like enterotoxins. The two tissue culture models are based on morphological changes that occur after the cell lines are exposed to CT (Donta et al. 1974; Sack and Sack 1975; Guerrant et al. 1974). Many immunological assays have been developed to detect CT; the simplest, which is based on enzyme-linked immunosorbent assays (ELISAs), uses the ability of CT (and related enterotoxins) to bind to GM1 ganglioside (Cuatrecasas 1973; Holmgren et al. 1973a; King and van Heyningen 1973; Hill et al. 1983; McCardell et al. 1984). Shah et al. (1982) have developed a sensitive solid-phase sandwich radioimmunoassay technique to detect either CT- or LT-producing colonies that contain mixed populations of bacteria. Shah and his coworkers (manuscript in preparation) have further refined this technique so that an ELISA may be performed on a filter placed upon the lysed colonies on a petri dish, thus avoiding the need for radioactivity.

With the isolation and identification of CT and LT and the emergence of recombinant DNA methodologies came the cloning of genes that encode for these enterotoxins (So et al. 1978). Using these methods, Hill et al. (1983) demonstrated that as few as 100 LT-producing strains of *E. coli* organisms in one gram of food could be detected without the need for prior enrichment. With this method the phenotype of the LT gene product need not be expressed, although radiation-handling laboratory facilities are required. A disadvantage of DNA and ELISA methods for detecting LT or CT is that the gene or its product may be incomplete and not biologically active. Recombinant DNA methodologies are not restricted to the detection of toxins produced by enteric bacteria. Although these methods serve well as screening methods, biological activity must be demonstrated in a tissue culture or in a whole animal model. The interested reader is directed to recent articles by Tucker (1984) and Levine et al. (1983).

Heat-Stable Enterotoxins

Some foodborne *E. coli* strains do not produce LT but cause illness by another type of mechanism: either a stable toxin (ST), or another invasive mechanism. The latter strains are known as enteropathogenic or enteroinvasive *E.*

coli (EPEC or EIEC) strains and do not elaborate LT or ST (Sack 1975). Unlike the LT produced by *E. coli*, ST maintains its biological activity after heating to 100°C and is of small (<3,000) molecular size (Field 1979; Staples et al. 1980; Alderete and Robertson 1978). ST binds to receptors other than those that bind LT or CT (Giannella et al. 1980) and stimulates the guanyl cyclase system rather than the adenyl cyclase system (Field 1979; Giannella and Drake 1979). *E. coli* produces several structurally different STs which also differ in host specificity (Burgess et al. 1978; Kapitany et al. 1979). *Klebsiella* species, *Enterobacter* species, *Y. enterocolitica*, and *V. cholerae* serogroup non-O1 also produce STs (Thorne and Gorbach 1979; Rao et al. 1979; Spira et al. 1979). ST, found in human intestinal isolates, is soluble in methanol and causes fluid accumulation in the intestines of infant mice, two traits which differentiate it from other STs involved in *E. coli* infections of pigs (Burgess et al. 1978). In human *E. coli* isolates, ST-producers may be further divided into two distinct classes, referred to as ST human and ST porcine, based upon DNA homology studies (Moseley et al. 1983; So and McCarthy 1980).

The standard assay for ST is the suckling mouse model, originally described by Dean et al. (1972). Kauffman (1981) conjugated the low molecular weight (2,000) *E. coli* ST (described by Staples et al. 1980) to a hapten and obtained antibodies directed against it. A radioimmunoassay test developed by Kauffman (1981) was followed in 1984 by a competitive ELISA procedure for the detection of *E. coli* ST-producers in humans (Shah et al. 1984). Cross-reactivity of the generated antibody with STs produced by genera of other enteric pathogens is currently unknown (Kauffman, personal communication). Genetic probes developed for the human *E. coli* STs (So and McCarthy 1980; Moseley et al. 1983) are specific for the *E. coli* ST human and ST porcine gene sequences (Moseley et al. 1982). Cross-reactivity with DNA sequences encoding for STs produced by genera of other pathogenic enteric bacteria is unknown (W. E. Hill, personal communication).

Invasive Enteric Pathogens

In contrast to enterotoxins which cause cells of the small intestine to secrete fluid and electrolytes, invasive microorganisms generally damage the intestinal mucosa of the colon, or large intestine. The damage caused by invasive enteric pathogens is a direct consequence of their invasion of cells and tissues of the intestinal epithelium. This type of infection is characteristic of such pathogens as *Shigella* sp., *Salmonella* sp., *V. parahaemolyticus*, *C. jejuni/coli*, *Y. enterocolitica* and the enteroinvasive *E. coli*, and is generally indicated by the presence of red blood cells and leukocytes in the stool. The animal models used to determine the potential virulence of foodborne bacterial genera range from the oral challenge of monkeys (LaBrec et al. 1964; Takeuchi 1967; Kinsey et al. 1976), and the injection of viable organisms into ligated rabbit ileal loops (Formal et al. 1961) to the oral challenge of starved, opiated (opium retarding intestinal peristalsis) guinea pigs (LaBrec et al. 1964). The Sereny (1957) test is a whole animal model that measures the ability of invasive *Shigella* species and enteroinvasive *E. coli* strains to cause a keratoconjunctivitis in adult guinea pigs or rabbits. The Sereny test correlates well with the virulence of shigella-like organisms but fails to detect the virulence of all pathogenic *Salmonella* strains and pathogenic strains of *Y. enterocolitica* (Voino-Yasenetsky and Bakacs 1977; Aulisio et al. 1983a). Aulisio et al. (1983b) demonstrated that a modification of the Sereny test, using adult mice in lieu of rabbits or guinea pigs, is a better model for predicting the pathogenic potential of *Y. enterocolitica* strains. However, like *Salmonella* strains in the original Sereny test, *Y. enterocolitica* strains do not cause a true keratitis in the mouse model such as that found with pathogenic *Shigella* strains (Voino-Yasenetsky and Bakacs 1977; Aulisio, personal communication; Piechaud et al. 1958). Tissue culture models have been developed to detect the invasion of either Henle or HeLa tissue culture cell lines for *Salmonella* sp., *Shigella* sp., and *Y. enterocolitica;* these may be routinely performed in food microbiology laboratories (Giannella et al. 1973; Hale and Bonventre 1979; Hale et al. 1979; Hale and Formal 1981; LaBrec et al. 1964; Ogawa et al. 1967; Lee et al. 1977). A relatively simple HeLa plaque assay, recently published by Oaks et al. (1985), is easy to read and perform.

Enteroinvasion appears to be plasmid-mediated rather than chromosomally linked. Strains of *Shigella flexneri* become avirulent, i.e., unable to penetrate epithelial cells, when they are cured of a 140 megadalton (Mdal) plasmid (Sansonetti et al. 1982). These authors also demonstrated lack of virulence in enteroinvasive strains of *E. coli* that were cured of the 140-Mdal plasmid. Transfer of the 140-Mdal plasmid from *S. flexneri* to cured enteroinvasive strains of *E. coli* or into a nonpathogenic strain of *E. coli* (K12) enables them to invade HeLa cells. Plasmids have been shown to be responsible for the virulence of *Shigella sonnei* (Kopecko et al. 1980: Sansonetti et al. 1980, 1981); *S. typhimurium* (Jones et al. 1982); *Shigella dysenteriae* (Watanabe et al. 1984; Watanabe and Timmis 1984; Watanabe and Nakamura 1985); *Y. enterocolitica* and *Y. pseudotuberculosis* (Gemski et al. 1980a, b; Zink et al. 1980; Portnoy et al. 1981).

A cytotoxin isolated from *S. dysenteriae* is enterotoxic (Eiklid and Olsnes 1983) and is elaborated by strains of *S. flexneri* and *S. sonnei* in smaller quantities (Keusch and Jacewicz 1977; O'Brien et al. 1977). Its role in the pathogenesis of shigellosis is as yet unknown, since strains of *S. dysenteriae*, which are noninvasive yet enterotoxin-producing, fail to induce illness in monkeys or human volunteers (Gemski et al. 1972; Levine et al. 1973). Pathogenicity of *Y. enterocolitica*, however, has been associated with the presence of the Vwa antigen, which in turn is dependent upon the microorganism possessing 42–44 Mdal plasmids (Aulisio et al. 1983a, b); these authors also correlated the presence of the Vwa antigen with that of the 42–44 Mdal plasmids and pathogenicity for the suckling mouse. *Y. enterocolitica* is the only organism in which the correlation of an antigen and the presence of specific plasmids, as determined by plasmid-specific DNA probes (Aulisio et al. 1983b), totally agrees with animal pathogenicity tests. Plasmids of various size have been found necessary for virulence, but no specific DNA probes have successfully detected the necessary DNA base sequences encoding for virulence. Animal models must be relied on to assess the virulence of food isolates that belong to these genera; the induction of diarrhea/dysentery is the only definitive method for determining the true pathogenic potential of food isolates. The use of animal models will become a necessity if attenuated bacterial vaccines (Levine et al. 1983) are found safe and effective and are used routinely to vaccinate the general population against bacterial pathogens. Care, however, must be observed in the choice of animal used, as some are resistant to various microbial pathogens (Webster 1924, 1933a, b; Schott 1932; Schutze et al. 1936; Hormaeche 1979; Robson and Vas 1972; Eisenstein et al. 1984).

The mechanisms responsible for the virulence of many microbes have been isolated and a variety of in vitro assays have been developed to detect these factors accurately. In many cases, however, a microbe may have a variety of virulence factors, all of which may be necessary for pathogenesis. It is hard to estimate the relative importance of one virulence factor over another, e.g., motility versus a strong adhesion. Although motility enhances the virulence of *V. cholerae* by aiding the microbes' penetration to the intestinal mucosa, it is not essential for effective colonization. New mechanisms of pathogenesis, attachment factors, and microbial factors that defeat host defense mechanisms are constantly being discovered. Currently, the only definitive method to determine the pathogenic potential of a food isolate may be the fulfillment of Koch's postulates in a suitable animal model.

REFERENCES

ALDERETE, J. F. and ROBERTSON, D. C. 1978. Purification and chemical characterization of the heat-stable enterotoxin produced by porcine strains of *E. coli*. *Infect. Immun.* 19: 1021–1030.

APHA. 1984. *Compendium of Methods for the Microbiological Examination of Foods.* American Public Health Association., Washington, DC.

ARCHER, D. L. 1984. Diarrheal episodes and diarrheal disease: Acute disease with chronic implications. *J. Food Prot.* 47: 322–328.

AULISIO, C. C. G., HILL, W. E., STANFIELD, J. T., and MORRIS, J. A. 1983a. Pathogenicity of *Yersinia enterocolitica* demonstrated in the suckling mouse. *J. Food Prot.* 46: 856–860.

AULISIO, C. C. G., HILL, W. E., STANFIELD, J. T., and SELLERS, R. L., JR. 1983b. Evaluation of virulence factor testing and characteristics of pathogenicity in *Yersinia enterocolitica*. *Infect. Immun.* 40: 330–335.

BARON, S., HOWIE, V., LANGFORD, M., MacDONALD, E. M., STANTON, G. J., REITMEYER, J., and WIEGENT, D. A. 1982. Induction of interferon by bacteria, protozoa and viruses: defensive role. *Tex. Rep. Biol. Med.* 41: 150–157.

BLACHMAN, U., GOSS, S. J., and PICKETT, M. J. 1974. Experimental cholera in the chinchilla. *J. Infect. Dis.* 129: 376–384.

BLAKE, P. A., WEAVER, R. E., and HOLLIS, D. G. 1980. Diseases of humans (other than cholera) caused by vibrios. *Ann. Rev. Microbiol.* 34: 341–367.

BUKHOLM, G. and DEGRE, M. 1983. Effect of human leukocyte interferon on invasiveness of *Salmonella* species in HEp-2 cell cultures. *Infect. Immun.* 42: 1198–1202.

BUKHOLM, G., BERDAL, B.P., HAUG, C., and DEGRE, M. 1984. Mouse fibroblast interferon modifies *Salmonella typhimurium* infection in infant mice. *Infect. Immun.* 45: 62–66.

BURGESS, M. N., BYWATER, R. J., COWLEY, C. M., MULLAN, N. A., and NEWSOME, P. M. 1978. Biological evaluation of a methanol-soluble, heat-stable *Escherichia coli* enterotoxin in infant mice, pigs, rabbits, and calves. *Infect. Immun.* 21: 526–531.

BURROWS, W., ELLIOTT, M. E., and HAVENS, I. 1947. Studies on immunity to Asiatic cholera. IV. The excretion of copra-antibody in experimental enteric cholera in the guinea pig. *J. Infect. Dis.* 81: 161–181.

CAMPBELL, P. A. 1976. Immunocompetent cells in resistance to bacterial infections. *Bacteriol. Rev.* 40: 284–313.

CLEMENTS, J. D. and FINKELSTEIN, R. A. 1978. Immunological cross-reactivity between heat-labile enterotoxins(s) of *Escherichia coli* and subunits of *Vibrio cholerae* enterotoxin. *Infect. Immun.* 21: 1036–1039.

COLLINS, F. M. and CARTER, P. B. 1974. Cellular immunity in enteric disease. *Am. J.Clin. Nutr.* 27: 1424–1433.

CUATRECASAS, P. 1973. Gangliosides and membrane receptors for cholera toxin. *Biochemistry* 12: 3558–3566.

DEAN, A. G., CHING, Y., WILLIAMS, R. G., and HARDEN, L. B. 1972. Test for *Escherichia coli* enterotoxin using infant mice: application in a study of diarrhea in children in Honolulu. *J. Infect. Dis.* 125: 407–411.

DENSEN, P. and MANDELL, G. I. 1980. Phagocyte strategy vs. microbial tactics. *Rev. Infect. Dis.* 2: 817–838.

DINARELLO, C. A. 1984. Interleukin-1 and the pathogenesis of the acute-phase response. *N. Engl. J. Med.* 311: 1413–1418.

DINGLE, J. A., BADGER, G. F., and JORDAN, W. S. 1964. *Illness in the Home: A Study of 25,000 Illnesses in a Group of Cleveland Families.* Western Reserve University Press, Cleveland, OH.

DONTA, S. T., SMITH, D. M., MOON, H. W., and WHIPP, S. C. 1974. Detection of heat-labile *Escherichia coli* enterotoxin with the use of adrenal cells in tissue culture. *Science* 183: 334–336.

DUTTA, N. K. and HABBU, K. 1955. Experimental cholera in infant rabbits: a method for chemotherapeutic investigation. *Br. J. Pharmacol.* 10: 153–159.

EBRINGER, A. 1983. The cross-tolerance hypothesis, HLA-B27 and ankylosing spondylitis. *Br. J. Rheumatol.* 22: 53–66.

EIKLID, K. and OLSNES, S. 1983. Animal toxicity of *Shigella dysenteriae* cytotoxin: evidence that the neurotoxic, enterotoxic, and cytotoxic activities are due to one toxin. *J. Immunol.* 130: 380–384.

EISENSTEIN, T. K., KILLAR, L. M., and SULTZER, B. M. 1984. Immunity to infection with *Salmonella typhimurium*: mouse-strain differences in vaccine- and serum-mediated protection. *J. Infect. Dis.* 150: 425–435.

EVANS, D. G., SILVER, R. P., EVANS, D. J., JR., CHASE, D. G., and GORBACH, S. L. 1975. Plasmid-controlled colonization factor associated with virulence in *Escherichia coli* enterotoxigenic for humans. *Infect. Immun.* 12: 656–667.

EVANS, D. G. and EVANS, D. J., JR. 1978. New surface-associated heat-labile colonization factor antigen (CFA/II) produced by enterotoxigenic *Escherichia coli* of serogroups O6 and O8. *Infect. Immun.* 21: 638–647.

EVANS, D. G., EVANS, D. J., JR., TJOA, W. S., and DUPONT, H. L. 1978. Detection and characterization of colonization factor of *Escherichia coli* isolated from adults with diarrhea. *Infect. Immun.* 19: 727–736.

FALCONI, G., CAMPA, A., SMITH, H., and SCOTT, G. M. 1984. *Bacterial and Viral Inhibition and Immunomodulation of Host Defences.* Academic Press, London.

FIELD, M. 1979. Mechanisms of action of cholera and *E. coli* enterotoxins. *Am. J. Clin. Nutr.* 32: 189–196.

FINKELSTEIN, R. A., SCIORTINO, C. V., and McINTOSH, M. A. 1983. Role of iron in microbe-host interactions. *Rev. Infect. Dis.* 5: S759–S777.

FOOD AND DRUG ADMINISTRATION. 1984. *Bacteriological Analytical Manual.* 6th ed. Association of Official Analytical Chemists, Arlington, VA.

FORMAL, S. B., KUNDEL, D., SCHNEIDER, H., KUNEV, N., and SPRINZ, H. 1961. Studies with *Vibrio cholerae* in the ligated loop of the rabbit intestine. *Br. J. Exp. Pathol.* 42: 504–510.

FRETER, R. 1980. Prospects for preventing association of harmful bacteria with host mucosal surfaces. In *Bacterial Adherence.* Beachey, E. H. (Ed.). Chapman Hall, London.

FRETER, R. and JONES, G. W. 1983. Models for studying the role of bacterial attachment in virulence and pathogensis. *Rev. Infect. Dis.* 5: S647–S658.

FRETER, R., ALLWEISS, B., O'BRIEN, P. C. M., HALSTEAD, S. A., and MACSAI, M. S. 1981a. Role of chemotaxis in the association of motile bacteria with intestinal mucosa: in vitro studies. *Infect. Immun.* 34: 241–249.

FRETER, R., O'BRIEN, P. C. M., and MACSAI, M. S. 1981b. The role of chemotaxia in the association of motile bacteria with intestinal mucosa: in vivo studies. *Infect. Immun.* 34: 234–240.

FRETER, R., BRICKNER, H., FEKETE, J., VICKERMAN, M. M., and CAREY, K. E. 1983. Survival and implantation of *Escherichia coli* in the intestinal tract. *Infect. Immun.* 39: 686–703.

GEMSKI, P., LAZERE, J. R., and CASEY, T. 1980a. Plasmid associated with pathogenicity and calcium dependency of *Yersinia enterocolitica. Infect. Immun.* 27: 682–685.

GEMSKI, P., LAZERE, J. R., CASEY, T., and WOHLHIETER, J. A. 1980b. Presence of a virulence-associated plasmid in *Yersinia pseudotuberculosis. Infect. Immun.* 28: 1044–1047.

GEMSKI, P., JR., TAKEUCHI, A., WASHINGTON, O., and FORMAL, S. B. 1972. Shigellosis due to *Shigella dysenteriae* 1: relative importance of mucosal invasion versus toxin production in pathogenesis. *J. Infect. Dis.* 126: 523–530.

GIANNELLA, R. A. and DRAKE, K. W. 1979. Effect of purified *E. coli* heat-stable enterotoxin on intestinal cyclic nucleotide metabolism and fluid secretion. *Infect. Immun.* 24: 19–23.

GIANNELLA, R. A., LUTTRELL, M., and DRAKE, K. 1980. Binding of pure *E. coli* heat-stable enterotoxin to isolated rat intestinal villus cells. *Clin. Res.* 28: 764.

GIANNELLA, R. A., WASHINGTON, O., GEMSKI, P., and FORMAL, S. B. 1973. Invasion of HeLa cells by *Salmonella typhimurium*: a model for the study of invasiveness of *Salmonella*. *J. Infect. Dis.* 128: 69–75.

GOTSCHLICH, E. C. 1983. Thoughts on the evolution of strategies used by bacteria for evasion of host defenses. *Rev. Infect. Dis.* 5: S778–S783.

GUBINA, M., ZAJC-SATLER, J., DRAGAS, A. Z., ZELEZNIK, Z., and MEHLE, J. 1982. Enterotoxin activity of *Campylobacter* species. In *Campylobacter: Epidemiology, Pathogenesis, and Biochemistry*. Newell, D. G. (Ed.). MTP Press, Hingham, MA.

GUERRANT, R. L., BRUNTON, L. L., SCHNAITMAN, T. C., REBUN, L. L., and GILMAN, A. C. 1974. Cyclic adenosine monophosphate and alteration of Chinese hamster ovary cell morphology: a rapid, sensitive in vitro assay for the enterotoxins of *Vibrio cholerae* and *Escherichia coli*. Infect. Immun. 10: 320–327.

HALE, T. L. and BONVENTRE, P. F. 1979. Shigella infection of Henle intestinal epithelial cells: role of the bacterium. *Infect. Immun.* 24: 879–886.

HALE, T. L. and FORMAL, S. B. 1981. Protein synthesis in HeLa or Henle 407 cells infected with *Shigella dysenteriae* 1, *Shigella flexneri* 2a, *Salmonella typhimurium* W118. *Infect. Immun.* 32: 137–144.

HALE, T. L., MORRIS, R. E., and BONVENTRE, P. F. 1979. Shigella infection of Henle intestinal epithelial cells: role of the host cell. *Infect. Immun.* 24: 887–894.

HILL, W. E., MADDEN, J. M., McCARDELL, B. A., SHAH, D. B., JAGOW, J. A., PAYNE, W. L., and BOUTIN, B. K. 1983. Foodborne enterotoxigenic *Escherichia coli*: detection and enumeration by DNA colony hybridization. *Appl. Environ. Microbiol.* 45: 1324–1330.

HOLMGREN, J., LONNROTH, I., and SVENNERHOLM, L. 1973a. Tissue receptor for cholera exotoxin: postulated structure from studies with GM1 ganglioside and related glycolipids. *Infect. Immun.* 8: 208–214.

HOLMGREN, J., SODERLIND, I., and WADSTROM, T. 1973b. Crossreactivity between heat-labile enterotoxin of *Vibrio cholerae* and *Escherichia coli* in neutralization tests in rabbit ileum and skin. *Acta Pathol. Microbiol. Scand. B* 81: 757–762.

HORMAECHE, C. E. 1979. Natural resistance to *Salmonella typhimurium* in different inbred mouse strains. *Immunology* 37: 311–318.

IGLEWSKI, B. H. and SADOFF, J. C. 1979. Toxin inhibitors of protein synthesis: production, purification, and assay of *Pseudomonas aeruginosa* toxin A. *Methods Enzymol.* 60: 780–793.

ISAACSON, R. E., NAGY, B., and MOON, H. W. 1977. Colonization of porcine small intestine by *Escherichia coli*: colonization and adhesion factors in pig enteropathogens that lack K88. *J. Infect. Dis.* 135: 531–539.

IZADKHAH, Z., MANDOL, A. D., and SONNENFELD, G. 1980. Effects of treatment of mice with sera containing gamma interferon on the course of infection with *Salmonella typhimurium*. *J. Interferon Res.* 1: 137–145.

JONES, G. W., ABRAMS, G. D., and FRETER, R. 1976. Adhesive properties of *Vibrio cholerae*: adhesion to isolated rabbit brush-border membranes and haemagglutinating activity. *Infect. Immun.* 14: 232–239.

JONES, G. W. and FRETER, R. 1976. Adhesion properties of *Vibrio cholerae*, nature of the interaction with isolated rabbit brush-border membranes and human erythrocytes. *Infect. Immun.* 14: 240–245.

JONES, G. W., RABERAT, D. K., SVINARICH, D. M., and WHITFIELD, H. J. 1982. Association of adhesive, invasive, and virulent phenotypes of *Salmonella typhimurium* with autonomous 60-megadalton plasmids. *Infect. Immun.* 38: 476–486.

JONES, G. W. and RUTTER, J. M. 1972. Role of the K88 antigen in the pathogenesis of neonatal diarrhea caused by *Escherichia coli* in piglets. *Infect. Immun.* 6: 918–927.

KAPITANY, R. A., FORSYTH, G. W., SCOOT, A., McKENZIE, S. F., and WORTHINGTON, R. W. 1979. Isolation and partial characterization of two different heat-stable enterotoxins produced by bovine and porcine strains of enterotoxigenic *E. coli*. *Infect. Immun.* 26: 173–177.

KAUFFMAN, P. E. 1981. Production and evaluation of antibody to the heat-stable enterotoxin from a human strain of enterotoxigenic *Escherichia coli*. *Appl. Environ. Microbiol.* 42: 611–614.

KAZMI, S. U., ROBERSON, B. S., and STERN, N. J. 1984. Animal-passed, virulence-enhanced *Campylobacter jejuni* causes enteritis in neonatal mice. *Curr. Microbiol.* 11: 159–164.

KEUSCH, G. T. and JACEWICZ, M. 1977. The pathogenesis of shigella diarrhea. VI. Toxin and antitoxin in *Shigella flexneri* and *Shigella sonnei* infections in humans. *J. Infect. Dis.* 135: 552–556.

KING, C. A. and VAN HEYNINGEN, W. E. 1973. Deactivation of cholera toxin by a sialidase-resistant monosialosyl-ganglioside. *J. Infect. Dis.* 127: 639–647.

KINSEY, M. D., FORMAL, S. B., DAMMIN, G. J., and GIANNELLA, R. A. 1976. Fluid and electrolyte transport in rhesus monkeys challenged intracecally with *Shigella flexneri* 2A. *Infect. Immun.* 14: 368–371.

KOPECKO, D. J., WASHINGTON, O., and FORMAL, S. B. 1980. Genetic and physical evidence for plasmid control of *Shigella sonnei* form I cell surface antigen. *Infect. Immun.* 29: 207–214.

KORNFELD, S. J. and PLAUT, A. G. 1981. Secretory immunity and bacterial IgA proteases. *Rev. Infect. Dis.* 3: 521–534.

LaBREC, E. H., SCHNEIDER, H., MAGNANI, T. J., and FORMAL, S. B. 1964. Epithelial cell penetration as an essential step in the pathogenesis of bacillary dysentery. *J. Bacteriol.* 88: 1503–1518.

LANKFORD, C. E. 1973. Bacterial assimilation of iron. *CRC Crit. Rev. Microbiol.* 2: 273–331.

LEE, W. H., McGRATH, P. P., CARTER, P. H., and EIDE, E. L. 1977. The ability of some *Yersinia enterocolitica* strains to invade HeLa cells. *Can. J. Microbiol.* 23: 1714–1722.

LeFEVRE, M. E., HAMMER, R., and JOEL, D. D. 1979. Macrophages of the mammalian small intestine: a review. *J. Reticuloendothelial Soc.* 26: 553–573.

LEVINE, M. M., DUPONT, H. L., FORMAL, S. B., HORNICK, R. B., TAKEUCHI, A., GANGAROSA, E. J., SNYDER, M. J., and LIBONATI, J. P. 1973. Pathogensis of *Shigella dysenteriae* 1 (Shiga) dysentery. *J. Infect. Dis.* 127: 261–270.

LEVINE, M. M., KAPER, J. B., BLACK, R. E., and CLEMENTS, M. L. 1983. New knowledge on pathogenesis of bacterial enteric infections as applied to vaccine development. *Microbiol. Rev.* 47: 510–550.

LEVINE, M. M., NALIN, D. R., HOOVER, D. L., BERGQUIST, E. J., HORNICK, R. B., and YOUNG, C. R. 1979. Immunity to enterotoxigenic *Escherichia coli*. *Infect. Immun.* 23: 729–736.

LUMISH, R. M., RYDER, R. W., ANDERSON, D. C., WELLS, J. G., and PUHR, N. 1980. Heat-labile enterotoxigenic *Escherichia coli* induced diarrhea aboard a Miami-based cruise ship. *Am. J. Epidemiol.* 111: 432–436.

MARTIN, S. P. and CHAUDHURI, S. N. 1952. Effect of bacteria and their products on migration of leukocytes. *Proc. Soc. Exp. Biol. Med.* 81: 286–288.

McCARDELL, B. A., MADDEN, J. M., and LEE, E. C. 1984. *Campylobacter jejuni* and *Campylobacter coli* production of a cytotonic toxin immunologically similar to cholera toxin. *J. Food Prot.* 47: 943–949.

MOON, H. W., NAGY, B., ISAACSON, R. E., and ØRSKOV, I. 1977. Occurrence of K99 antigen on *Escherichia coli* isolated from pigs and colonization of pig ileum by K99+ enterotoxigenic *E. coli* from calves and pigs. *Infect. Immun.* 15: 614–620.

MOSELEY, S. L., ECHEVERRIA, P., SERIWATANA, J., TIRAPAT, C., CHAICUMPA, W., SAKULDAIEARA, T., and FALKOW, S. 1982. Identification of enterotoxigenic *Escherichia coli* by colony hybridization using three enterotoxin gene probes. *J. Infect. Dis.* 145: 863–869.

MOSELEY, S. L., HARDY, J. W., HUQ, M. I., ECHEVERRIA, P., and FALKOW, S. 1983. Isolation and nucleotide sequence determination of a gene encoding a heat-stable enterotoxin of *Escherichia coli*. *Infect. Immun.* 39: 1167–1174.

NALIN, D. R., LEVINE, R. J., LEVINE, M. M., HOOVER, D., BERGQUIST, E., LIBONATI, J., ALAM, J., and HORNICK, R. B. 1978. Cholera, non-vibrio cholera, and stomach acid. *Lancet* ii: 856–859.

OAKS, E. V., WINGFIELD, M. E. and FORMAL, S. B. 1985. Plaque formation by virulent *Shigella flexneri*. *Infect. Immun.* 48: 124–129.

O'BRIEN, A. D., THOMPSON, M. R., GEMSKI, P., DOCTOR, B. P., and FORMAL, S. B. 1977. Biological properties of *Shigella flexneri* 2A toxin and its serological relationship to *Shigella dysenteriae* 1 toxin. *Infect. Immun.* 15: 796–798.

OGAWA, H., NAKAMURA, A., NAKAYA, R., MISE, K., HONJO, S., TAKASAKA, M., FUJIWARE, T., and IMAIZUMI, K. 1967. Virulence and epithelial cells invasiveness of dysentery bacilli. *Jpn. J. Med. Sci. Biol.* 20: 315–328.

O'GRADY, F. and SMITH, H. 1981. *Microbial Perturbation of Host Defenses.* Academic Press, London.

ØRSKOV, I. and ØRSKOV, F. 1966. Episome-carried surface antigen K88 of *Escherichia coli*. I. Transmission of the determinant of the K88 antigen and influence on the transfer of chromosomal markers. *J. Bacteriol.* 96: 69–75.

ØRSKOV, I., ØRSKOV, F., SMITH, H. W., and SOJKA, W. J. 1975. The establishment of K99, a thermolabile, transmissible, *Escherichia coli* K antigen, previously called "Kco," possessed by calf and lamb enterotoxigenic strains. *Acta Pathol. Microbiol. Scand. Sect. B* 83: 31–36.

PIECHAUD, M., SZTURM-RUBINSTEN, S., and PIECHAUD, D. 1958. Evolution histologique de la kerato-conjonctivite a bacilles dysenteriques du cobaye. *Ann. Inst. Pasteur* 94: 298–309.

PORTNOY, D. A., MOSELEY, S. L., and FALKOW, S. 1981. Characterization of plasmids and plasmid-associated determinants of *Yersinia enterocolitica* pathogenesis. *Infect. Immun.* 31: 775–782.

PRIZONT, R. and REED, W. P. 1980. Possible role of colonic content in the mucosal association of pathogenic shigella. *Infect. Immun.* 29: 1197–1199.

RAO, M. C., GUANDALINI, S., LAIRD, W., and FIELD, M. 1979. Effects of heat-stable enterotoxin of *Yersinia enterocolitica* on ion transport and cyclic guanosine 3′,5′-monophosphate metabolism in rabbit ileum. *Infect. Immun.* 26: 875–878.

ROBINS-BROWNE, R. M., RABSON, A. R., and KOORNHOF, H. J. 1979. Generalized infection with *Yersinia enterocolitica* and the role of iron. *Contrib. Microbiol. Immunol.* 5: 277–282.

ROBSON, H. G. and VAS, S. I. 1972. Resistance of inbred mice to *Salmonella typhimurium. J. Infect. Dis.* 126: 378–386.

ROWLAND, M. G. M., COLE, T. J., TULLY, M., DOLBY, J. M., and HONOUR, P. 1980. Bacteriostasis of *Escherichia coli* by milk. VI. The in-vitro bacteriostatic property of Gambian mother's milk in relation to the in-vivo protection of their infants against diarrhoeal disease. *J. Hyg. (London)* 85: 405–413.

RUIZ-PALACIOS, G. M., TORRES, J., TORRES, N. I., ESCAMILLA, E., RUIZ-PALACIOS, B., and TAMAYO, J. 1983. Cholera-like enterotoxin produced by *Campylobacter jejuni*: characterization and clinical significance. *Lancet* ii: 250–251.

SACK, D. A. and SACK, R. B. 1975. Test for enterotoxigenic *Escherichia coli* enterotoxin in Y-1 adrenal cells in miniculture. *Infect. Immun.* 11: 334–336.

SACK, R. B. 1975. Human diarrheal disease caused by enterotoxigenic *E. coli. Ann. Rev. Microbiol.* 29: 333–353.

SACK, R. B. and CARPENTER, C. C. J. 1969. Experimental canine cholera. I. Development of the model. *J. Infect. Dis.* 119: 138–149.

SANDEFUR, P. D. and PETERSON, J. W. 1977. Neutralization of *Salmonella* toxin-induced elongation of Chinese hamster ovary cells by cholera antitoxin. *Infect. Immun.* 15: 988–992.

SANDERS, A. C., BRYAN, F. L., OLSON, J. C., JR., and MADDEN, J. M. 1984. Foodborne illness—suggested approaches for the analysis of foods and specimens obtained in outbreaks. In *Compendium of Methods for the Microbiological Examination of Foods*, 2nd ed. Speck M. L. (Ed.). American Public Health Association, Washington, DC.

SANSONETTI, P., DAVID, M., and TOUCAS, M. 1980. Correlation entre la perte d'ADN plasmidique et le passage de la phase I virulente a la phase II avirulente chez *Shigella sonnei. CR Seances Acad. Sci.* (III) 290(D): 879–882.

SANSONETTI, P. J., D'HAUTEVILLE, FORMAL, S. B., and TOUCAS, M. 1982. Plasmid-mediated invasiveness of "shigella-like" *Escherichia coli. Ann. Microbiol. (Paris)* 133A: 351–355.

SANSONETTI, P. J., KOPECKO, D. J., and FORMAL, S. B. 1981. *Shigella sonnei* plasmids: evidence that a large plasmid is necessary for virulence. *Infect. Immun.* 34: 75–83.

SCHOTT, R. B. 1932. The inheritance of resistance to *Salmonella aertrycke* in various strains of mice. *Genetics* 17: 203–229.

SCHUTZE, H., GORER, P. A., and FINLAYSON, M. H. 1936. The resistance of four mouse lines to bacterial infections. *J. Hyg. (Camb.)* 36: 37–49.

SERENY, B. 1957. Experimental keratoconjunctivitis shigellosa. *Acta Microbiol. Acad. Sci. Hung.* 4: 367–376.

SHAH, D. B., KAUFFMAN, P. E., BOUTIN, B. K., and JOHNSON, C. H. 1982. Detection of heat-labile-enterotoxin-producing colonies of *Escherichia coli* and *Vibrio cholerae* by solid-phase sandwich radioimmunoassays. *J. Clin. Microbiol.* 16: 504–508.

SHAH, D. B., WIMSATT, J. C., and KAUFFMAN, P. E. 1984. Enzyme linked immunosorbent assay (ELISA). In *Bacteriological Analytical Manual.* 6th ed. Association of Official Analytical Chemists, Arlington, VA.

SIMPSON, L. M. and OLIVER, J. D. 1983. Siderophore production by *Vibrio vulnificus. Infect. Immun.* 41: 644–649.

SMITH, H. 1958. The use of bacteria grown in vivo for studies on the basis of their pathogenicity. *Ann. Rev. Microbiol.* 12: 77–102.

SMITH, H. 1976. Survival of vegetative bacteria in animals. *Symp. Soc. Gen. Microbiol.* 26: 299–326.

SMITH, H. 1982. The role of microbial interactions in infectious disease. *Philos. Trans. R. Soc. London Ser. B* 297: 551–561.

SMITH, H. 1983. The elusive determinants of bacterial interference with non-specific host defences. *Phil. Trans. R. Soc. London Ser. B* 303: 99–113.

SMITH, H. W. and LINGGOOD, M. A. 1971. The transmissible nature of enterotoxin production of a human enteropathogenic strain of *Escherichia coli. J. Med. Microbiol.* 4: 301–305.

SO, M., DALLAS, W. S., and FALKOW, S. 1978. Characterization of an *Escherichia coli* plasmid encoding for synthesis of heat-labile toxin: molecular cloning of the toxin determinant. *Infect. Immun.* 21: 405–411.

SO, M. and McCARTHY, B. J. 1980. Nucleotide sequence of the bacterial transposon Tn1681 encoding a heat-stable (ST) toxin and its identification in enterotoxigenic *Escherichia coli* strains. *Proc. Natl. Acad. Sci. USA* 77: 4011–4015.

SPIK, G., CHERON, A., MONTREUIL, J., and DOLBY, J. M. 1978. Bacteriostasis of a milk-sensitive strain of *Escherichia coli* by immunoglobulins and iron-binding proteins in association. *Immunology* 35: 663–671.

SPIRA, W., DANIEL, R. R., AHMED, Q. S., HUQ, A., YUSUF, A., and SACK, D. A. 1979. Clinical features and pathogenicity of O group 1, Non-agglutinating *Vibrio cholerae* and other vibrios isolated from cases of diarrhea in Dacca, Bangladesh. In *Proceedings of the 14th Joint Conference on Cholera*, U.S.-Japan Coop., Sept. 27–29, 1978, Karatsu, Japan.

SPIRA, W. M., SACK, R. B., and FROELICH, J. L. 1981. Simple adult rabbit model for *Virbrio cholerae* and enterotoxigenic *Escherichia coli* diarrhea. *Infect. Immun.* 32: 739–747.

SPIRA, W., SACK, D., SANYAL, S., MADDEN, J., and McCARDELL, B. 1983. Description of a possible new extracellular virulence factor in non-toxigenic *V. cholerae* O-1. Abstr. 19th U.S.-Japan Joint Conf. Cholera. Bethesda, MD.

STAPLES, S. J., ASHER, S. E., and GIANNELLA, R. A. 1980. Purification and characterization of heat-stable enterotoxin produced by a strain of *E. coli* pathogenic for man. *J. Biol. Chem.* 255, 4716–4721.

SUGARMAN, B. 1983. Zinc and infection. *Rev. Infect. Dis.* 5: 137–147.

SUSSMAN, M. 1974. Iron and infection. In *Iron in Biochemistry and Medicine*. Jacobs, A. and Worwood, M. (Ed.). Academic Press, New York.

TAGLIABUE, A., NENCIONI, L., VILLA, L., KEREN, D. F., LOWELL, G. H., and BORASCHI, D. 1983. Antibody-dependent cell-mediated antibacterial activity of intestinal lymphocytes with secretory IgA. *Nature* 306: 184–186.

TAKEUCHI, A. 1967. Electron microscopic studies of experimental salmonella infection. I. Penetration into the intestinal epithelium by *Salmonella typhimurium. Am. J. Pathol.* 50: 109–136.

THOMAS, L. V., CRAIOTO, A., SCOTLAND, S. M., and ROWE, B. 1982. New fimbrial antigenic type (E8775) that may represent a colonization factor in enterotoxigenic *Escherichia coli* in humans. *Infect. Immun.* 35: 1119–1124.

THORNE, G. M., DENEKE, C. F., and GORBACH, S. L. 1979. Hemagglutination and adhesiveness of toxigenic *Escherichia coli* isolated from humans. *Infect. Immun.* 23: 690–699.

THORNE, G. M. and GORBACH, S. L. 1979. New bacterial enterotoxins and human diarrheal diseases. In *Infections of the GI Tract. Clinics in Gastroenterology 8*: 3. Lambert, H. P. (Ed.). Saunders, Philadelphia, PA.

TUCKER, J. B. 1984. Gene machines: the second wave. *High Technol.* March: 50–61.

UCHIDA, T. 1983. Diphtheria toxin. *Pharmacol. Ther.* 19: 107–122.

UJIIYE, A. and KOBARI, K. 1970. Protective effect on infections with *Vibrio cholerae* in suckling mice caused by the passive immunization with milk of immune mothers. *J. Infect. Dis.* 121: S50–S55.

VANZANT, F. R., ALVAREZ, W. C., EUSTERMAN, G. B., DUNN, H. L., and BERKSON, J. 1932. The normal range of gastric acidity from youth to old age. *Arch. Int. Med.* 49: 345–359.

VOINO-YASENETSKY, M. V. and BAKACS, T. 1977. Conjunctival and intravesical challenge of guinea pigs with salmonellae. In *Pathogenesis of Intestinal Infections.* Voino-Yasenetsky, M. V. and Bakacs, T. (Ed.). Akademiae Kaido, Budapest.

WALKER, W. A. and ISSELBACHER, K. J. 1977. Intestinal antibodies. *N. Engl. J. Med.* 297: 767–773.

WATANABE, H. and NAKAMURA, A. 1985. Large plasmids associated with virulence in *Shigella* species have a common function for epithelial cell penetration. *Infect. Immun.* 48: 260–262.

WATANABE, H., NAKAMURA, A., and TIMMIS, K. N. 1984. Small virulence plasmid of *Shigella dysenteriae* 1 strain W30864 encodes a 41,000-dalton protein involved in formation of specific lipopolysaccharide side chain of serotype 1 isolates. *Infect. Immun.* 46: 55–63.

WATANABE, H. and TIMMIS, K. N. 1984. A small plasmid in *Shigella dysenteriae* 1 specifies one or more functions essential for O-antigen production and bacterial virulence. *Infect. Immun.* 43: 391–396.

WEBSTER, L. T. 1924. Microbic virulence and host susceptibility in paratyphoid-enteritidis infection of white mice. IV. The effect of selective inbreeding on host resistance. *J. Exp. Med.* 39: 879–886.

WEBSTER, L. T. 1933a. Inherited and acquired factors in resistance to infection. I. Development of resistant and susceptible lines of mice through selective breeding. *J. Exp. Med.* 57: 793–817.

WEBSTER, L. T. 1933b. Inherited and acquired factors in resistance to infection. II. A comparison of mice inherently resistant or susceptible to *Bacillus enteritidis* infection with respect to various routes and types of infection. *J. Exp. Med.* 57: 819–843.

ZINK, D. L., FEELEY, J. C., WELLS, J. G., VANDERZANT, C., VICKERY, J. C., ROOF, W. D., and O'DONOVAN, G. A. 1980. Plasmid-mediated tissue invasiveness in *Yersinia enterocolitica*. *Nature* 283: 224–226.

15

Detection and Quantitation of Foodborne Pathogens and Their Toxins: Gram-Negative Bacterial Pathogens

Michael P. Doyle

University of Wisconsin-Madison
Madison, Wisconsin

INTRODUCTION

Several gram-negative bacteria are now recognized agents of foodborne disease. Those of major interest include: *Salmonella* spp., *Campylobacter jejuni*, *Yersinia enterocolitica*, colohemorrhagic *Escherichia coli*, *Vibrio parahaemolyticus*, and *Vibrio cholerae*. Present concern indicates that detecting small numbers of these pathogens in foods is often important. To accomplish this, culture conditions specific for each organism must be used. To decrease detection time, improved methods are evolving that combine appropriate culture procedures with pathogen-specific antibodies or genetic probes. This chapter will focus on some of the most recently reported information and procedures regarding the detection of gram-negative bacterial pathogens in foods.

SALMONELLA SPP.

Five steps are common to most culture methods for isolating and identifying salmonellae in foods. These are: (a) preenrichment of the food sample in a nutritious, nonselective broth; (b) selective enrichment in a broth that allows salmonellae to grow but suppresses the growth of competing bacteria; (c) isolation of *Salmonella* by streaking onto selective plating agar; (d) biochemical characterization of isolates; and (e) serological confirmation of biochemically screened isolates (Andrews 1985). However, only the first two steps of conventional culture methods have application to new, rapid methods for salmonellae detection. Hence, only these two steps will be discussed. Detailed methodology for the latter three steps has been described elsewhere (Andrews et al. 1984; Fagerberg and Avens 1976; Poelma et al. 1984).

Preenrichment

A primary function of preenrichment is to rehydrate cells of *Salmonella* that have been dehydrated during food processing (Andrews 1985). The importance of rehydration for enchancing the recovery of salmonellae has been well-documented (Andrews et al. 1983; van Schothorst et al. 1979). During preenrichment injured cells are restored to a stable physiological condition and then grow on the nutrients present in the medium.

Preenrichment media are generally nutritionally complex and include: lactose broth, Trypticase soy broth, reconstituted nonfat dry milk, nutrient broth, and buffered peptone water. Results of previous studies suggest that the choice of preenrichment medium is not critical for recovery and that media of low and high nutritive capacity are equally effective for detection of salmonellae in raw and processed foods (D'Aoust 1984a; D'Aoust and Maishment 1979; Poelma et al. 1981). Traditionally, preenrichment requires incubating cultures at 35 to 37°C for 16 to 24 hr, and attempts to shorten the incubation period have led to conflicting reports (D'Aoust 1984a). A shortened ($\leq$ 6 hr) preenrichment is desirable because it allows presumptive identification one day earlier than with standard cultural methods; however, short preenrichment results in unacceptably high numbers of false-negative samples (D'Aoust 1981; D'Aoust and Maishment 1979). Studies with pure cultures have shown that a 6-hr incubation period is not sufficient time for resuscitation of injured cells in lactose or tryptone soya broths (van Schothorst and van Leusden 1972). Hence, it appears that salmonellae detection procedures requiring the presence of large numbers of salmonellae ($\geq$ 10^5

CFU/mL) cannot use a preenrichment method of ≤6 hr without resulting in an unacceptably high number of false-negative samples.

Selective Enrichment

Of the many selective enrichment media that have been developed for isolating *Salmonella*, selenite cystine broth and tetrathionate broth are the most widely used. These media allow salmonellae to grow but restrict the growth of other competing bacteria. Omitting the preenrichment step and suspending food samples directly in selective enrichment media (direct enrichment) would greatly reduce detection time. This approach is recommended for the analysis of meats and animal products that are raw and may contain high numbers of competing microorganisms (Andrews et al. 1984; D'Aoust 1984a; USDA 1974). It was thought that salmonellae may be overgrown by the competing microflora during the preenrichment (Andrews 1985). However, results of studies done on raw meats indicate substantially greater *Salmonella* recovery from samples submitted to preenrichment than direct enrichment (Edel and Kampelmacher 1973).

Selective enrichment cultures are generally incubated for 16 to 24 hr at 35–37 or 43°C. Several studies have shown greater salmonellae recovery from high-moisture foods in which selective enrichment media were incubated at 43°C than at 35–37°C (Kafel and Bryan 1977; Morris and Dunn 1970; Silliker and Gabis 1974; van Schothorst and van Leusden 1975). However, one report indicates that some strains of *Salmonella* cannot grow in Mueller-Kauffman tetrathionate broth incubated at 43°C (McCoy 1962). Nonetheless, several organizations recommend incubation of tetrathionate broth at 43°C. Results of a recently reported 6-year study involving 22 laboratories in which 2085 *Salmonella*-contaminated low- and high-moisture foods were tested, indicated that selective enrichment of high-moisture foods in tetrathionate brilliant green broth (TBG) at 43°C was markedly more sensitive for *Salmonella* detection than enrichment in selenite cystine broth (SC) at 35°C (D'Aoust 1984b). Enrichment in TBG and SC identified 92 and 63%, respectively, of contaminated samples when enrichment cultures were plated on both bismuth sulfite agar and brilliant green sulfa agar. With low-moisture foods, TBG rates of isolation were only a few percent better than SC.

Three recent studies have shown that the incubation period for selective enrichment may be successfully shortened to 6 to 8 hr. D'Aoust et al. (1983) obtained identical recovery rates for *Salmonella* from feeds and feed ingredients following overnight preenrichment in nutrient broth and short (6 hr) or overnight incubation in TBG and SC. Entis et al. (1982) analyzed naturally and artificially contaminated foods by the hydrophobic grid-membrane filter technique using overnight preenrichment in nutrient broth and a 6-hr selective enrichment in TBG and SC, and identified *Salmonella* in 97.8% of the samples that were positive by a standard culture procedure. Rappold et al. (1984) compared the recovery of *Salmonella* from dry foods enriched in tetrathionate broth or modified Rappaport broth (Vassiliadis et al. 1981) for 8 or 24 hr. All 27 samples were positive after 8 and 24 hr of incubation in modified Rappaport broth, whereas 24 and 27 samples were positive after 8 and 27 hr, respectively, in tetrathionate broth. Hence, there may be potential for reducing the incubation time of selective enrichment for conventional culture methods and possibly for rapid methods. However, for those rapid methods that require 10^6 to 10^7 *Salmonella* per milliliter of medium to assure detection, Robison and Flowers (1985) have found that 16 hr of incubation in selective enrichment media are necessary.

Innovative Detection or Isolation Procedures

Several innovative procedures have recently been developed for detecting salmonellae in foods. Notable examples include the hydrophobic grid-membrane filtration technique (Entis et al. 1982), the DNA-DNA hybridization test (Fitts 1985; Fitts et al. 1983), and enzyme immunoassay procedures (Flowers 1985; Mattingly 1984; Mattingly and Gehle 1984; Mattingly et al. 1985; Swaminathan et al. 1985). All are shorter tests than conventional culture procedures; however, all first require preenrichment and selective enrichment of samples before being applied. These procedures are discussed in Chapters 5, 12, and 13.

CAMPYLOBACTER JEJUNI

Campylobacter jejuni is a relatively fragile bacterium that is quite sensitive to drying, 21% oxygen (Koidis and Doyle 1983), storage at 25°C, acidic conditions, disinfectants, and heat (Doyle 1984b). Hence, it is unlikely that large numbers of the organism would be present in food under normal holding conditions. Because of the organism's great sensitivity to environmental conditions outside of the confines of its host, for best recovery of the small numbers of *C. jejuni* likely to be present in food, isolation procedures must utilize conditions that, most importantly, promote the organism's survival and also allow its growth.

Four important components of an isolation procedure should be considered when identifying a method to recover *C. jejuni* from foods. These include: (a) conditions for handling and storage of specimens, (b) enrichment procedures, (c) selective plating media, and (d) microaerobic conditions for culturing the organism.

Handling and Storage of Specimens

Methods for sampling, transporting, and storing specimens are extremely important yet often are the least considered components of a procedure for isolating *C. jejuni* from foods. Because of the organism's fragility, improper handling of specimens before testing can negate the value of a sensitive isolation procedure.

Koidis and Doyle (1983) found that survival of *C. jejuni* is greatly influenced by temperature and atmospheric oxygen. Temperature is the most influential factor, with death occurring eight times more rapidly at 25°C than at 4°C. Survival is greater in an oxygen-free environment (100% N_2) than in the presence of any level of oxygen, i.e., 5, 21, or 100% O_2. Additionally, adding 0.01% sodium bisulfite to the medium further enhances *Campylobacter* survival. When these *Campylobacter* survival-promoting conditions are combined, i.e., storing *C. jejuni* at 4°C in an oxygen-free medium containing 0.01% sodium bisulfite, the organism will survive ten times longer than when the same strain is held in a bisulfite-free medium exposed to air at 25°C.

Koidis and Doyle (1984) applied these survival-promoting conditions to raw milk samples inoculated with large numbers of *C. jejuni*. *Campylobacter* survival was twice as long in milk supplemented with 0.01% sodium bisulfite and maintained in the presence of 100% N_2 compared to milk containing no added bisulfite and maintained in air. Although not quite as effective as a survival-promoting agent, supplementing raw milk with 0.15% sodium thioglycollate (an oxygen scavenger) served as a practical alternative to exchanging the milk-holding environment with nitrogen. Hence, milk samples to be transported and assayed at a later date would best be held refrigerated (4°C) and supplemented with 0.01% sodium bisulfite and either 0.15% sodium thioglycollate or an atmosphere of 100% N_2.

Meats and solid food specimens should also be refrigerated and stored in an atmosphere of 100% N_2. Alternatively, storing meat samples at 4°C with an equal amount of Cary-Blair diluent results in little change in *Campylobacter* viability during 14 days of storage, and may be used as a transport and storage procedure (Stern and Kotula 1982). Freezing food specimens should be avoided as this treatment substantially reduces the incidence of *C. jejuni* detection (Blankenship et al. 1982; Stern and Kotula 1982).

Enrichment Procedures

Because only small numbers of *C. jejuni* may be present in foods, an enrichment procedure is often required to detect the organism. This is illustrated by results of a study by Park et al. (1981) in which using an enrichment procedure resulted in detecting approximately twice as many *Campylobacter*-positive poultry carcasses than was identified by direct plating onto selective agar.

Several enrichment procedures have been developed for isolating *C. jejuni* from foods or feces (Acuff et al. 1982; Barot and Bokkenheuser 1984; Blaser et al. 1979; Bolton and Robertson 1982; Doyle and Roman 1982a, b; Hänninen 1982; Lander 1982; Lovett et al. 1983; Martin et al. 1983; Park et al. 1981, 1983; Rosef 1981; Rothenberg et al. 1984; Tanner and Bullin 1977; Wesley et al. 1983). However, a comprehensive study has not been done to compare the efficacy of the different procedures in recovering *Campylobacter* from inoculated or naturally contaminated foods. Hence, presently it is not possible to identify any single method as being the best for isolating *C. jejuni* from a wide variety of foods. This discussion will focus on several of the more promising enrichment procedures for isolating *C. jejuni* from foods.

The procedure of Park et al. (1981; 1983) has been shown to be useful for isolating *C. jejuni* from naturally contaminated poultry carcasses. The procedure is sensitive, reportedly being effective in detecting *Campylobacter* when as few as 0.2 *C. jejuni* cell is present per gram of food in the presence of 10^4 to 10^6 contaminants per gram. It requires that each chicken be washed in nutrient broth; that the nutrient broth be filtered through cheesecloth and centrifuged; and that the sediment be suspended in enrichment broth. The enrichment medium is then incubated for 48 hr at 42°C in a microaerobic environment maintained in an anaerobic incubator or under a constant flow of 5% O_2, 10% CO_2, 85% N_2 (5 to 7 mL/min) bubbled into the broth. After incubation, enrichment culture is either filtered through a 0.65-μm membrane and then plated onto Skirrow's agar or streaked directly onto Skirrow's agar.

Lovett et al. (1983) modified the Park et al. procedure and applied the technique to the isolation of *C. jejuni* from raw milk. The procedure is sensitive, being able to recover < 1 *C. jejuni*/mL of raw milk having aerobic plate counts of 10^4 to 10^6 CFU/mL, and was used to identify two *C. jejuni*-positive milk samples from bulk tanks of 195 different farms. The protocol for the procedure is as follows. A 40-g sample of milk is centrifuged and the pellet is suspended in enrichment medium. This medium is incubated at

42°C under a constant flow (10 mL/min) of gas (5% O_2, 10% CO_2, 85% N_2) bubbled into the broth. After 24 hr of incubation, 5 mL of enrichment culture is filtered through a 0.65-μm membrane. Both filtered and unfiltered enrichment broths are streaked onto Skirrow's agar supplemented with ferrous sulfate, sodium metabisulfite, and pyruvate (each at a concentration of 0.25 g/L).

Acuff et al. (1982) evaluated an enrichment procedure for recovery of *C. jejuni* from turkey eggs and meat. Inoculation studies indicated a minimum level of sensitivity of 3 to 33 cells per gram of egg or muscle. The procedure is not complicated. It involves diluting 50 grams of eggs or 40 grams of muscle 1:10 with enrichment broth, holding the broth first at 4°C for 12 hr and then at 42°C for 48 hr in a microaerobic environment, and then streaking enrichment cultures onto selective agar. This procedure was used successfully to detect *C. jejuni* in poultry giblets (Christopher et al. 1982).

Wesley et al. (1983) developed a selective enrichment procedure for isolating *C. jejuni* from poultry products. The method is sensitive, being able to recover as few as 0.4 cell/g of poultry product for nine *C. jejuni* strains evaluated, and reportedly represses the growth of *Pseudomonas aeruginosa* which is commonly associated with poultry products. For solid meat tissue, the procedure involves adding the poultry sample to 50 ml of 0.1% peptone; hand-massaging samples; placing 10 mL of rinse fluid in 100 mL of enrichment broth; and incubating the enrichment culture in a horizontally-positioned modified milk dilution bottle containing a microaerobic atmosphere. The cultures are incubated statically at 42°C for 48 hr and then streaked onto selective agar. A study was done to compare the efficacy of this procedure to that of the original enrichment procedure of Park et al. (1981) for isolating *C. jejuni* from retail cut-up chicken and chicken parts. Of 50 samples evaluated, *C. jejuni* was recovered from 25 samples by the Wesley et al. (1983) procedure and from 6 samples by the Park et al. (1981) procedure.

Bolton and Robertson (1982) developed an enrichment medium (Preston medium) that greatly increased the isolation of *C. jejuni* from fecal specimens. Comparing isolation rates of *Campylobacter* from bovine, ovine, porcine, and avian fecal specimens by direct plating onto Skirrow's medium and Preston medium to enrichment in Preston medium, substantially more cultures were positive by enrichment. The Preston enrichment medium detected 46.5% *Campylobacter*-positive specimens, whereas direct plating onto Skirrow's or Preston medium detected 13.5 and 29% *Campylobacter*-positive specimens, respectively. Preston broth was originally composed of nutrient broth No. 2 (Oxoid) supplemented with 5% lysed horse blood, polymyxin B (5 IU/mL), rifampicin (10 μg/mL), trimethoprim (10 μg/mL), and actidione (100 μg/mL). Broth (10 mL) was distributed into 6 in × 5/8 in tubes and incubated for 24 hr, apparently at 43°C and without a microaerobic atmosphere. The broth was later modified (Bolton et al. 1983) to include 0.025% each FeSO$_4$·7H$_2$O, sodium metabisulfite, and sodium pyruvate, and was distributed in 5-mL portions into 1/4-oz screw-capped bottles.

Rosef (1981) developed an enrichment procedure that effectively isolated *C. jejuni* from the gallbladder of pigs. The enrichment medium is composed of "Lab lemco" powder (Oxoid), peptone, yeast extract, sodium chloride, rezasurin, vancomycin (10 μg/mL), trimethoprim lactate (5 μg/mL), and polymyxin B (2.5 IU/mL). Cultures are incubated at 42°C for 48 hr under microaerobic conditions. Rosef and Kapperud (1983) also used this procedure to isolate *C. jejuni* from house flies and detected the organism in 28.4% of 518 flies tested. Garcia et al. (1985) found the procedure to be quite useful for isolating campylobacters from slaughter cattle. They detected *C. jejuni* and *C. coli* in 50 and 1, respectively, of 100 animals tested. *C. jejuni* was isolated 40.2% more frequently by the enrichment technique than by direct plating.

Doyle and Roman (1982b) developed a direct enrichment procedure that can recover small numbers of *C. jejuni*, *C. coli*, and *Campylobacter laridis* from raw milk, raw ground beef, and chicken skin having aerobic plate counts of 10^5 to 10^9 CFU/g. The procedure is effective in recovering as few as 0.1 to 0.4 cell of *Campylobacter* per gram of food. The assay includes a selective enrichment medium composed of brucella broth, 7% lysed horse blood, 0.3% sodium succinate, 0.01% cysteine hydrochloride, vancomycin (15 μg/mL), trimethoprim (5 μg/mL), polymyxin B (20 IU/mL), and cycloheximide (50 μg/mL) that is inoculated with 10 or 25g of food and incubated with agitation (100 gyrations/min) under microaerobic conditions (5% O$_2$, 10% CO$_2$, 85% N$_2$) at 42°C for 16 to 18 hr. The enrichment medium is held in a 250-mL sidearm, capped Erlenmeyer flask that is evacuated three times to 20 in. Hg and replaced with the microaerobic gas mixture. After incubation, the culture is plated [0.1 mL and 0.1 mL each of two serial dilutions (1:10)] onto Campy-BAP for isolation and identification of *Campylobacter*.

Using this procedure, Doyle and Roman (1982a) isolated *C. jejuni* from one of 108 raw milk samples obtained from bulk tanks of grade A dairy farms. Doyle (1984a) has also used this procedure to isolate *C. jejuni* from the surface of 2 of 226 eggs from hens identified as *C. jejuni*-fecal excreters. This procedure was also used by a group of nine laboratories participating in a national survey to identify the prevalence of *C. jejuni* and *C. coli* in retail cuts of meat and poultry (Stern et al. 1985). A total of 2,160 retail samples were assayed and campylobacters were isolated from 4.7% of beef flank steak, 5.0% of pork chops, 8.1% of lamb stew meat, 29.7% of broiler chickens, 3.6% of ground beef, and 4.2% of pork sausage.

Rothenberg et al. (1984) compared the efficacy of the Doyle and Roman procedure with the modified Park et al. (1983) enrichment method, and found the Doyle and Roman procedure had a slightly higher isolation rate and greater selectivity in recovering *C. jejuni* from inoculated poultry carcasses. Similarly, Heisick et al. (1984) reported slightly better recovery of *C. jejuni* from inoculated hamburger by the Doyle and Roman procedure (69% positive tests) than by the modified Park et al. method (Lovett et al. 1983) (57% positive tests). Fricker (1984) compared the effectiveness of different enrichment procedures in recovering *C. jejuni* and *C. coli* from naturally contaminated chicken giblets. Of 198 samples examined, 177 were found to contain *Campylobacter* and enrichment procedures using Preston medium and Doyle and Roman medium were superior, with each facilitating the isolation of *Campylobacter* from 176 samples.

Selective Plating Media

Following any enrichment procedure, the enrichment culture must be plated on a selective medium to isolate *C. jejuni*. Many different media have been purposed for selective isolation of *Campylobacter*; however, the efficacy of four such media has been well-documented. Of these, three are widely used, including: (a) Skirrow's medium (Skirrow 1977), composed of blood agar base or brucella agar, 5 to 7% lysed horse blood, vancomycin (10 μg/mL), polymyxin B (2.5 IU/mL), and trimethoprim (5 μg/mL); (b) Butzler's medium (Lauwers et al. 1978), composed of Columbia agar base or blood agar base, 5 to 7% sheep blood, bacitracin (25 IU/mL), novobiocin (5 μg/mL), actidione (50 μg/mL), colistin (10 units/mL), and cephalothin (15 μg/mL) or cephazolin (15 μg/mL); and (c) Blaser-Wang's or Campy BAP medium (Blaser et al. 1979), composed of brucella agar or blood agar base, 10% sheep blood, vancomycin (10 μg/mL), trimethoprim (5 μg/mL), polymyxin B (2.5 IU/mL), amphotericin B (2 μg/mL), and cephalothin (15 μg/mL).

A fourth medium, Preston agar (Bolton and Robertson 1982) of which the composition has been described earlier except that 1.2% New Zealand agar is included, is not as widely used as the three media described above; however, Preston agar has been reported to be more selective and sensitive in isolating *C. jejuni* and related campylobacters than the other three selective plating media (Bolton and Robertson 1982; Bolton et al. 1983). Butzler et al. (1983) and Goossens et al. (1983) have recently described a medium, Butzler's medium Virion, composed of Columbia agar base, cefoperazone (15 μg/mL), rifampicin (10 μg/mL), colistin (10 IU/mL), and amphotericin B (2μg/mL), which also deserves consideration. This medium is more selective than Butzler's original medium in repressing growth of contaminants and allowing better recognition of *Campylobacter* colonies. Consideration should also be given to a recently reported blood-free selective plating medium (CCD agar) developed by Bolton et al. (1984) which contains nutrient broth, charcoal, ferrous sulfate, sodium pyruvate, casein hydrolysates, cefazolin (10 μg/mL), and sodium deoxycholate. Bolton et al. (1984) found CCD agar to be as effective as Preston agar in isolating *C. jejuni* from human feces, but CCD agar was less selective.

Using the appropriate selective plating medium is very important to the success of an enrichment procedure. Enrichment procedures utilizing membrane filtration following enrichment incubation generally do not require a highly selective plating agar, because most of the competing microbial flora are retained by the filter. However, those procedures involving direct plating following incubation require use of a selective plating medium that represses the growth of competing microbes but allows the growth and isolation of *Campylobacter*.

Results of many studies comparing the selectivity and isolation rates of *C. jejuni* by the different selective agars have been reported (Billingham 1981; Bolton and Robertson 1982; Bolton et al. 1983, 1984; Butzler et al. 1983; Fricker 1984; Goossens et al. 1983; Patton et al. 1981; Stern 1982; Weber et al. 1983). The most thorough study (Bolton et al. 1983) comparing Skirrow's, Butzler's original, Blaser-Wang's, and Preston media resulted in Preston medium not only being the most selective in repressing growth of contaminants, but also being the most sensitive by isolating *C. jejuni* from the greatest number of fecal and drain effluent specimens (250 isolations from 653 specimens). Blaser-Wang's medium was second best in isolating *Campylobacter* (227 isolations from 653 specimens) but allowed more contaminants to grow than either Butzler's or Skirrow's medium. Butzler's medium was the second most selective medium in repressing contaminant growth, but was the least effective in isolating *C. jejuni* (203 isolations from 653 specimens).

Fricker (1984) compared the effectiveness of Preston medium and Blaser-Wang medium in isolating *Campylobacter* from enrichments of naturally contaminated chicken giblets. He found that Preston medium was slightly more effective in recovering campylobacters than Blaser-Wang medium, although the difference was not significant. A study by Stern (1982) compared the sensitivity and selectivity of modified Skirrow's (supplemented with 15 μg of cephalothin/mL), Blaser-Wang's, and Butzler's original media for recovery of inoculated *C. jejuni* from ground beef. He observed Blaser-Wang's medium was most sensitive for recovery and Butzler's medium was most selective.

Microaerobic Conditions

The ideal concentrations of oxygen and carbon dioxide for the growth of *C. jejuni* are 3 to 5% and 2 to 10%, respectively. Hence, the microaerobic growth requirements of *C. jejuni* should be considered in culturing the organism. An evacuation-replacement or continuous flow percolation procedure in which the atmosphere of the environment is replaced with a gas mixture of 5% O_2, 10% CO_2, 85% N_2 is considered optimal for this purpose. Bolton and Coates (1983) have compared several other microaerobic systems for the culture of *C. jejuni* and related campylobacters. The systems tested included two commercial gas generating envelopes, the candle jar technique, and an evacuation-replacement procedure using 10% carbon dioxide in nitrogen as the replacement gas mixture. The two commercial gas generating systems (Oxoid BR56 and BBL Campy Pak II envelopes) and the evacuation-replacement procedure were approximately equivalent in promoting development of colonies of campylobacters on nonselective medium. The candle jar technique gave significantly reduced counts for most of the strains tested, indicating this technique is inferior to the others for isolating *Campylobacter*.

YERSINIA ENTEROCOLITICA

Many studies have shown that *Y. enterocolitica* is present in a wide variety of foods; however, most food isolates are avirulent. Because the presence of avirulent *Y. enterocolitica* in foods is of little public health concern, interest in procedures to detect the organism primarily focuses on isolating and identifying virulent strains. Some of the early procedures used to isolate *Y. enterocolitica* from foods were not able to recover low levels of clinical strains, because many clinical strains, including those of serotype O:8, are sensitive to selective agents commonly used in isolation procedures (Lee et al. 1980) or because of overgrowth by competing bacteria during several weeks of cold enrichment.

More recently, three approaches have been reported which appear to have potential in detecting small numbers of virulent *Y. enterocolitica* in foods. These include: (a) an enrichment-alkali (KOH) postenrichment treatment procedure, (b) a two-step enrichment procedure, and (c) a DNA colony hybridization procedure.

Enrichment-Alkali Postenrichment Treatment Procedure

The purpose of enrichment is to promote the growth of both small numbers and injured cells of *Y. enterocolitica* that may be present in food. To accomplish this, enrichment of food samples has generally been done in a nonselective medium, such as phosphate-buffered saline (PBS). To promote the growth of *Y. enterocolitica*, which is a psychrotroph, among other microbial competitors present in foods, enrichment cultures are often incubated for 2 to 4 weeks at 4°C. Although *Y. enterocolitica* generally grows well under these conditions, certain other competing microorganisms may also proliferate. Hence, a postenrichment medium or treatment is needed to select for *Y. enterocolitica*.

Aulisio et al. (1980) observed that many strains of *Y. enterocolitica* and *Yersinia pseudotuberculosis* are more tolerant to exposure to dilute alkali than most other *Enterobacteriaceae*. They subsequently used this principle to develop a postenrichment treatment to select for yersiniae, which involved exposing samples of cultures grown in enrichment broth to 0.5% potassium hydroxide (KOH) before plating onto selective agar. The treatment successfully eliminates most background contaminants and allows a fourfold increase in the recovery of *Y. enterocolitica*.

Doyle et al. (1981) confirmed the usefulness of the alkali postenrichment treatment procedure when they evaluated the efficacy of different procedures for detecting *Y. enterocolitica* on naturally contaminated porcine tongues. Cold enrichment of tongues in PBS followed by treatment with dilute KOH detected the most *Y. enterocolitica* [12 isolates; 5 were virulent (4 of serotype O:8 and 1 of serotype O:3)], whereas cold enrichment alone only recovered two isolates (1 was virulent; serotype O:8).

In contrast, Schiemann (1983a) and Ratnam et al. (1983) reported the alkali postenrichment treatment was not highly successful in recovering *Y. enterocolitica* from enrichments of inoculated foods or fecal specimens, respectively. In both studies, test specimens were exposed to 0.5% KOH for several minutes (ca. 5 min). This is too long. Doyle and Hugdahl (1983) determined the sensitivity of 22 different strains of *Y. enterocolitica* to different concentrations of KOH and found that only a 15-sec exposure to 0.5% KOH reduced the surviving population of *Y. enterocolitica* by an average of 1.5 $\log_{10}$, with a single, most sensitive strain experiencing an approximate 3-$\log_{10}$ decrease. A 4-min exposure to 0.5% KOH is generally too severe of a treatment for recovering many strains of *Y. enterocolitica*, hence a 15-sec exposure time is recommended.

Although enrichment of foods at 4°C for 2 to 4 weeks combined with a KOH postenrichment treatment is a successful technique for isolating virulent *Y. enterocolitica*, a 2- to 4-week cold enrichment procedure is not amenable to routine testing of foods. To improve upon this, Doyle and Hugdahl (1983) developed a 1- to 3-day enrichment-KOH postenrichment treatment procedure that is as effective in recovering *Y. enterocolitica* from meats as a cold enrichment-KOH postenrichment treatment procedure. The shortened procedure consists of enriching 1.0- and 25-gram samples of food in PBS at 25°C. After incubation (48 and 72 hr for 1.0-gram samples and 24 and 48 hr for 25-gram samples), 0.5-mL portions of enrichment culture are treated with 4.5 mL of 0.25% KOH for 2 min or 0.5% KOH for 15 sec, and 0.1-mL portions of treated culture are plated onto selective agar. In a study comparing *Y. enterocolitica*-isolation rates from naturally contaminated porcine tongues, the organism (including virulent strains of serotype O:5,27) was isolated from the tongues at similar rates by both shortened enrichment and cold enrichment procedures (Doyle and Hugdahl 1983).

Two-Step Enrichment Procedure

A two-step enrichment procedure, involving both a preenrichment and selective enrichment step, was developed and shown by Schiemann (1982) to be a promising method to recover *Y. enterocolitica* from foods. Schiemann evaluated several different combinations of preenrichment and selective enrichment media and conditions, and found that the enrichment system with the widest selectivity was preenrichment at 4°C with either phosphate-buffered saline for 14 days or yeast extract-rose bengal broth (YER) for 9 days followed by selective enrichment in bile-oxalate-sorbose broth (BOS) at 22°C for 5 days. Schiemann (1983b) later modified this procedure and recommended a shortened method which includes preenrichment in Trypticase soy broth at 22°C for 1 day and then at 2 to 4°C for 4 to 7 days followed by selective enrichment in BOS at 22°C for 3 to 5 days.

Strains of serotype O:5,27 do not grow well in BOS; however, for some unknown reason, the addition of 2.5% sodium chloride to BOS improves the growth of these strains (Schiemann 1982). Unfortunately, some strains of other serotypes, including O:3, are salt sensitive in this medium (Schiemann 1982). Hence, both types of BOS media (with and without 2.5% NaCl) must be used for detection of the different serotypes of virulent strains that may be present in foods.

DNA Colony Hybridization

Using a portion of the virulence plasmid (Zink et al. 1978) present in a pathogenic strain of *Y. enterocolitica* as a genetic probe, Hill et al. (1983) developed a DNA colony hybridization technique to detect virulent *Y. enterocolitica* in food. The procedure involves inoculating 0.1 mL of a particular dilution of food sample onto a sterile nitrocellulose filter that had been placed on plate count agar. The plates are incubated for 48 hr at 26°C, and the colonies are lysed by exposure to 0.5M NaOH. Filters are air-dried (30 min) then baked for 2 hr at 80°C.

For DNA hybridization, (^{32}P) radiolabeled DNA fragments are added to the filter and incubated for 18 hr at 37°C. Filters are then washed and allowed to dry overnight. Autoradiograms are made by exposing the filter to X-ray film for 1 to 3 days at −70°C. Using this procedure, Hill et al. (1983) were able to detect small numbers of a virulent strain of *Y. enterocolitica* in an inoculated homogenate of scallops. The DNA colony hybridization procedure can detect pathogenic *Y. enterocolitica* in foods without the need for enrichment.

Selective Isolation Media

Several selective isolation agar media have been used for isolating *Y. enterocolitica* from food homogenates or enrichment cultures; however, best isolation rates have generally been with cefsulodin-irgasan-novobiocin (CIN) (Devenish and Schiemann 1981; Schiemann 1979) and MacConkey agars (Doyle and Hugdahl 1983; Harmon et al. 1983; Mehlman et al. 1978). Many studies have shown the superiority of CIN agar in isolating *Y. enterocolitica* (Fossepre et al. 1983; Harmon et al. 1983; Helstad et al. 1983; Ratnam et al. 1983). Not only is this medium highly selective in restricting the growth of many background colonies, but *Y. enterocolitica* is easily differentiated because of the bacterium's distinctive colonial morphology. A typical colony of *Y. enterocolitica* develops on CIN agar as a dark red "bull's eye" surrounded by a transparent border. In contrast, MacConkey agar is less selective for *Y. enterocolitica* than CIN agar, and *Yersinia* colonies are not easily distinguished from other enterics that have the same nonpigmented to pinkish, smooth colonial morphology as *Y. enterocolitica*.

Doyle and Hugdahl (1983) compared the efficacy of CIN and MacConkey agars for isolating *Y. enterocolitica* from enrichment cultures of porcine tongues. They isolated the organism from 25 tongues 94 times by different combinations of enrichment-postenrichment treatments. Forty isolations were made from the same combinations of treatments by both CIN and MacConkey agars, 30 isolations were made only by MacConkey agar, and 24 were made only by CIN agar. Virulent strains (serotype O:5,27) were isolated from the same enrichment-postenrichment treatments by both media five times, eight times by MacConkey agar only, and four times by CIN agar only. Results of this study suggest that both media should be used in combination when attempting to isolate *Y. enterocolitica* from food enrichments.

Testing for Virulence

Several in vitro tests have been developed to differentiate virulent from avirulent strains of *Y. enterocolitica*. Examples include: (a) the presence of virulence-specific plasmids (40 to 48 and 82 megadaltons) (Kay et al. 1982; Zink et al. 1978, 1980), (b) calcium-dependent growth of virulent strains on magnesium oxalate agar at 37°C (Berche and Carter 1982; Brubaker 1983;

Gemski et al. 1980), (c) autoagglutination of virulent strains grown at 35–37°C in tissue culture medium (Laird and Cavanaugh 1980; Skurnik et al. 1984), (d) agglutination with a "virulence-specific" antiserum (WA-SAA) (Doyle et al. 1982), and (e) colony morphology on Trypticase soy agar when grown at 37°C for 24 hr (Lazere and Gemski, 1983). All of the above tests are useful for presumptively identifying strains that are virulent; however, studies by Kay et al. (1983) and Chang et al. (1984) comparing different tests for detecting virulent *Y. enterocolitica* revealed that the virulence potential of a *Y. enterocolitica* isolate cannot always be identified by these in vitro methods. There are apparent pathogenicity differences among many *Y. enterocolitica* strains likely because of differences in the virulence factors they possess. Hence no single current assay can definitively identify the virulence potential of all strains of *Y. enterocolitica*.

COLOHEMORRHAGIC *ESCHERICHIA COLI* (*E. COLI* O157:H7)

Escherichia coli O157:H7 has recently been associated with foodborne outbreaks of hemorrhagic colitis (Riley et al. 1983) and has been linked to cases of hemolytic uremic syndrome (Karmali et al. 1983). Ground beef has been implicated as a vehicle of transmission in foodborne outbreaks. The organism has been shown to produce a Vero cell cytotoxin (Johnson et al. 1983) and culture filtrate of *E. coli* O157:H7 produces colonic and renal lesions in mice following intraperitoneal or intravenous injection (Berry et al. 1984). The colonic hemorrhage produced in humans and mice by *E. coli* O157:H7 cultures and culture filtrates, respectively, is uniquely different from the syndromes produced by other types of known pathogenic *E. coli*.

E. coli O157:H7 is also different from most other *E. coli* in certain growth and physiological characteristics, hence many procedures commonly used to detect *E. coli* in foods will not detect *E. coli* O157:H7. For example, traditional detection procedures for *E. coli* in foods use an incubation temperature in the range of 44.5 to 45.5°C to select for the organism. *E. coli* O157:H7 does not grow well, if at all, within 48 hr in this temperature range (Doyle and Schoeni 1984). Additionally, the organism responds differently than most *E. coli* in a recently developed rapid fluorogenic assay which uses the compound 4-methylumbelliferone glucuronide (MUG) as an indicator to detect *E. coli* (Feng and Hartman, 1982). In this assay, MUG is hydrolyzed by glucuronidase, an enzyme present in most *E. coli* strains, to yield a fluorogenic product. All of the five *E. coli* O157:H7 strains tested were negative by this assay (Doyle and Schoeni 1984).

A property that may be useful in screening specimens for *E. coli* O157:H7 is the organism's inability to ferment sorbitol. Most (93%) strains of *E. coli* ferment sorbitol within 24 hr; however, *E. coli* O157:H7 does not (Johnson et al. 1983; Riley et al. 1983; Wells et al. 1983). This property has been used successfully to screen *E. coli* isolates from stool specimens to detect *E. coli* O157:H7 (Harris et al. 1985). The screening procedure involves transferring typical *E. coli* isolates obtained from standard enteric media to a medium composed of 1% sorbitol and Bacto-purple agar base. Sorbitol-negative isolates are confirmed as *E. coli* by biochemical tests and serotyped with O157- and H7-specific antisera. A limitation of this procedure is that 7% of *E. coli* of human origin do not ferment sorbitol, hence there are likely to be many sorbitol-negative isolates that are not *E. coli* O157:H7. This is indeed supported by the study of Harris et al. (1985) who found only two *E. coli* O157:H7 isolates in a total of 106 sorbitol-negative *E. coli* isolates obtained from stool specimens.

Because of the problems and limitations of presently available procedures for detecting *E. coli* O157:H7 in foods, better procedures for recovering this organism are needed.

VIBRIO PARAHAEMOLYTICUS

Special consideration should be given to two characteristics of *V. parahaemolyticus* for its successful isolation from seafoods. These include: (a) the organism's sensitivity to cold stress (Clark 1977; Johnson and Liston 1973; Lamprecht 1980; Ma-Lin and Beuchat 1980; Matches et al. 1971) and (b) its halophilic growth and survival requirement (Lee 1972). To avoid cold stress, samples should be assayed as soon as possible after receipt, and preferably should not be frozen (Lamprecht 1980; Matches et al. 1971). If samples are to be stored, they should be held under moderate refrigeration (ca. 10°C) to reduce the tendency for overgrowth of *V. parahemolyticus* by indigenous microflora (Twedt et al. 1984). Because of the organism's growth requirement for sodium chloride, culture media should contain NaCl, usually about 3%. Additionally, because of osmotic fragility, *V. parahaemolyticus* cells are readily inactivated in distilled water (Lee 1972), hence all diluents should also contain 2 to 3% NaCl.

Preenrichment of samples in a nonselective medium has been recommended for detecting injured *V. parahaemolyticus* in refrigerated or frozen seafood (Ray et al. 1978). Such samples are first cultured overnight at 35°C in Trypticase soy broth containing 3% NaCl and then transferred to a selective medium, such as glucose salt Teepol broth, for selective enrichment (overnight, 35°C) (Twedt et al. 1984). When one is not concerned about detecting injured cells of *V. parahaemolyticus*, food specimens are inoculated directly into selective enrichment medium. Following enrichment, cultures are streaked onto thiosulfate citrate bile salts sucrose (TCBS) agar (Kobayashi et al. 1963) for isolation of typical colonies of *V. parahaemolyticus*. This medium inhibits most of the other bacterial species comprising the fecal flora primarily because of the presence of bile salts and the highly alkaline pH of 8.6 (Joseph et al. 1982). *V. parahaemolyticus* grows extremely well at pH 8.6, which is within the organism's optimal pH range for growth. Good differentiation of *Vibrio* species is provided by the sucrose reaction. *Vibrio cholerae* and *Vibrio alginolyticus* ferment sucrose, producing yellow colonies indicated by a color change in the brom thymol blue and thymol blue included in the medium. *V. parahaemolyticus* does not ferment sucrose on TCBS agar and hence produces a bluish or blue-green colony. Isolates are confirmed by biochemical and serological tests which have been described by Twedt et al. (1984). Generally, a most probable number determination is done on food samples using the above cultural procedures to enumerate the organism.

The Kanagawa phenomenon is generally used as an indicator of pathogenicity of *V. parahaemolyticus* isolates. The Kanagawa reaction tests for a specific heat stable hemolysin that is detected on a special high-salt human blood agar formulated by Wagatsuma (1968). A positive Kanagawa reaction is indicated by β-hemolysis in the medium in less than 24 hr when incubated at 35°C. A positive reaction correlates closely with pathogenicity of *V. parahaemolyticus*, as indicated by the studies of Sakazaki et al. (1968) who reported that 96.5% (2655 out of 2720) of strains isolated from human patients was Kanagawa-positive. In contrast, isolates recovered from seafoods are almost always (<1 to 2%) Kanagawa-negative (Ayres and Barrow 1978; Bockemuhl and Triemer 1974; Sakazaki et al. 1968; Sutton 1974).

VIBRIO CHOLERAE

A good selective enrichment broth has not been developed for *V. cholerae*. However, the organism grows best in an alkaline medium, hence this property is used to advantage in most isolation procedures for *V. cholerae*. Alkaline peptone water (APW) provides suitable enrichment at 35°C for incubation periods of 6 to 8 hours, but other competing microflora may overgrow *V. cholerae* during longer enrichment periods (Bushnell 1984). Bushnell (1984), in a comprehensive study, compared different enrichment procedures currently used for isolating *V. cholerae* from food. He found APW to be as good or, in most instances, better than the eight other broths evaluated in isolating the organism from oysters. However, he did note that all broths would have given better recovery of *V. cholerae* if they had been more selective because all of the broths supported luxuriant growth of the natural flora of oysters. Hence, a better, more selective enrichment medium is needed.

Several selective plating media have been used for isolating *V. cholerae* following enrichment (Bushnell 1984); however, the three media generally recommended are TCBS agar, gelatin agar, and gelatin phosphate salt (GPS) agar (Madden et al. 1984; Twedt et al. 1984). TCBS agar is a selective medium, whereas gelatin agar and GPS agar are nonselective media. *V. cholerae* will typically appear as large yellow (sometimes green if they are late sucrose fermenters) colonies on TCBS or as transparent colonies surrounded by a cloudy ring on gelatin or GPS agars. Rennels et al. (1980) compared the efficacy of TCBS agar with gelatin agar for detecting *V. cholerae* in stool specimens by direct plating and, in some instances, following enrichment, and found TCBS agar detected 99% of *V. cholerae*-positive stools, whereas gelatin agar identified only 80%. Similarly, Bushnell (1984) reported TCBS agar to be reliable in isolating *V. cholerae* from oysters following enrichment. Hence, TCBS agar should be one of at least two plating media for isolating *V. cholerae* from foods (Twedt et al. 1984).

Colonies typical of *V. cholerae* on agar plates are confirmed by biochemical and serological tests, and biotyped (Madden et al. 1984; Twedt et al. 1984).

Cholera Toxin Detection

Many different procedures may be used to test confirmed isolates of *V. cholerae* for their ability to produce enterotoxin or cytotoxin (Lai 1980). Tissue culture assays using Y-1 mouse adrenal cells (Madden et al. 1984; Sack and Sack 1975) or Chinese hamster ovary cells (Guerrant et al. 1974) are typically used for detection of toxin. Monolayers of the tissue culture cells are prepared in microtiter plates and culture filtrates of *V. cholerae* isolates are applied to cells. After overnight incubation, cells are examined microscopically for morphologic changes. If cholera enterotoxin is present, Y-1 mouse adrenal cells round up, whereas Chinese hamster ovary cells elongate. If cholera cytotoxin is present, Y-1 mouse adrenal cells are killed, lysed, and often detached from the microtiter plate (Madden et al. 1984). Each toxin may also be detected with antisera specific for the toxin by an enzyme-linked immunosorbent assay or radioimmunoassay (Madden et al. 1984; Twedt et al. 1984).

CONCLUSION

Within the past 3 to 5 years, substantial progress has been made in perfecting methods to detect many of the gram-negative bacterial pathogens associated with foods; however, additional improvements are still needed. There is a continuing need for more rapid, sensitive tests to detect these pathogens as well as their virulence-specific properties which may be used to differentiate pathogenic from nonpathogenic strains. For many of the gram-negative pathogens, such as *C. jejuni*, additional research is needed to identify virulence factors responsible for pathogenicity. There is little doubt that with the technology to prepare antigen-specific monoclonal antibodies and pathogen-specific gene probes, and the likelihood of additional major technological advances in developing means to detect virulent microorganisms, procedures for detecting pathogens in foods will continue to evolve to more rapid, simple, and reliable tests.

REFERENCES

ACUFF, G. R., VANDERZANT, C., GARDNER, F. A., and GOLAN, F. A. 1982. Evaluation of an enrichment-plating procedure for recovery of *Campylobacter jejuni* from turkey eggs and meat. *J. Food Prot.* 45: 1276–1278.

ANDREWS, W. H. 1985. A review of culture methods and their relation to rapid methods for the detection of *Salmonella* in foods. *Food Technol.* 39(3): 77–82.

ANDREWS, W. H., POELMA, P. L., and WILSON, C. R. 1984. Isolation and identification of *Salmonella* species. In *Bacteriological Analytical Manual.* 6th ed. Association of Official Analytical Chemists, Arlington, VA.

ANDREWS, W. H., WILSON, C. R., and POELMA, P. L. 1983. Improved *Salmonella* species recovery from nonfat dry milk pre-enriched under reduced rehydration. *J. Food Sci.* 48: 1162–1165.

AULISIO, C. C. G., MEHLMAN, I. J., and SANDERS, A. C. 1980. Alkali method for recovery of *Yersinia enterocolitica* and *Yersinia pseudotuberculosis* from foods. *Appl. Environ. Microbiol.* 39: 135–140.

AYRES, P. A. and BARROW, G. I. 1978. The distribution of *Vibrio parahaemolyticus* in British coastal waters: report of a collaborative study 1975–1976. *J. Hyg.* 80: 281–294.

BAROT, M. S. and BOKKENHEUSER, V. D. 1984. Systematic investigation of enrichment media for wild-type *Campylobacter jejuni* strains. *J. Clin. Microbiol.* 20: 77–80.

BERRY, J. T., DOYLE, M. P., and HIGLEY, N. A. 1984. Cytotoxic activity of *Escherichia coli* O157:H7 culture filtrate on the mouse colon and kidney. *Curr. Microbiol.* 11: 335–342.

BERCHE, P. A. and CARTER, P. B. 1982. Calcium requirement and virulence of *Yersinia enterocolitica*. *J. Med. Microbiol.* 15: 277–284.

BILLINGHAM, J. D. 1981. A comparison of two media for the isolation of *Campylobacter* in the tropics. *Trans. Roy. Soc. Trop. Med. Hyg.* 75: 645–646.

BLANKENSHIP, L. C., CRAVEN, S. E., CHIU, J. Y., and KRUMM, G. W. 1983. Sampling methods and frozen storage of samples for detection of *Campylobacter jejuni* on freshly processed broiler carcasses. *J. Food Prot.* 46: 510–513.

BLASER, M. J., BERKOWITZ, I. D., LAFORCE, F. M., CRAVENS, J., RELLER, L. B., and WANG, W.-L. W. 1979. Campylobacter enteritis: clinical and epidemiologic features. *Ann. Intern. Med.* 91: 179–185.

BOCKEMUHL, J. and TRIEMER, A. 1974. Ecology and epidemiology of *Vibrio parahaemolyticus* on the coast of Logo. *Bull. Wld. Hlth. Org.* 51: 353–360.

BOLTON, F. J. and COATES, D. 1983. A comparison of microaerobic systems for the culture of *Campylobacter jejuni* and *Campylobacter coli.* *Eur. J. Clin. Microbiol.* 2: 105–110.

BOLTON, F. J., COATES, D., HINCHLIFFE, P. M., and ROBERTSON, L. 1983. Comparison of selective media for isolation of *Campylobacter jejuni/coli.* *J. Clin. Pathol.* 36: 78–83.

BOLTON, F. J., HUTCHINSON, D. N., and COATES, D. 1984. Blood-free selective medium for isolation of *Campylobacter jejuni* from feces. *J. Clin. Microbiol.* 19: 169–171.

BOLTON, F. J. and ROBERTSON, L. 1982. A selective medium for isolating *Campylobacter jejuni/coli.* *J. Clin. Pathol.* 35: 462–467.

BRUBAKER, R. R. 1983. The Vwa$^+$ virulence factor of yersiniae: the molecular basis of the attendant nutritional requirement for Ca^{++}. *Rev. Infect. Dis.* 5: S748–S758.

BUSHNELL, R. 1984. Evaluation of media for the isolation of *Vibrio cholerae* from food. *Food Technol. Aust.* 36: 223–226.

BUTZLER, J.-P., DEBOECK, M., and GOOSSENS, H. 1983. New selective medium for isolation of *Campylobacter jejuni* from faecal specimens. *Lancet* i: 818.

CHANG, M. T., SCHINK, J., SHIMOAKA, J., and DOYLE, M. P. 1984. Comparison of three tests for virulent *Yersinia enterocolitica.* *J. Clin. Microbiol.* 20: 589–591.

CHRISTOPHER, F. M., SMITH, G. C., and VANDERZANT, C. 1982. Examination of poultry giblets, raw milk and meat for *Campylobacter fetus* subsp. *jejuni.* *J. Food Prot.* 45: 260–262.

CLARK, A. G. 1977. Survival of *Vibrio parahaemolyticus* after chilling in transport media: an explanation for divergent findings. *Appl. Environ. Microbiol.* 34: 597–599.

D'AOUST, J.-Y. 1981. Update on preenrichment and selective enrichment conditions for detection of *Salmonella* in foods. *J. Food Prot.* 44: 369–374.

D'AOUST, J.-Y. 1984a. *Salmonella* detection in foods: present status and research needs for the future. *J. Food Prot.* 47: 78–81.

D'AOUST, J.-Y. 1984b. Effective enrichment-plating conditions for detection of *Salmonella* in foods. *J. Food Prot.* 47: 588–590.

D'AOUST, J.-Y., BECKERS, H. J., BOOTHROYD, M., MATES, A., McKEE, C. R., MORAN, A. B., SADO, P., SPAIN, G. E., SPERBER, W. H., BASSILIADIS, P., WAGNER, D. E., and WIBERT, C. 1983. ICMSF methods studies. XIV. Comparative study on recovery of *Salmonella* from refrigerated preenrichment and enrichment broth cultures. *J. Food Prot.* 46: 391–399.

D'AOUST, J.-Y. and MAISHMENT, C. 1979. Preenrichment conditions for effective recovery of *Salmonella* in foods and feed ingredients. *J. Food Prot.* 42: 153–157.

DEVENISH, J. A. and SCHIEMANN, D. A. 1981. An abbreviated scheme for identification of *Yersinia enterocolitica* isolated from food enrichments on CIN (cefsulodin-irgasan-novobiocin) agar. *Can. J. Microbiol.* 27: 937–941.

DOYLE, M. P. 1984a. Association of *Campylobacter jejuni* with laying hens and eggs. *Appl. Environ. Microbiol.* 47: 533–536.

DOYLE, M. P. 1984b. *Campylobacter* in foods. pp. 163–180. In *Campylobacter Infection in Man and Animals*. Butzler, J.-P. (Ed.). CRC Press, Boca Raton, FL.

DOYLE, M. P. and HUGDAHL, M. B. 1983. Improved procedure for recovery of *Yersinia enterocolitica* from meats. *Appl. Environ. Microbiol.* 45: 127–135.

DOYLE, M. P., HUGDAHL, M. B., CHANG, M. T., and BERRY, J. T. 1982. Serological relatedness of mouse-virulent *Yersinia enterocolitica*. *Infect. Immun.* 37: 1234–1240.

DOYLE, M. P., HUGDAHL, M. B., and TAYLOR, S. L. 1981. Isolation of virulent *Yersinia enterocolitica* from porcine tongues. *Appl. Environ. Microbiol.* 42: 661–666.

DOYLE, M. P. and ROMAN, D. J. 1982a. Prevalence and survival of *Campylobacter jejuni* in unpasteurized milk. *Appl. Environ. Microbiol.* 44: 1154–1158.

DOYLE, M. P. and ROMAN, D. J. 1982b. Recovery of *Campylobacter jejuni* and *Campylobacter coli* from inoculated foods by selective enrichment. *Appl. Environ. Microbiol.* 43: 1343–1353.

DOYLE, M. P. and SCHOENI, J. L. 1984. Survival and growth characteristics of *Escherichia coli* associated with hemorrhagic colitis. *Appl. Environ. Microbiol.* 48: 855–856.

EDEL, W. and KAMPELMACHER, E. H. 1973. Comparative studies on the isolation of "sublethally injured" salmonellae in nine European laboratories. *Bull. Wld. Hlth. Org.* 48: 167–174.

ENTIS, P., BRODSKY, M. H., SHARPE, A. N., and JARVIS, G. A. 1982. Rapid detection of *Salmonella* spp. in food by use of the ISO-GRID hydrophobic grid membrane filter. *Appl. Environ. Microbiol.* 43: 261–268.

FAGERBERG, D. J. and AVENS, J. S. 1976. Enrichment and plating methodology for *Salmonella* detection in food. A review. *J. Food Technol.* 39: 628–646.

FENG, P. C. S. and HARTMAN, P. A. 1982. Fluorogenic assays for immediate confirmation of *Escherichia coli*. *Appl. Environ. Microbiol.* 43: 1320–1329.

FITTS, R. 1985. Development of a DNA-DNA hybridization test for the presence of *Salmonella* in foods. *Food Technol.* 39(3): 95–102.

FITTS, R., DIAMOND, M., HAMILTON, C., and NERI, M. 1983. DNA-DNA hybridization assay for detection of *Salmonella* spp. in foods. *Appl. Environ. Microbiol.* 46: 1146–1151.

FLOWERS, R. S. 1985. Comparison of rapid *Salmonella* screening methods and the conventional culture method. *Food Technol.* 39(3): 103–108.

FOSSEPRE, J. M., LOGGHE, G. N., DECLERCQ, P. R., and VANLANDUYT, H. W. 1983. Evaluation of 4 different methods for the isolation of *Yersinia enterocolitica* from faeces. *Abstr. Annu. Meet. Am. Soc. Microbiol.*, C153, p. 337.

FRICKER, C. R. 1984. Procedures for the isolation of *Campylobacter jejuni* and *Campylobacter coli* from poultry. *Intl. J. Food Microbiol.* 1: 149–154.

GARCIA, M. M., LIOR, H., STEWART, R. B., RUCKERBAUER, G. M., TRUDEL, J. R. R., and SKLJAREVSKI, A. 1985. Isolation, characterization, and serotyping of *Campylobacter jejuni* and *Campylobacter coli* from slaughter cattle. *Appl. Environ. Microbiol.* 49: 667–672.

GEMSKI, P., LAZERE, J. R., and CASEY, T. 1980. Plasmid associated with pathogenicity and calcium dependency of *Yersinia enterocolitica*. *Infect. Immun.* 27: 682–685.

GOOSSENS, H., DEBOECK, M., and BUTZLER, J.-P. 1983. A new selective medium for the isolation of *Campylobacter jejuni* from human feces. *Eur. J. Clin. Microbiol.* 2: 389–394.

GUERRANT, R. L., BRUNTON, L. L., SCHNAITMAN, T. C., REBHUN, L. I., and GILMAN, A. G. 1974. Cyclic adenosine monophosphate and alteration of Chinese hamster ovary cell morphology: a rapid, sensitive *in vitro* assay for the enterotoxins of *Vibrio cholerae* and *Escherichia coli*. *Infect. Immun.* 10: 320–327.

HÄNNINEN, M.-L. 1982. Comparison of four enrichment media in the recovery of *Campylobacter jejuni*. *Acta Vet. Scand.* 23: 425–437.

HARMON, M. C., YU, C. L., and SWAMINATHAN, B. 1983. An evaluation of selective differential plating media for the isolation of *Yersinia enterocolitica* from experimentally inoculated fresh ground pork homogenate. *J. Food Sci.* 48: 6–9.

HARRIS, A. A., KAPLAN, R. L., GOODMAN, L. J., DOYLE, M., LANDAU, W., SEGRETI, J., MAYER, K., and LEVIN, S. 1985. Results of a twelve month stool survey for *Escherichia coli* O157:H7-use of a screening method. *J. Infect. Dis.* 152:775–777.

HEISICK, J., LANIER, J., and PEELER, J. T. 1984. Comparison of enrichment methods and atmosphere modification procedures for isolating *Campylobacter jejuni* from foods. *Appl. Environ. Microbiol.* 48: 1254–1255.

HELSTAD, A. G., CHRISTENSON, E., DODGE, L., and ARCHER, J. 1983. Comparison of three agar media for the isolation of *Yersinia* from human fecal specimens. *Abstr. Annu. Meet. Am. Soc. Microbiol.* C152, p. 337.

HILL, W. E., PAYNE, W. L., and AULISIO, C. C. G. 1983. Detection and enumeration of virulent *Yersinia enterocolitica* in food by DNA colony hybridization. *Appl. Environ. Microbiol.* 46: 636–641.

JOHNSON, H. C. and LISTON, J. 1973. Sensitivity of *Vibrio parahaemolyticus* to cold in oysters, fish fillets and crabmeat. *J. Food Sci.* 38: 437–441.

JOHNSON, W. M., LIOR, H., and BEZANSON, G. S. 1983. Cytotoxic *Escherichia coli* O157:H7 associated with haemorrhagic colitis in Canada. *Lancet* i: 76.

JOSEPH, S. W., COLWELL, R. R., and KAPER, J. B. 1982. *Vibrio parahaemolyticus* and related halophilic vibrios. *CRC Rev. Microbiol.* 10: 77–124.

KAFEL, S. and BRYAN, F. L. 1977. Effects of enrichment media and incubation conditions on isolating salmonellae from ground-meat filtrate. *Appl. Environ. Microbiol.* 34: 285–291.

KARMALI, M. A., PETRIC, M., STEELE, B. T., and LIM, C. 1983. Sporadic cases of haemolytic-uraemic syndrome associated with faecal cytotoxin and cytotoxin-producing *Escherichia coli* in stools. *Lancet* i: 619–620.

KAY, B. A., WACHSMUTH, K., and GEMSKI, P. 1982. New virulence-associated plasmid in *Yersinia enterocolitica*. *J. Clin. Microbiol.* 15: 1161–1163.

KAY, B. A., WACHSMUTH, K., GEMSKI, P., FEELEY, J. C., QUAN, T. J., and BRENNER, D. J. 1983. Virulence and phenotypic characterization of *Yersinia enterocolitica* isolated from humans in the United States. *J. Clin. Microbiol.* 17: 128–138.

KOBAYASHI, T., ENOMOTO, S., SAKAZAKI, R., and KUWABARA, S. 1963. A new selective isolation medium for pathogenic vibrios: TCBS agar. *Jpn. J. Bacteriol.* 18: 387–391.

KOIDIS, P. and DOYLE, M. P. 1983. Survival of *Campylobacter jejuni* in the presence of bisulfite and different atmospheres. *Eur. J. Clin. Microbiol.* 2: 384–388.

KOIDIS, P. and DOYLE, M. P. 1984. Procedure for increased recovery of *Campylobacter jejuni* from inoculated unpasteurized milk. *Appl. Environ. Microbiol.* 47: 455–460.

LAI, C.-Y. 1980. The chemistry and biology of cholera toxin. *CRC Rev. Biochem.* 9: 171–206.

LAIRD, W. J. and CAVANAUGH, D. C. 1980. Correlation of autoagglutination and virulence of yersiniae. *J. Clin. Microbiol.* 11: 430–432.

LAMPRECHT, E. C. 1980. Survival of *Vibrio parahaemolyticus* during freezing. *J. Sci. Food Agr.* 31: 1309–1312.

LANDER, K. P. 1982. A selective, enrichment and transport medium for campylobacters. p. 77. In *Campylobacter-Epidemiology, Pathogenesis and Biochemistry*. Newell, D. G. (Ed.). MTP Press Ltd, Lancaster, England.

LAUWERS, S., DEBOECK, M., and BUTZLER, J.-P. 1978. Campylobacter enteritis in Brussels. *Lancet* i: 604–605.

LAZERE, J. R. and GEMSKI, P. 1983. Association of colony morphology with virulence of *Yersinia enterocolitica*. *FEMS Microbiol. Lett.* 17: 121–126.

LEE, J. S. 1972. Inactivation of *Vibrio parahaemolyticus* in distilled water. *Appl. Microbiol.* 23: 166–167.

LEE, W. H., HARRIS, M. E., MCCLAIN, D., SMITH, R. E., and JOHNSTON, R. W. 1980. Two modified selenite media for the recovery of *Yersinia enterocolitica* from meats. *Appl. Environ. Microbiol.* 39: 205–209.

LOVETT, J., FRANCIS, D. W., and HUNT, J. M. 1983. Isolation of *Campylobacter jejuni* from raw milk. *Appl. Environ. Microbiol.* 46: 459–462.

MADDEN, J. M., McCARDELL, B. A., and BOUTIN, B. K. 1984. Isolation and identification of *Vibrio cholerae*. In *Bacteriological Analytical Manual*. 6th ed. Association of Official Analytical Chemists, Arlington, VA.

MA-LIN, C. F. A. and BEUCHAT, L. R. 1980. Recovery of chill-stressed *Vibrio parahaemolyticus* from oysters with enrichment broths supplemented with magnesium and iron salts. *Appl. Environ. Microbiol.* 39: 179–185.

MARTIN, W. T., PATTON, C. M., MORRIS, G. K., POTTER, M. E., and PUHR, N. D. 1983. Selective enrichment broth medium for isolation of *Campylobacter jejuni*. *J. Clin. Microbiol.* 17: 853–855.

MATCHES, J. R., LISTON, J. and DANEAULT, L. P. 1971. Survival of *Vibrio parahaemolyticus* in fish homogenate during storage at low temperatures. *Appl. Microbiol.* 21: 951–952.

MATTINGLY, J. A. 1984. An enzyme immunoassay for the detection of all *Salmonella* using a combination of a myeloma protein and a hybridoma antibody. *J. Immunol. Meth.* 73: 147–156.

MATTINGLY, J. A. and GEHLE, W. D. 1984. An improved enzyme immunoassay for the detection of *Salmonella*. *J. Food Sci.* 49: 807–809.

MATTINGLY, J. A., ROBISON, B. A., BOEHM, A., and GEHLE, W. D. 1985. Use of monoclonal antibodies for the detection of *Salmonella* in foods. *Food Technol.* 39(3): 90–94.

McCOY, J. H. 1962. The isolation of salmonellae. *J. Appl. Bacteriol.* 25: 213–224.

MEHLMAN, I. J., AULISIO, C. C. G., and SANDERS, A. C. 1978. Problems in the recovery and identification of *Yersinia* from food. *J. Assoc. Off. Anal. Chem.* 61: 761–771.

MORRIS, G. K. and DUNN, C. G. 1970. Influence of incubation temperature and sodium heptadecylsulfate (Tergitol No. 7) on the isolation of salmonellae from pork sausage. *Appl. Microbiol.* 20: 192–195.

PARK, C. E., STANKIEWICZ, Z. K., LOVETT, J., and HUNT, J. 1981. Incidence of *Campylobacter jejuni* in fresh eviscerated whole market chickens. *Can. J. Microbiol.* 27: 841–842.

PARK, C. E., STANKIEWICZ, Z. K., LOVETT, J., HUNT, J., and FRANCIS, D. W. 1983. Effect of temperature, duration of incubation, and pH of enrichment culture on recovery of *Campylobacter jejuni* from eviscerated market chickens. *Can. J. Microbiol.* 19: 803–806.

PATTON, C. M., MITCHELL, S. W., POTTER, M. E., and KAUFMANN, A. F. 1981. Comparison of selective media for primary isolation of *Campylobacter fetus* subsp. *jejuni*. *J. Clin. Microbiol.* 13: 326–330.

POELMA, P. L., ANDREWS, W. H., and SILLIKER, J. H. 1984. *Salmonella*. In *Compendium of Methods for the Microbiological Examination of Foods*. 2nd ed. Speck, M. L. (Ed.). American Public Health Association, Washington, DC.

POELMA, P. L., ANDREWS, W. H., and WILSON, C. R. 1981. Comparison of methods for the isolation of *Salmonella* species from lactic casein. *J. Food Sci.* 46: 804–809.

RAPPOLD, H., BOLDERDIJK, R. F., and DE SMEDT, J. M. 1984. Rapid cultural method to detect *Salmonella* in foods. *J. Food Prot.* 47: 46–48.

RATNAM, S., LOOI, C. L., and PATEL, T. R. 1983. Lack of efficacy of alkali treatment for isolation of *Yersinia enterocolitica* from feces. *J. Clin. Microbiol.* 18: 1092–1097.

RAY, B., HAWKINS, S. M., and HACKNEY, C. R. 1978. Method for the detection of injured *Vibrio parahaemolyticus* in seafoods. *Appl. Environ. Microbiol.* 35: 1121–1127.

RENNELS, M. B., LEVINE, M. M., DAYA, V., ANGLE, P., and YOUNG, C. 1980. Selective vs. nonselective media and direct plating vs. enrichment technique in isolation of *Vibrio cholerae:* recommendations for clinical laboratories. *J. Infect. Dis.* 142: 328–331.

RILEY, L. W., REMIS, R. S., HELGERSON, S. D., MCGEE, H. B., WELLS, J. G., DAVIS, B. R., HEBERT, R. J., OLCOTT, E. S., JOHNSON, L. M., HARGETT, N. T., BLAKE, P. A., and COHEN, M. L. 1983. Hemorrhagic colitis associated with a rare *Escherichia coli* serotype. *N. Engl. J. Med.* 308: 681–685.

ROBISON, B. J. and FLOWERS, R. S. 1985. Optimization of selective enrichment conditions for detection of salmonellae by enzyme immunoassay. *Abst. Annu. Meet. Am. Soc. Microbiol.* P32, p. 256.

ROSEF, O. 1981. Isolation of *Campylobacter fetus* subsp. *jejuni* from the gallbladder of normal slaughter pigs, using an enrichment procedure. *Acta Vet. Scand.* 22: 149–151.

ROSEF, O. and KAPPERUD, G. 1983. House flies (*Musca domestica*) as possible vectors of *Campylobacter fetus* subsp. *jejuni. Appl. Environ. Microbiol.* 45: 381–383.

ROTHENBERG, P. J., STERN, N. J., and WESTHOFF, D. C. 1984. Selected enrichment broths for recovery of *Campylobacter jejuni* from foods. *Appl. Environ. Microbiol.* 48: 78–80.

SACK, D. A. and SACK, R. B. 1975. Test for enterotoxigenic *Escherichia coli* using Y1 adrenal cells in miniculture. *Infect. Immun.* 11: 334–336.

SAKAZAKI, R., TAMURA, K., KATO, T., OBARA, Y., YAMAI, S., and HOBO, K. 1968. Studies on the enteropathogenic, facultatively halophilic bacteria, *Vibrio parahaemolyticus.* III. Enteropathogenicity. *Jpn. J. Med. Sci. Biol.* 21: 325–331.

SCHIEMANN, D. A. 1979. Synthesis of a selective agar medium for *Yersinia enterocolitica. Can. J. Microbiol.* 25: 1298–1304.

SCHIEMANN, D. A. 1982. Development of a two-step enrichment procedure for recovery of *Yersinia enterocolitica* from food. *Appl. Environ. Microbiol.* 43: 14–27.

SCHIEMANN, D. A. 1983a. Alkalotolerance of *Yersinia enterocolitica* as a basis for selective isolation from food enrichments. *Appl. Environ. Microbiol.* 46: 22–27.

SCHIEMANN, D. A. 1983b. Comparison of enrichment and plating media for recovery of virulent strains of *Yersinia enterocolitica* from inoculated beef stew. *J. Food Prot.* 46: 957–964.

SILLIKER, J. H. and GABIS, D. A. 1974. ICMSF method studies. V. The influence of selective enrichment media and incubation temperatures on the detection of salmonellae in raw frozen meats. *Can. J. Microbiol.* 20: 813–816.

SKIRROW, M. B. 1977. Campylobacter enteritis: a "new" disease. *Br. Med. J.* 2: 9–11.

SKURNIK, M., BÖLIN, I., HEIKKINEN, H., PIHA, S., and WOLF-WATZ, H. 1984. Virulence plasmid-associated autoagglutination in *Yersinia* spp. *J. Bacteriol.* 158: 1033–1036.

STERN, N. J. 1982. Selectivity and sensitivity of three media for recovery of inoculated *Campylobacter fetus* subsp. *jejuni* from ground beef. *J. Food Safety* 4: 169–175.

STERN, N. J., HERNANDEZ, M. P., BLANKENSHIP, L., DEIBEL, K. E., DOORES, S., DOYLE, M. P., NG, H., PIERSON, M. D., SOFOS, J. N., SVEUM, W. H., and WESTHOFF, D. C. 1985. Prevalence and distribution of *Campylobacter jejuni* and *Campylobacter coli* in retail meats. *J. Food Prot.* 48: 595–599.

STERN, N. J. and KOTULA, A. W. 1982. Survival of *Campylobacter jejuni* inoculated into ground beef. *Appl. Environ. Microbiol.* 44: 1150–1153.

SUTTON, R. G. A. 1974. Some quantitative aspects of *Vibrio parahaemolyticus* in oysters in the Sydney area. In *International Symposium on Vibrio parahaemolyticus*. Fujino, T., Sakaguchi, G., Sakazaki, R., and Takeda, Y. (Ed.). Saikon Publishing Co., Tokyo.

SWAMINATHAN, B., ALEIXO, J. A. G., and MINNICH, S. A. 1985. Enzyme immunoassays for *Salmonella*: one-day testing is now a reality. *Food Technol.* 39(3): 83–89.

TANNER, E. I. and BULLIN, C. H. 1977. Campylobacter enteritis. *Br. Med. J.* 2: 579.

TWEDT, R. M., MADDEN, J. M., and COLWELL, R. R. 1984. *Vibrio*. In *Compendium of Methods for the Microbiological Examination of Foods*. Speck, M. L. (Ed.). American Public Health Association, Washington, DC.

USDA. 1974. *Microbiology Laboratory Guidebook*. Animal and Plant Health Inspection Service, U.S. Dept. of Agric., Washington, DC.

VAN SCHOTHORST, M. and VAN LEUSDEN, F. M. 1972. Studies on the isolation of injured salmonellae from foods. *Zbl. Bakteriol. Hyg. I. Abt. Orig. A* 221: 19–29.

VAN SCHOTHORST, M. and VAN LEUSDEN, F. M. 1975. Comparison of several methods for the isolation of salmonellae from egg products. *Can. J. Microbiol.* 21: 1041–1045.

VAN SCHOTHORST, M., VAN LEUSDEN, F. M., DEGIER, E., RIJNIERSE, V. F. M., and VEEN, A. J. D. 1979. Influence of reconstitution on isolation of *Salmonella* from dried milk. *J. Food Prot.* 42: 936–937.

VASSILIADIS, P., TRICHOPOULOS, D., PAPADAKIS, J., KALAPO-THAKI, V., ZAVITSANOS, X., and SERIE, C. 1981. *Salmonella* isolation with Rappaport's enrichment medium of different compositions. *Zbl. Bakteriol. Mikrobiol. Hyg. I. Abt. Orig. B* 173: 382–389.

WAGATSUMA, S. 1968. A medium for the test of the hemolytic activity of *Vibrio parahaemolyticus. Media Circle* 13: 159–161.

WEBER, A., LEMBKE, C., SCHÄFER, R., and BERGMANN, I. 1983. Vergleichende Anwendung von zwei Selektivnährböden zur Isolierung von *Campylobacter jejuni* aus Kotproben von Tieren. *Zbl. Vet. Med. B* 30: 175–179.

WELLS, J. G., DAVIS, B. R., WACHSMUTH, I. K., RILEY, L. W., REMIS, R. S., SIKOLOW, R., and MORRIS, G. K. 1983. Laboratory investigation of hemorrhagic colitis associated with a rare *Escherichia coli* serotype. *J. Clin. Microbiol.* 18: 512–520.

WESLEY, R. D., SWAMINATHAN, B., and STADELMAN, W. J. 1983. Isolation and enumeration of *Campylobacter jejuni* from poultry products by a selective enrichment method. *Appl. Environ. Microbiol.* 46: 1097–1102.

ZINK, D. L., FEELEY, J. C., VANDERZANT, C., VICKERY, J. C., and O'DONOVAN, G. A. 1978. Possible plasmid-mediated virulence in *Yersinia enterocolitica. Trans. Gulf Coast Mol. Biol. Conf.* 3: 156–163.

ZINK, D. L., FEELEY, J. C., WELLS, J. G., VANDERZANT, C., VICKERY, J. C., ROOF, W. D., and O'DONOVAN, G. A. 1980. Plasmid-mediated tissue invasiveness in *Yersinia enterocolitica. Nature* 283: 224–226.

16

Detection and Quantitation of Gram-Positive Nonsporeforming Pathogens and Their Toxins

R. W. Bennett

Food and Drug Administration
Washington, D.C.

INTRODUCTION

Essential in the diagnosis of foodborne illnesses are meaningful interviews with the victims, and the gathering and analyzing of epidemiologic data. Incriminated foods should be collected correctly and examined by effective laboratory methods. The proper choice of methods for the detection and quantitation of the suspect pathogens depends, in part, on the epidemiologic findings. Three foodborne pathogens, *Staphylococcus aureus*, *Streptococcus* (enterococci), and *Listeria monocytogenes*, exhibit vastly different characteristics in causing human illness as well as requirements for their recovery, isolation, and identification.

SOME ASPECTS OF PATHOGENS

Bacterial foodborne illness can be classified into two types: intoxications caused by the ingestion of food containing preformed toxin due to bacterial growth in the food, and foodborne infections caused by the ingestion of food containing viable bacteria that establish themselves in the host, grow, and cause pathological problems. Species of *Salmonella* and *Shigella*, which the host acquires by ingesting contaminated food, are examples of organisms that cause foodborne illness of the infection type. Botulism and staphylococcal enterotoxemia are examples of foodborne bacterial intoxications.

Staphylococcus aureus

Staphylococcal food poisoning is an intoxication whose onset, in terms of symptoms, is usually rapid. In many cases it is acute, depending on individual susceptibility to the toxin, the amount of contaminated food eaten, the amount of toxin in the food ingested and the general health of the victim. The most common symptoms are nausea, vomiting, retching, abdominal cramping, and prostration. Some individuals may not demonstrate all the symptoms associated with the illness (Bergdoll 1979). In more severe cases, headache, muscle cramping, and transient changes in blood pressure and pulse rate may occur. Bergdoll (1979) gives a detailed account of symptoms and victims' responses to the illness. Recovery generally takes two days. However, it is not unusual for complete recovery to take three days and, in severe cases, longer. Death from staphylococcal food poisoning is infrequent although such cases have occurred among the elderly, infants, and the severely debilitated. Staphylococcal foodborne illness, once considered the most prevalent foodborne illness in the U.S. (Brachman et al. 1976), is currently estimated to be the second most prevalent (Bennett 1982), but the true incidence is unknown for a number of reasons. These include: poor response by victims to interviews conducted by health officials; misdiagnosis due to symptoms similar to those of other types of food poisoning (such as the vomiting caused by *Bacillus cereus* emetic toxin); inadequate collection of samples for laboratory analysis; and improper laboratory examination.

In the United States from 1969 to 1973, there were 499 outbreaks attributed to staphylococcal food poisoning (Bergdoll 1979), and from 1975 to 1981, 223 confirmed staphylococcal food poisoning outbreaks.

Staphylococci exist in or on air, dust, sewage, water, milk, food, food equipment, environmental surfaces, humans, and animals. Humans and animals are the primary reservoirs for bacterial growth. The organisms are present in the nasal passages and throat and on the hair and skin of more than 50% of healthy individuals (Bergdoll 1979). The incidence is even higher for those who associate with or who come into contact with sick persons and hospital environments (Abramson 1973). Although food handlers are usually the main source of food contamination in food poisoning outbreaks, equipment and environmental surfaces can also be sources of contamination. Detailed accounts of the sources of staphylococcal contamination are given by Bergdoll (1979) and Bryan (1978). Like other foodborne illnesses, staphylococcal food poisoning can be thought of as the interaction of agent (toxin), host, and environment (Bryan 1979b).

Foods most often incriminated in staphylococcal foodborne disease in the United States are meats and meat products, poultry, baked foods, and salads (including poultry, fish, egg, and potato salads). However, it is not uncommon for other foods to be vehicles of staphylococcal foodborne disease. Often several foods are implicated in food poisoning outbreaks because of cross contamination from a single source. Specific and general categories of foods incriminated in staphylococcal food poisoning outbreaks in the United States between 1975 and 1981 are shown for comparative purposes (Table 16.1).

Listeria monocytogenes

An example of a foodborne bacterium that invades and multiplies in the intestinal mucosa and in other tissues of animals and human hosts is *Listeria monocytogenes*. Human infection was first described by Nyfeldt (1929), when this organism was isolated from the blood of three patients with an infectious mononucleosis-like syndrome (Siegel and Nelson, 1981). In succeeding years, this organism has been implicated as the etiologic agent in a multiplicity of clinical syndromes. Currently, the major impact of the organism as a pathogen is in its ability to produce septicemia and meningitis in newborns, the elderly, and debilitated and otherwise immunocompromised persons. This coccal-bacillary Gram-positive organism observed in infected tissues and in fluids or on primary isolation has often been mistaken for diphtheroids and discarded as a contaminant by inexperienced laboratory personnel. The far-reaching consequences of listeric infections have been reviewed meticulously by Gray and Killinger (1966) and more recently by Ralovich (1984).

The incidence of listeric infection is difficult to ascertain, except in symptomatic instances, since some evidence of an asymptomatic carrier state exists. In one Swedish study, 3000 subjects free of clinical disease exhibited a fecal carriage rate which varied from 1% in a group of hospitalized adults

Table 16.1. Foods Incriminated in Staphylococcal Food Poisoning Outbreaks in the United States, 1975 to 1981

Foods	1975	1976	1977	1978	1979	1980	1981	Total/ product
Beef	2	2	1	0	2	0	3	10
Lamb	0	0	1	0	0	1	0	2
Ham	16	3	9	10	8	3	8	57
Pork	2	0	1	0	0	1	2	5
Sausage	0	1	1	0	0	1	1	4
Chicken	0	2	3	0	1	2	3	11
Turkey	1	1	1	0	3	3	4	14
Other meat	2	2	0	0	1	2	1	8
Shellfish	0	0	1	0	0	0	0	1
Other fish	2	0	0	0	0	0	1	3
Dairy products	0	0	1	0	0	0	3	4
Baked foods	1	2	1	0	0	3	7	14
Fruits and vegetables	0	1	0	0	0	0	1	2
Potato salad	1	1	1	1	2	3	0	9
Poultry, fish, egg salad	6	0	1	1	2	1	2	13
Other salads	1	3	0	5	1	0	2	12
Mexican foods	1	0	0	0	0	0	0	1
Multiple foods	8	3	1	4	5	5	1	27
Other foods	1	5	1	0	1	0	0	8
Unknown	1	0	1	2	7	2	5	18
Total out- breaks/yr	45	26	25	23	33	27	44	

(*From Centers for Disease Control 1976; 1977; 1979; 1981a, b; 1983 a, b*)

to 26% in a group of household contacts of patients with proven disease (Siegel and Nelson 1981).

Listeria monocytogenes is widely distributed in nature. It has been isolated from numerous species of mammals and fowl, trout, ticks, crustaceans, water, sewage, silage, and soil (Gray and Killinger 1966). The relationship between the disease in humans and animals has still not been totally understood, particularly with respect to the source of infection in animals. In view of the possibility of foodborne infection in humans, milk as a possible vehicle is of particular importance. Substantial evidence has been presented indicating that infected animals may secrete *Listeria* spp. with their milk. As a consequence, special attention is also being given to milk products such as cheese. In mid-1983, 49 individuals in Massachusetts acquired listeriosis. Fourteen of the 49 (29%) died. This episode was traced to the consumption of pasteurized 2% milk (Fleming et al. 1985). Although the majority of cases seem to be sporadic, a number of outbreaks have been attributed to the ingestion of contaminated coleslaw (Schlech et al. 1983) as well as raw milk. However, in other cases, suspicion has been cast on cream, sour milk, and cottage cheese (Bryan 1979a). Most evidence, including the occurrence of gastrointestinal symptoms at the outset of bacteremic illness (Nieman and Lober 1980), points to the intestine as the usual portal of entry into the tissues (Barza 1985). It has been found in the intestinal tract of humans and animals. Egg-product plant and slaughterhouse workers have been shown to harbor *L. monocytogenes* at rates from 10–30%.

Streptococcus Species (Enterococci)

Perhaps the most controversial of all disputed food poisoning agents are the fecal streptococci (Foster 1973). While the term "enterococci" is not acceptable for classification, it is used as a collective term for *Streptoccocus faecalis* and *Streptococcus faecium* (Bryan 1979b). The incubation period and clinical symptoms of the "fecal strep" food poisoning syndrome have been summarized by Jay (1978) from five reported outbreaks in which fecal streptococci were implicated. The incubation periods ranged from 2–22 hr after ingestion of the food. Dack (1963) reported that the incubation period as well as symptoms of streptococcal food poisoning mimicked those of *Clostridium perfringens* and *Bacillus cereus* food poisoning. Hobbs et al. (1953) reported that the incubation period for *C. perfringens* food poisoning ranged from 8–22 hr with symptoms of acute abdominal pain, diarrhea, nausea, and occasional vomiting. The duration was a day or less. Unsuccessful attempts to reproduce these symptoms by feeding streptococci to human volunteers have been made by several investigators. However, a number of accounts of food poisoning caused by the enterococci have been reviewed by Deibel and Silliker (1963) and Jay (1978). The causative strains are undoubtedly weak pathogens as suggested by the large numbers of organisms associated with vehicle foods. In 1981, one reported outbreak (CDC 1983a, b) involving 24 individuals occurred, while no outbreaks were reported for the years 1979 and 1980.

Enterococci are commonly isolated from foods and from food processing and service establishments (Bryan 1979a). Vehicle foods of streptococcal food poisoning include turkey dressing, cured ham, barbequed beef, Vienna sausage, cheese, evaporated milk, and turkey à la king and others (Jay 1978). Other foods which have been reviewed by Bryan (1979a) include commercially frozen fruits, fruit juices, vegetables, ready-to-eat meats, frozen meat pies and prepared dinners, ground beef, beef and pork sausage, meat and fish, pork, chickens, turkeys, spray-dried whole egg powder, pecan nutmeats, raw and pasteurized milk, barley, malt kernels and instant malted milk powder, lobster and fish.

METHODS FOR *LISTERIA*

L. monocytogenes usually grows well on most of the commonly employed bacteriological media after initial isolation. Considerable evidence suggests that with both natural and experimental infections initial isolation is not always successful (Gray and Killinger 1966). The earlier techniques proven to be most successful for the isolation of *L. monocytogenes* generally involve tissue maceration. These bacteria are often contained in the focal lesions of infected tissue.

Cultivation and Isolation

Listeria monocytogenes strains have no special nutritional requirements. They grow readily on either nutrient agar, serum agar, or blood agar. An agar containing tryptose provides improved cultivation conditions (Ralovich 1984). On agar or agar containing blood, *Listeria* spp. can hardly, if at all, be distinguished from other bacteria such as streptococci. The essence of the stereomicroscopic examination is that in oblique, transmitted light, *Listeria* spp. colonies exhibit an unevenly glittering blue surface.

Primary Cultivation and Enrichment

Primary cultivation and enrichment procedures are applicable to samples that most probably are not contaminated with bacteria other than *Listeria* spp. These may include cerebrospinal fluid, blood, non-decomposing postmortem specimens, liver, spleen, brain, lymph node, placenta, and meconium (Ralovich 1984).

In the primary cultivation of *Listeria* spp., blood containing Holman medium (Ralovich 1984) or tryptose phosphate broth (TPB) can be used with relatively good results. Fluid media tend to have an advantage over solid media because the semianaerobic conditions enhance the multiplication of the facultatively anaerobic *Listeria* spp. This is particularly useful if one is isolating the organism from pathological materials. Incubation is carried out at 35–37°C. Transfer of growth from the fluid medium onto a solid medium such as serum or blood agar can generally be made after 1–2 days incubation in the fluid medium. Colonies develop on the solid medium after an incubation period of 24–48 hr.

Selective cultivation. A selective cultivation procedure might be more applicable to samples or specimens also containing miscellaneous bacteria other than *Listeria* spp. Examples of such specimens might be feces, throat or vaginal secretions, food, fodder, sewage, soil, decomposing postmortem specimens, as well as any other specimens not sampled under aseptic conditions. In addition to the use of selective enrichment, cold cultivation ("cold enrichment" method at 4°C), with subsequent inoculation of Trypaflavine-Nalidixic Acid Serum Agar (TNSA) plates, should provide for the adequate isolation of *Listeria* spp. Some homogenization procedures for solid specimens have been reported by Ralovich (1984). Samples can be aseptically placed in blood-containing Holman medium or in tryptose phosphate broth and incubated in the refrigerator at 4°C for 3 months (if necessary). According to Ralovich (1984), the first subcultures are made 2–3 weeks after initial cultivation in broth medium and subsequently at weekly or monthly intervals. This prolonged incubation at 4°C hinders the proliferation of many other bacteria but will not inhibit the multiplication of *Listeria*. While this procedure is certainly not recommended for prompt diagnosis, it is highly suitable for the screening of specimens. TPB and Holman blood media can be even more selective if polymyxin B is added. TNSA can be applied in the subculturing protocol.

For more rapid results, a medium containing acridine dye and nalidixic acid should be employed. One of the best selective enrichment media is Levinthal broth containing trypaflavine and nalidixic acid. With this medium, the cultivation period is approximately a week. Initial incubation (first two days) is accomplished at 37°C and prolonged incubation at room temperature.

As a solid selective medium, the selectivity of TNSA can be enhanced by adding polymyxin B. In this medium, trypaflavine can be replaced by other acridine dyes such as xanthacridine, acriflavine, or proflavinhemisulfate. TNSA plates can be inoculated from a fluid or from selective enriching medium. Additionally, samples can be inoculated directly onto this medium. These plates are incubated at 35–37°C for 24 hr and then read. After being read, the plates should be kept at room temperature for an additional day for further observation. On a medium containing 5% sheep or horse blood, the virulent strains of *Listeria* spp. produce a beta-type hemolysis; avirulent strains are not hemolytic. However, hemolysis sometimes does not develop for several days. On TNSA medium, *Listeria* spp. produce their bluish-green colonies exhibiting the characteristic, unevenly glittering surface. Formulations for media discussed above appear in the review of Ralovich (1984).

Still other media formulations have been successfully used in the cultivation of *L. monocytogenes*: e.g. trypticase soy broth supplemented with 0.6% yeast extract containing acriflavine HCl (15 mg/L), naladixic acid (14 mg/L), and cycloheximide (50 mg/L) as an enrichment medium (Lovett et al. 1985). Direct streaking procedures or transfers from enrichment broth onto McBride agar (McBride 1960; Gray and Killinger 1966; Lovett et al. 1985) or onto a modified McBride agar (Francis et al. 1984) have also been used.

Verification Tests

When colonies suspected to be *L. monocytogenes* are observed on solid medium, they should be tested for catalase production; only those that split H_2O_2 are to be isolated by smearing on agar and blood agar plates (Ralovich 1984). After incubation (35–37°C for 24–48 hr), the colonies should be tested for catalase production. Catalase positive isolates should be inoculated into dextrose-free broth containing 0.5% agar to check motility. Motile strains typically exhibit characteristic "umbrella" growth. Motility can be demonstrated under the microscope. *Listeria* spp. show characteristic tumbling and rotating movement. *Listeria monocytogenes* are short, Gram-positive rods when stained specimens are observed microscopically. Preliminary diagnosis of *L. monocytogenes* should be corroborated by a detailed biochemical examination. In addition to observing colonies for hemolysin production, catalase production, absence of oxidase, motility, and other verification can also be employed. Additional tests and results are: indole production (−); urea hydrolysis (−); nitrate reduction (−); methyl red reaction (+); Voges-Proskauer reaction (+); H_2S production (−); esculin hydrolysis (+); citrate utilization (−); gelatin liquefaction (−); and carbohydrate fermentation. Typical *L. monocytogenes* ferment glucose, rhamnose, and amylose but not mannitol.

Biological Indications

Infections in the mouse, chinchilla, and embryonic chicken have been tried with varying degrees of success. Early attempts at pathogenicity testing have been documented by Gray and Killinger (1966). More recently applied biological tests include inoculation of *L. monocytogenes* culture material into the conjunctival sac of the guinea pig or young rabbit, resulting in production of keratoconjunctivitis; lethality from septicemia in mice; and induced infection of the chick embryo (Ralovich 1984).

Serological Confirmation

Early attempts to confirm *L. monocytogenes* serologically were, generally, not successful. Agglutination tests showed cross reactions between the O agglutinins of *L. monocytogenes* with Lancefield's group D streptococci and also with *Staphylococcus aureus*. In precipitation tests, cross reactions have been noted between the precipitinogens of *L. monocytogens* and antibodies for *Streptococcus faecalis* and *L. monocytogenes*. Other serological systems, such as complement fixation, offer promise in the serological identification of *L. monocytogenes*; however, cross reactions with other bacteria can occur. These findings suggest that extreme caution should be exercised in the diagnosis of listeric infection based only on serological results. The many attempts at diverse serological assays have been reviewed by Gray and Killinger (1966). More recently, Donnelly and Baigent (1985) have noted the limitation of the rapid identification of *L. monocytogenes* in food samples because of cross reactivity with *S. aureus* and other micrococci. Additionally, these authors suggest using automated fluorescent antibody techniques employing flow cytometry for the serological identification of *L. monocytogenes*.

METHODS FOR ENTEROCOCCI

The enterococci are members of the genus *Streptococcus*. They are Gram-positive, catalase negative cocci that form long or short chains. They are classified in the Lancefield's serologic group D, although other streptococcal species (*S. bovis*, *S. equinus* and *S. avium*) also belong to this serological group. Thus, the five recognized species of group D streptococci now constitute these three species in addition to *S. faecalis* and *S. faecium*, the enterococci. Two varieties of *S. faecalis* (*S. faecalis* var. *liquefaciens* and *S. faecalis* var. *zymogenes*) and one of *S. faecium* (*S. faecium* var. *durans*) have been proposed; in reality, these are two biotypes based on proteolytic and hemolytic characteristics (Deibel and Hartman 1984). The proteolytic characteristic appears to be stable while hemolysin demonstration is unstable and is often lost on laboratory media during subculture.

Sherman (1937) distinguished enterococci from other group D streptococci on the basis of their capacity to grow in the presence of 6.5% NaCl at a pH of 9.6 at temperatures of 10°C and 45°C and to withstand a temperature of 60°C for 30 min. According to Deibel (1964), some strains of enterococci may fail to produce positive results by one or more of these criteria.

As a result of their relatively high heat resistance, streptococci may survive traditional milk pasteurization procedures. *S. faecium* is markedly heat tolerant and it is a spoilage agent in marginally processed hams (Deibel and Hartman 1984). Additionally, most of the enterococci are resistant to freezing.

The enterococci may be identified by their physiological and serological characteristics; however, no trait(s) will establish definitive identification. Serological identity appears to be more consistent than identification on laboratory media.

Isolation and Enumeration

Numerous methods have been proposed for the isolation and enumeration of the enterococci. According to deFigueiredo and Jay (1976), most procedures employ presumptive media followed by confirmatory tests. Azide, tellurite, bile, neomysin taurocholate, Tween 80 selenite, NaCl, phenylethyl alcohol, and thallium have been used in media as selective agents. Both selectivity and quantitative recovery are less than ideal (Deibel and Hartman 1984).

KF streptococcal agar medium has been accepted by many industrial firms and regulatory agencies for quantitative estimation of enterococci in nondairy foods. The KG agar medium is recommended by the Association of Food and Drug Officials of the U.S.A. (1966) as well as by the American Public Health Association (Deibel and Hartman 1984). KF agar medium is a selective, differential medium that contains sodium azide as the major selective agent and triphenyltetrazolium chloride (TTC) for differential purposes (Kenner et al. 1961). The medium also contains a relatively high concentration of maltose (2.0%) and a small amount of lactose (0.1%). Most, but not all, streptococci ferment these sugars (Deibel and Hartman 1984). *S. faecalis* and its varieties produce a deep red color when TTC is reduced to its formazan derivative. Other group D species, including *S. salvarius* and *S. mitis*, are not as reductive, thereby producing light pink colonies.

KF agar contains azide which is inhibitory to many strains of *S. bovis* and *S. equinus*. In consequence, an alternative medium, gentamicin-thallous-carbonate (GTC), has been proposed by Donnelly and Hartman (1978) that permits the recovery of a wide variety of enterococci from foods (Thian and

Hartman 1981). The incubation period for GTC agar is 18 hr, while KF agar requires 48 hr.

Confirmation procedures for the identity of enterococci may be conducted by using "Sherman tests" (Sherman 1937), by growth in EVA broth (Litsky et al. 1955), or by one of the recently developed procedures such as tyrosine decarboxylase activity (Lee 1972). EVA broths in combination with azide dextrose have been employed by a number of investigators. Comparative studies with five media on the recovery of fecal streptococci from various food products showed that while thallous acetate medium yielded the highest counts, it was the least selective (Pavlova et al. 1972).

Presumptive Characterization

If confirmation of identity is desirable, a number of typical colonies should be picked and transferred to brain heart infusion broth (incubate at 35°C for 18–24 hr). Microscopic slides should be prepared to observe typical morphology by Gram staining. Colonies should be grown on bile-esculin agar (Facklam and Moody, 1970) if necessary. Test for growth in BHI broth containing 6.5% NaCl (incubation at 35°C for 72 hr). Test for growth at 45°C in BHI tempered in an air incubator prior to incubation. If growth in the salt-containing medium and at 45°C are to be determined, subcultures should be inoculated prior to testing for catalase to avoid contamination introduced by peroxide (Deibel and Hartman 1984). Rapid identification kits (Watkins et al. 1980) for the enterococci are commercially available and have been used with some success.

Serological Identification

If serological confirmation of enterococci is necessary, commercial grouping sera are available. The sources for grouping sera have been described by Deibel and Hartman (1984). It is sometimes difficult to demonstrate the presence of group D antigen in some strains of group D streptococci. In such circumstances, the method of group extraction (Elliott et al. 1977) may be necessary in defining strain association with the group D. The demonstration of serological group D reaction will definitively identify the isolate as an enterococcus (Deibel and Hartman 1984).

According to de Figueiredo and Jay (1976), one of the most rapid techniques reported for the enumeration of enterococci is a membrane filter fluorescent antibody test which Pugsley and Evison (1975) employed to detect enterococci in water in 10–12 hr. However, its applicability to a wide variety of food awaits testing.

METHODS FOR *STAPHYLOCOCCUS AUREUS* AND ITS TOXINS

The methods employed for recovery, enumeration, and isolation of *Staphylococcus aureus* are dependent, in part, on the purpose of conducting the analysis. Foods which are incriminated in food poisoning outbreaks frequently contain large numbers of staphylococci which may not require highly sensitive methods for their recovery. However, in some cases, viable *S. aureus* may not be detected in the incriminated food due to stress factors such as subsequent heat treatment or other handling procedures that may have rendered the organism nonviable. More sensitive methods might be required to study and evaluate staphylococcal contamination in insanitary processing or post-process handling. In these situations, small populations of *S. aureus* could develop. In food and food ingredients, *S. aureus* may not be the predominant organism; therefore, selective inhibitory media should be used.

Selective media contain various toxic chemicals which may inhibit *S. aureus* to some extent. More importantly, these toxic chemicals inhibit the growth of competitive organisms. While the use of selective agents may have an effect on stressed *S. aureus* in processed foods, a relatively toxic medium has definite advantage in preventing, to some extent, overgrowth of *S. aureus* by competing bacterial flora.

Recovery and Enumeration

Direct plating and enrichment isolation are the most commonly used techniques for retrieving *S. aureus* from foods. Enrichment procedures may be either selective (AOAC 1984) or nonselective (Heidelbaugh et al. 1973). Nonselective enrichment procedures are used primarily for the detection of injured cells which may be inhibited by toxic chemicals in selective enrichment media. Enumeration of *S. aureus* by enrichment isolation may be done by determining either an indicated number or most probable number (MPN). Commonly applied MPN procedures are the three tube (3 tubes of each dilution) and five tube (5 tubes of each dilution) methods (AOAC 1984; Heidelbaugh et al. 1973).

Direct plating for the enumeration of *S. aureus* is suitable for the analysis of foods in which more than 100 *S. aureus* cells/g are expected (Bennett 1984b). Food samples may be subjected to a variety of media in various ways in applying the direct plating technique. Surface spreading, drop plates and pour plates have been used in direct plating procedures. Of these, surface spreading has the advantage of allowing one to observe typical colonial morphology. The principal advantage of the pour plate technique is that larger volumes of samples can be used (Tatini et al. 1984). While both enrichment and direct plating techniques can be used, it is generally felt that plate count procedures are more precise and provide a more meaningful indication of the level of contamination. However, stress factors (e.g., smoking, heating, fermentation, drying, aging) may have reduced the original population of S. aureus. Some useful screening approaches for detecting the organism in processed food have been described by Tatini et al. (1984).

Isolation and Identification

Basic characteristics of the staphylococci for their successful isolation in the presence of other species are: the ability to grow in the presence of the toxic chemicals incorporated into the various selective media, their morphological appearance (both typical and atypical), the ability to ferment certain carbohydrates, and the ability to mount certain enzyme reactions. Media used in the recovery and enumeration of S. aureus may employ some of these diagnostic features for S. aureus identification (Tatini et al. 1984).

Laboratory media. A number of media have been developed for the isolation and enumeration of S. aureus. They differ primarily in the nature of the selective agents used (ICMSF 1978). The two selectively toxic chemicals most frequently used in media for the isolation of staphylococci are sodium chloride (NaCl) and potassium tellurite (K_2TeO_3). Various concentrations of these chemicals have been used ranging from 5.5–10% NaCl and from 0.025–0.05% K_2TeO_3. Other chemicals, such as ammonium sulfate, sorbic acid, glycine, lithium chloride, and polymyxin frequently are combined with NaCl and K_2TeO_3. Sodium azide alone or in combination with neomycin has also been used in selective media (Tatini et al. 1984).

Of the media formulated for the isolation and recovery of staphylococci, Baird-Parker (1965) agar appears to be the most widely used as a direct plating medium. Five media, Baird-Parker medium, Tellurite Polymyxin Egg-Yolk Agar (Crisley et al. 1964, 1965), Kranep Agar (Sinell and Baumgart 1967), Phenolphthalein Diphosphate Agar (Barber and Kuper 1951; Hobbs et al. 1968), and Milk Salt Agar after use of an enrichment procedure (Nefedjeva 1964), have been described by ICMSF (1978). All of the media have certain advantages as well as disadvantages. Baird-Parker medium has the following advantages: (1) selectivity; (2) no inhibition of injured staphylococci; and (3) ease of recognition of S. aureus colonies. It has been approved for use by the Association of Official Analytical Chemists (AOAC 1984). This medium is also recommended by the International Organization of Standardization and by the United States Department of Agriculture. In many countries it is commercially available as a dehydrated powder. A shortcoming, however, is that it is rather expensive. Furthermore, once poured into plates, the complete medium must be used within 24–48 hr. If it contains pyruvate, longer periods of storage reduce its selectivity. Loss of quality has also been noted after prolonged storage of the medium in powdered form. However, this effect can be reversed by adding a 20% solution of sodium pyruvate to the prepared medium to obtain a final concentration of 1% pyruvate (Collins-Thompson et al. 1974). To overcome the pyruvate stability problem, it is recommended that a stable (pyruvate-free) version of the original medium be used. Plates of pyruvate-free Baird-Parker medium can be stored at 4°C for up to 28 days. Before use, 0.5 mL of a 20% (w/v) solution of sodium pyruvate is spread over the surface of the plates, which are dried at 50°C prior to inoculation (ICMSF 1978). S. aureus colonies on Baird-Parker agar are usually 1.5 mm in size, jet black to dark grey, smooth, convex, have entire margins, an off-white edge, and may show an opaque zone and/or clear halo extending beyond the opaque zone. Plating procedures for the isolation and enumeration of staphylococci have been detailed by ICMSF (1978), Tatini et al. (1984), and Bennett (1984b).

S. aureus may be present in foods in larger numbers than are recovered by conventional media containing selective agents (Ray 1979). Sublethally injured or otherwise stressed cells are present in semipreserved or preserved food. It is important that methods also be used which will detect injured organisms. Since S. aureus cells which have been allowed to repair can again produce enterotoxin, they must be considered a potential cause of staphylococcal food poisoning (Smith et al. 1983).

The isolation and subsequent enumeration of injured S. aureus is dependent on the recovery media. Most selective media are acceptable for enumeration and isolation of nondebilitated cells but all too often are toxic for the growth of stressed cells. Consequently, preenrichment procedures have been developed to retrieve stressed and injured cells. An update on current resuscitation methods for the recovery of stressed S. aureus from foods was recently reported by Lancette (1985).

A number of repair selective procedures for the revival of injured and stressed S. aureus are currently being used. One method is recommended for testing processed foods likely to contain a small population of injured cells (Tatini et al. 1984). Another commonly used selective enrichment procedure (Armijo et al. 1957) is recommended for raw foods or unprocessed foods expected to contain < 100 S. aureus/g in the presence of large numbers of competing organisms. For this purpose, the procedure using the 3 or 5 tube most probable number (MPN) should be employed. The MPN procedure conforms to the AOAC (1984) method and directions for performance of the procedure are described in detail by Tatini et al. (1984) and Bennett (1984b). Procedures and characteristic reactions on media used for the isolation of *S. aureus* have been summarized by Bryan (1976).

Ancillary tests.   The staphylococci produce a large number of enzymes, toxins, and other metabolites. Many of these are substances that enable the organism to hydrolyze proteins, carbohydrates, and fats in order to obtain essential nutrients for its survival and proliferation. Some of the metabolites are also important in bacterial resistance to drugs and determine their function in pathogenicity. Some of the many metabolites synthesized by *S. aureus* have been used for identification of the bacteria. Ancillary to the coagulase test is the microscope slide test for thermostable nuclease (TNase) production developed by Lachica et al. (1972). This method is rapid and is claimed to be as specific as the coagulase reaction. Additionally, it is considerably less subjective than the coagulase test in that a positive reaction involves a color change of the medium from blue to bright pink. The test is not intended to act as a substitute for the coagulase test; however, it is recommended that 2 + coagulase reactions be supported by a positive TNase test before being considered confirmatory for *S. aureus* (ICMSF 1978).

Staphylococcal coagulase is an extracellular enzyme that accelerates the clotting of plasma. Citrated, oxalate, or heparinized human, pig, and rabbit plasma are most susceptible to coagulase, but horse, dog, goat, calf, donkey, and goose plasmas also are clotted by this enzyme. The coagulating principle, coagulase thrombin, is the result of the interaction of coagulase-reacting factor in plasma (Bryan 1976). Detailed reviews of coagulase have been published (Elek 1959; Tager and Drummond 1965).

Deoxyribonuclease is an enzyme produced by most strains of *S. aureus* which catalyzes the polymerization of deoxyribonucleic acid. In 1956, Cunningham et al. established that staphylococcal deoxyribonuclease (DNase) possessed remarkable heat stability. Earlier studies did not clearly distinguish between normal DNase activity or heat stable DNase. Lachica et al. (1971) recommended that heat-stable nuclease be referred to as thermonuclease (TNase). Other organisms as reported by Tatini et al. (1984) have been shown to produce TNase.

Recently, the American Public Health Association (Tatini et al. 1984) recommended a procedure which allows for the direct enumeration of coagulase and TNase positive *S. aureus* on Baird-Parker agar containing rabbit plasma-fibrinogen tellurite to which 0.5 mL 20% pyruvate (Hauschild et al. 1979) has been added just prior to use. All black colonies showing the opaque fibrin halos (coagulase positive) that surround the colonies (Julseth and Dudley 1973; Hauschild et al. 1979; Boothby et al. 1979) are counted. The plates can then be exposed to 65°C for 2 hr and TNase tested by an overlay of each plate with 10 mL melted toluidine blue DNA agar. After the required incubation (37°C, 4 hr), all colonies showing pink halos against a blue background are counted as TNase positive. Similar results can be obtained on Baird-Parker agar without egg yolk if pork plasma-fibrinogen overlay agar is used (Hauschild et al. 1979). To enumerate, all colonies that show both fibrin halos (coagulase positive) and also pink halos (TNase positive) times the dilution factor represent the number of *S. aureus*/g or mL of the product analyzed. This procedure has been detailed by Tatini et al. (1984) and is recommended for raw and processed foods.

While methodology for the direct enumeration of coagulase and TNase positive *S. aureus* is applicable in many situations, the tube coagulase test using commercially available rabbit plasma with ethylenediamine-tetraacetic acid (EDTA) appears to be the most commonly used in most laboratories. The interpretation of the tube coagulase test with regard to clot formation and its significance as to the degree of clot formation have been problems for many years. Many investigators consider any degree of clotting (Turner and Schwartz 1958) to be considered a positive test. Sperber and Tatini (1975) reported that only a firm clot (4+ reaction) should be considered positive. They also indicated that the cause of ambiguous coagulase reactions may be linked to the source of plasma. Still other investigators have proposed subjective clot interpretations of 3+, 4+ ratings (Baer et al. 1976; Rayman et al. 1975) and ratings of 2+, 3+, 4+ (Thatcher and Clark 1968; ICMSF 1978). AOAC (Tatini et al. 1984) recommends that a 3+ or 4+ clot formation should be deemed a positive coagulase reaction for *S. aureus* (Rayman et al. 1975; Sperber and Tatini 1975). Small or poorly organized clots (1+ and 2+) ought to be confirmed by ancillary tests. Similarly, the FDA *Bacteriological Analytical Manual* (Bennett 1984b) recommends that only a firm clot (4+ reaction) be considered positive and that partial clots (2+ and 3+ reactions) be tested further (Sperber and Tatini 1975). AOAC (1984) recommends that any degree of clotting be considered a positive coagulase reaction. The various studies on coagulase and their reactions have been reviewed by Sperber (1976).

If anomalies are encountered which might cause doubt as to the identification of *Staphylococcus* spp., additional testing may be required to establish the species or its potential for causing staphylococcal foodborne illness. Tests which might be helpful are microscopic examination, susceptibility to lysostaphin, catalase activity, anaerobic utilization of glucose, and mannitol and bacteriophage sensitivity. The bacteriophage typing of *S. aureus* may be useful in elucidating the epidemiology of staphylococcal food poisoning outbreaks. The ancillary tests have been described in detail (Tatini et al. 1984; Bennett 1984b) and the salient characteristics of *S. aureus* have been summarized (Bryan 1976).

Relationship to enterotoxigenicity. The early indications that all pathogenic staphylococci produced coagulase was followed by the discovery that all enterotoxigenic staphylococci also produced coagulase (Sperber 1976). Many investigators have tried to find biochemical or physiological properties of *S. aureus* that correlate with toxin production. Production of coagulase and TNase as common characteristics of *S. aureus* have been shown to correlate well with enterotoxigenicity (Tatini et al. 1976). However, other studies have shown that most nontoxigenic strains also produce these enzymes. Sperber and Tatini (1975) examined 145 toxigenic and 190 nontoxigenic strains, and all produced TNase. Similar results have been reported by Niskanen (1977).

   To correlate enterotoxigenicity with the conventional ancillary tests used for identification of *Staphylococcus aureus*, Bennett et al. (1985) evaluated 151 strains of staphylococci from foods. These strains were examined for enterotoxin production, colonial morphology on Baird-Parker agar, coagulase activity using the tube test with rabbit and pig plasma, TNase production, lysostaphin sensitivity, and anaerobic utilization of glucose and mannitol. Enterotoxins A,B,C,D, and E were produced singly or in combination by 100 of the *S. aureus* strains; 51 strains produced no enterotoxin. False negative rates in identifying the enterotoxigenic group as typical *S. aureus* were 11% on Baird-Parker Agar; 8% for coagulase activity with Difco rabbit plasma; 7% for TNase production; 4% for lysostaphin sensitivity; and 2% and 4%, respectively, for the anaerobic utilization of glucose and mannitol. In all cases, the reactions of the enterotoxigenic and nonenterotoxigenic strains of *S. aureus* varied by only 12% or less. As a consequence, none of these tests are reliable for differentiating toxigenic from nontoxigenic *S. aureus*.

   Other properties of *S. aureus*, such as pigment and hemolysin production (Feldman 1946), protein A (Forsgren 1970), and gelatin hydrolysis (Stone 1936), used either alone or in combination, have not served to establish whether an *S. aureus* isolate is enterotoxigenic or not. Therefore, direct testing for toxin production is the only reliable way for screening *S. aureus* for enterotoxigenicity (Meyer et al. 1982). Many investigators insist on isolating and enumerating only typical *S. aureus* from plating media, although instability has been shown in certain physiological traits demonstrated by this species. Variability has been attributed to both physiologic and genetic factors. The frequency with which physiological traits may change and the elements stimulating such change have not been clearly demonstrated (Tatini et al. 1984). While employing the various plating media and ancillary tests for the enumeration and identification of *S. aureus*, consideration should be given to the possibility of variation in certain physiologic traits. Certain of the usual diagnostic features characteristic of the species may or may not be displayed in a given instance (Tatini et al. 1984). Bennett et al. (1986b) tabulated (Table 16.2) some of the characteristics of enterotoxigenic *S. aureus* isolated

Table 16.2. Biological Confirmation of Enterotoxigenicity of Some Isolates Demonstrating Characteristics which Differ from Typical *Staphylococcus aureus*

Strain designation	Aberrant characteristic(s)	Enterotoxin serotype produced	Bioassay in kittens No. ill/No. injected
GF-9	Atyp. colony[a]	C[b]	2/3
GF-36	Coag-[c]; TNase-[d]; Man-[e]	B/C	1/1
GF-38	Man-; Glu[f]	C	1/1
GF-63	Man-; Glu	C	1/1
GF-74	Atyp. colony	B	1/1
GF-77	Atyp. colony; TNase-; Lyso-[g]	A	1/1
GF-78	Atyp. colony; TNase-; Coag-	A	1/1
GF-83	Atyp. colony	A	1/1
GF-84	Atyp. colony	B	1/1
GF-119	TNase-	A	1/1
GF-133	Atyp. colony	A/D	1/3
GF-189	Coag-; Man-	E	1/1

[a]Atypical colony formation on Baird-Parker agar.
[b]Reacts with antibodies to one or more of the staphylococcal enterotoxins A–E.
[c]Coag- = coagulase negative applying the 1–4+ in all plasmas studied.
[d]TNase- = negative for the demonstration of thermostable nuclease (TNase).
[e]Man- = negative for the anaerobic utilization of mannitol.
[f]Glu- = negative for the anaerobic utilization of glucose.
[g]Lyso- = nonsensitivity to lysostaphin.
(*From Bennett et al. 1986b*)

from foods. These isolates demonstrated characteristics which differed from typical *S. aureus*.

Enterotoxin Production and Detection

Media and methods. A number of laboratory media and procedures have been proposed for the production of enterotoxin. A rather detailed account of such media proposals has been presented previously (Bergdoll 1972, 1979).

Of these media, brain heart infusion has been shown to be a simple and adequate media. Other media such as 3.0% NZ amine A (pancreatic digest of casein) containing 1% yeast extract appears to be comparable (Bergdoll 1972). Of the methods described by Casman and Bennett (1963) for the laboratory production of enterotoxin, cultivation of suspect staphylococcal isolates on semisolid BHI agar (0.7%), pH 5.3, is simple and can be conducted in any laboratory because it does not require the use of special apparatus. This method of enterotoxin production has been studied collaboratively (Bennett and McClure 1976) and adopted by AOAC as an official method (AOAC 1984). The details of this method have been described previously (Bergdoll and Bennett 1976, 1984; Bennett and McClure 1976; Bennett 1984a). Earlier, a number of investigators reported good yields of enterotoxin using BHI as growth medium (Casman and Bennett 1963; Genigeorgis and Sadler 1966), whereas others (Reiser and Weiss 1969) have reported poor yields. It has been observed that these differences in enterotoxin production yield in BHI differ from the same manufacturer as well as from BHI lots of different manufacturers. Recently, these differences have not been observed frequently. Suggestions for the use of still other media of various formulations and modifications for the production of the staphylococcal enterotoxins have already been reviewed by Bergdoll (1972). Of the various methods described for routine laboratory production of high yields of enterotoxin (Casman and Bennett 1963; Donnelly et al. 1967; Hollander 1965; Jarvis and Lawrence 1970), the cellophane-over-agar (Jarvis and Lawrence 1970) and the cellophane sac method of Donnelly et al. (1967) appear to be the most simple when working with enterotoxigenic strains which yield very small amounts of enterotoxin. However, in studies in which low toxin producing staphylococci were evaluated, the semisolid BHI method (Casman and Bennett 1963) was highly satisfactory when the BHI supernatants were tested for the presence of enterotoxin the microslide gel double diffusion test. In using simultaneous growth-toxin concentration methods (e.g., methods utilizing cellophane) for the production of enterotoxin, the less sensitive optimum sensitivity plate (OSP) method of Robbins et al. (1974) can be used for serological determination of the enterotoxigenicity of staphylococcal isolates (Bergdoll and Bennett 1984). Brain heart infusion broth at pH 5.5, in shake flasks, has also been widely used with success (Casman and Bennett 1963). The shake flask method requires 24 hr incubation, whereas the BHI semisolid agar method requires 48 hr incubation.

Enterotoxin isolation methods for foods. A wide variety of foods can provide a highly nutritious menstruum for the growth of staphylococci. Under optimal conditions of time, temperature, pH, a_w, and atmospheric conditions, these organisms can proliferate rapidly with subsequent production of enterotoxin. Factors and conditions which might influence staphylococcal growth and toxin production have been reviewed by a number of investigators (Ashton and Evancho 1973; Bryan 1976; Tatini 1973; Niskanen 1977; Bergdoll 1979).

The foods generally involved in staphylococcal food poisonings are usually high in protein and thus subject to contamination after cooking (Bryan 1976). However, staphylococcal growth is not always limited to such foods or food mixtures. In the U.S. during the period from 1975 to 1981 (Table 16.1), ham caused the largest number (57) of staphylococcal food poisoning outbreaks. Other foods which caused a significant number of outbreaks during this same period were baked goods, turkey, salads (including poultry, fish, and egg mixtures), and beef. A similar pattern of food vehicles incriminated in food poisoning outbreaks during the period from 1961 to 1973 have been summarized by Bryan (1976).

Currently, five enterotoxins (serotypes A,B,C,D, and E) have been established as serological entities to which antibodies have been produced. Of these enterotoxins, serotypes A and D or A/D combinations appear to cause foodborne intoxication at a greater frequency (Table 16.3) than do enterotoxin serotypes B and C. Serotype A occurs with the greatest frequency (Casman et al. 1967; Simkovicova and Gilbert 1971; Toshach and Thorsteinson 1972; Gilbert and Wieneke 1973). More recently, studies on *S. aureus* growth and toxin production in nitrogen-packed sandwiches (Bennett and Amos 1982) and growth of *S. aureus* and toxin production in imitation cheeses (Bennett and Amos 1983) correlated the time of appearance of detectable toxin with staphylococcal populations. These studies indicated that staphylococcal enterotoxin serotypes A and D are produced earlier or in the presence of fewer staphylococci than are serotypes B and C. Furthermore, the higher frequency of enterotoxin serotypes A and D in food poisoning outbreaks may be due, in part, to their earlier production in some foods. The methods chosen for the routine separation and subsequent serological detection of the staphyococcal enterotoxins from foods are certainly dependent on the amount of enterotoxin required to cause human intoxication. In a study by Dangerfield (1973) using human volunteers, the amount of purified enterotoxin required to cause illness was 3.5 μg in a 70 kg man. These studies were conducted only with adult males, who might be less sensitive than other members of the population. Other members of the population, such as children and women, who weigh less, may respond to smaller amounts of enterotoxin. Based on the small amounts of enterotoxin recovered from foods causing food poisoning, it is thought that 1 μg or less can cause symptoms of staphylococcal intoxication. In two food poisoning outbreaks, one involving cheese and the other salami, there was an indication that those who became ill may have consumed less than 1 μg of enterotoxin A (Bergdoll 1972). While this kind of information may be useful to manufacturers of

Table 16.3. Effect of Elution Buffer Composition[a] on the Recovery of *Staphylococcus aureus* Enterotoxins in Food Poisoning Samples by CMC-22[b] Column Chromatography

Food (100 g)	Elution buffer		Enterotoxin type(s) detected
	0.2M/pH 7.4 (150 ml)	0.05M/pH 6.5 (200 ml)	
Ham	+[c]	+	A
Cheese	+	+	A
Salami	+	+	A
Macaroni salad	+	+	A
Turkey	+	+	A
Powdered milk	+	+	A
Chicken salad	NU[d]	+	A/C
Baked beans	NU	+	D
Spaghetti	NU	+	D
Chili	NU	+	D
Tuna	NU	+	B
Beef stew	NU	+	A
Cube steak	NU	+	A/E
Bar-B-Q pork	NU	+	A
Turkey pieces	NU	+	A
Turkey dressing	NU	+	A
Turkey gravy	NU	+	A
Mashed potatoes	NU	+	A
Turkey broth	NU	+	A
Turkey salad	NU	+	D
Ground turkey	NU	+	D
Ham and cheese sandwich	NU	+	A
Ham	NU	+	A/B
Cooked ground beef	NU	+	A
Turkey slices	NU	+	A
Turkey dressing	NU	+	A
Banana cream pie	NU	+	A
Cooked taco mixture	NU	+	A
Chicken salad sandwiches	NU	+	D
Chicken croquettes	NU	+	A

[a]Sodium phosphate-sodium chloride buffer of varying ionic concentrations (0.5M, 0.2M) and pH (6.5 and 7.4), respectively.
[b]Carboxymethyl cellulose, physical variant 22.
[c](+) Denotes a visible line of precipitation by slide test.
[d]Elution conditions not used (NU).
(*From Bennett et al. 1986a*)

food products, any detectable amount of enterotoxin in a food product which has caused foodborne illness is considered in violation of the Federal Food, Drug, and Cosmetic Act (1979).

In the development of methods for the separation and detection of the enterotoxins, attempts have been made to employ highly sensitive techniques in which food extracts can be tested directly without such pretreatments as partial purification of the toxin, isolation of the toxin from insoluble food proteins, or concentration of food extracts. The reverse passive hemagglutination method is sufficiently sensitive to detect 1 μg of enterotoxin B in an extract from 100 g of food (Silverman et al. 1968). However, some investigators (Bergdoll 1972; Bennett et al. 1973) have encountered false positive reactions with this method. To eliminate the interfering materials which give rise to false positive reactions with the reversed passive hemagglutination test, food extracts must be subjected to some degree of purification (Bergdoll 1972).

A number of procedures for the extraction and isolation of enterotoxins from foods have been proposed. The various aspects, such as procedural extraction steps, minimum enterotoxin detection, serological detection method application, and foods evaluated, have been reviewed (Niskanen 1977). In all of these studies, direct precipitation of antigen and antibody in gels was used for the detection of staphylococcal enterotoxins A and B in foods to which enterotoxins had been added or foods incriminated in food poisoning outbreaks. These studies employed the double gel diffusion tube test (Read et al. 1965a, b; Hall et al. 1965). Other equally elaborate enterotoxin extraction and separation procedures (Casman and Bennett 1965; Stojanow and Schenk 1967; Zehren and Zehren 1968; Mahnke et al. 1970; Barber and Deibel 1972; Gilbert et al. 1972; Reiser et al. 1974; Niskanen 1977) for foods utilized the microslide gel double diffusion test for the detection of enterotoxin.

While it has been the aim of such methods as radioimmunoassay (RIA) as well as enzyme linked immunosorbent assay (ELISA) systems to detect enterotoxins directly in food extracts, few systems have been proposed which employ very simple sample extractions without sacrificing method sensitivity and/or specificity. While all of these food extraction method/serological detection systems have certain specific advantages as well as some disadvantages, only a few which utilize ion exchange materials for the adsorption of the toxin as a partial purification step have been employed widely in the analysis of foods incriminated in food poisoning outbreaks. Of these methods, that of Casman and Bennett (1965), which uses column chromatography employing carboxymethyl cellulose (CMC) ion exchanger, and that of Reiser et al. (1974), employing CG50 ion exchange resin by batch adsorption of the toxin, are the most popular. More recently, a modification of the Casman-Bennett method has been proposed which increases the efficiency of toxin recovery by greater selection of the toxin from food proteins during desorption of the toxin from CMC column chromatography (Bennett et al. 1986a). These chromatographic conditions can be used for the detection of 0.0006 μg of enterotoxin/g of food and have been successfully applied for the detection of enterotoxin in a wide variety of foods incriminated in food poisoning outbreaks (Table 16.3). Both of these extraction-concentration methods are recommended for routine use and have been described in detail by Bergdoll and Bennett (1984). The modified Casman and Bennett method (Bennett 1984b) is the official AOAC method for the extraction and separation of staphylococcal enterotoxins from foods as described by Bennett and McClure (1980), with their subsequent serological detection by the microslide gel double diffusion test as described by Bennett and McClure (1976) and Bergdoll and Bennett (1984). Both methods are of approximately equivalent efficiency, although the toxin adsorption batch method (Reiser et al. 1974) requires less time to obtain the analytical results.

Biological methods. Although the human is a most exquisite model for demonstrating staphylococcal intoxication, this species is seldom used for such experimental endeavors. Occasionally, humans have been used to study the symptomatic effects of this type of bacterial intoxication (Dack 1956; Dangerfield 1973). Many models, such as pigs, frogs, fish, kittens and cats, monkeys, nematodes, protozoa, insects, and bull spermatozoa, have been studied in an attempt to find an inexpensive bioassy system. Tissue cultures have also been employed to study the enterotoxins. Of all animals studied, only kittens (Dolman and Wilson 1940), rhesus monkeys (Surgalla et al. 1953), and chimpanzees have been shown to be of sufficient sensitivity. Of these, kittens and monkeys have been used with the greatest frequency for studying the biological activities of the enterotoxins.

Kittens. Intraperitoneal or intravenous injection of kittens or cats (Dolman and Wilson 1940; Hammon, 1941) have proven to be successful in the bioassay of toxin. Of the routes of administration, the intravenous route is the most commonly used. If one analyzes a culture filtrate for the presence of toxin, it is necessary to inactivate substances (e.g., hemolysins) which may evoke symptoms similar to those caused by the enterotoxins when administered by parenteral routes (Bergdoll 1972). The two primary approaches to the inactivation of metabolites which may produce similar symptoms with the enterotoxin are 20–30 minute boiling or digestion with trypsin (Denny and Bohrer 1963) or pancreatin (Casman and Bennett 1963), since the enterotoxins are resistant to proteolytic digestion. Generally, kittens will produce an emetic response when 1 μg/mL of enterotoxin is injected intravenously. However, cats are relatively insensitive to enterotoxin C and require larger amounts of enterotoxin to achieve an emetic response (Bergdoll 1972). Kittens have been used widely for determining the presence of unidentified enterotoxins (Casman et al. 1967), for thermal inactivation studies (Read and Bradshaw 1966; Denny et al. 1966; Tatini 1976), and for checking the toxicity of purified enterotoxins (Bergdoll 1979).

Monkeys. The feeding of young monkeys has been successful in demonstrating the biological effects of the staphylococcal enterotoxins. While most studies have been conducted with rhesus monkey, cynamologous monkeys have also been used. Either monkey type provides reliable results since the enterotoxin is the only biologically active component which causes emesis when administered by the oral route (Surgalla et al. 1953). Dosing monkeys with solutions of enterotoxins is done by catheter. Generally, animals are observed for 5 hr for emesis. Some investigators also observe the animals for diarrhea (Schantz et al. 1965). Monkeys can be fed a relatively large amount (e.g., 1L or more) of culture supernatant containing enterotoxin by concentrating the material to be tested. The feeding of concentrated supernatants has resulted in demonstrating enterotoxigenicity of *S. aureus* strains which produce enterotoxins in very small or trace amounts. Monkeys are not only expensive to purchase but also to maintain. Additionally, they may become resistant to the enterotoxin with repeated use.

Serological methods. Since the staphylococcal enterotoxins are simple proteins of reasonably good antigenicity, specific antibodies can be produced against them in various animals. The earlier methods for the detection and identification of the enterotoxins have been reviewed (Bergdoll 1972; Minor and Marth 1972; Sommerfeld and Terplan 1975; Niskanen 1977; Bergdoll 1979). A number of these methods have been compared for reliability and specificity (Table 16.4) (Bennett et al. 1973). While all of the earlier data generated use polyclonal antibodies, some of the more recent methods use monoclonal antibodies. The discussion of serological methods will be limited primarily to some of the widely used current methods and more recently proposed approaches for the detection of the staphylococcal enterotoxins.

Hemagglutination. Agglutination (Morse and Mah 1967; Johnson et al. 1967; Silverman et al. 1968) has been proposed as a means of detecting enterotoxins. Of the several variant methods, reverse passive hemagglutination (Silverman et al. 1968) showed some promise with regard to sensitivity and relative ease of execution. With this system, specific antibodies to the staphylococcal enterotoxins are absorbed to sheep red blood cells treated with tannic acid. Other investigators have substituted bisdiazotized benzidene (Bergdoll et al. 1976) for tannic acid. When such treated cells are added to enterotoxin, cell agglutination takes place. Serial twofold dilutions of *S. aureus* culture fluids or food extracts can be prepared in tubes or microtiter plates; added to them is a standard volume and concentration of sheep red blood cells sensitized with antibody. The system is rotated carefully and

Table 16.4. Evaluation of Some Serological Methods for *Staphylococcus aureus* Enterotoxin Detection Specificity and Cross Reactivity

Culture fluids	Strain designation	Entero-toxin Type(s)	Micro-slide (1)		Micro-slide(2)		RIA[a]		RPHA (1)[a]		RPHA (2)	
			A	B	A	B	A	B	A	B	A	B
Culture fluids containing enterotoxins A and B	262 (S6)	A,B	+	+	+	+	+	+	+	+	+	+
	485	A,B,C	+	+	+	+	+	+	+	+	+	+
	243	B	−	+	NL[c]	+	−	+	−	+	±[b]	+
	Staph I	C	−	−	−	−	−	−	+	+	+	+
	789	F	−	−	−	−	−	−	−	−	−	−
	BHIB (con-trol)		−	−	−	−	−	−	−	+	±	±
Antisera to enterotoxins A and B vs. culture fluids[d] from nonenterotoxigenic staphylococci	298		−	−	−	−	−	−	−	−	−	+
	R-124		−	−	−	−	−	−	−	−	−	+
	D-87		−	−	−	−	−	−	−	−	−	+
	R-121		−	−	−	−	−	−	−	−	±[b]	±
	W-46		−	−	−	−	−	−	−	−	−	+
	785		−	−	−	−	−	−	−	−	−	+

Table 16.4. (*Continued*)

Culture fluids	Strain designation	Entero-toxin Type(s)	Micro-slide (1) A	B	Micro-slide (2) A	B	RIA[a] A	B	RPHA (1)[a] A	B	RPHA (2) A	B
Antiserum to enterotoxin	196E			−		−	−	−	−		±	±[b]
B vs. culture fluids[e] con-	D510[d]			−		−	−	−		+		+
taining enterotoxin A	267			−		−	−	−	−		±	+
	787			−		−	−	−				+
	786			−		−	−	−		+	+	+
	265-I			−		−			−		+	+
	S-100									+		+
	743									+	+	+

[a]Radioimmunoassay (RIA); reversed passive hemagglutination (RPHA). (1) and (2) refer to results for Laboratory 1 and Laboratory 2.

[b]Double sign represents results obtained in two different trials with RPHA (2).

[c]No lines of precipitation observed (NL).

[d]500X concentrated culture fluids negative for enterotoxin types A and B by immunodiffusion test.

[e]400X concentrated culture fluids negative for enterotoxin type B by immunodiffusion test.

(*From Bennett et al. 1973*)

placed at room temperature for approximately 2 hr. If enterotoxin is present, the cells agglutinate. It takes 1–2 days to obtain results. Although this approach appeared to be highly sensitive, a number of investigators (Bennett et al. 1973; Bergdoll 1979) experienced nonspecific reactions (Table 16.4) with this procedure. Another problem is that antibodies in some sera fail to react with red blood cells (Bergdoll et al. 1976; Bergdoll 1979). Considerable treatment of food extracts was required to eliminate nonspecific reactions due to food proteins (Reiser et al. 1974). Yamada et al. (1977) applied the RPHA method using formalized sheep red blood cells sensitized with affinity chromatography fractionated immunoglobulins of anti A-E rabbit hyperimmune sera to the A-E toxins. The formalized sheep red blood cells sensitized with these immunoglobulins showed a high degree of specificity with no nonspecific reactions to food ingredients or cross reactions among enterotoxin serotypes. Yamada et al. (1977) reported a minimum detection of enterotoxin in foods by this method to be 0.01 µg/g without concentration of the food extracts. This test is reported to detect as little as 0.0015 µg enterotoxin/mL. However, highly specific antiserum must be used to eliminate nonspecific hemagglutination. It is difficult to determine whether hemagglutination is due to enterotoxin or other antigen impurities, since there is no way to compare test results directly with a control in contrast to radial serological systems such as the Ouchterlony plate technique (Bergdoll et al. 1965) or the microslide gel diffusion test (Casman and Bennett 1963; Casman et al. 1969). Consequently, this method, as it is currently performed, is not recommended as reliable for the detection of staphylococcal enterotoxins.

Precipitation in gels. A number of quantitative methods which utilize linear migration of the antibody and the enterotoxin have been proposed. They include the Oudin single gel diffusion tube test, Oakley double gel diffusion tube test, and a miniaturized system—the capillary tube test (Fung and Wagner 1971; Gandhi and Richardson 1971; Fung 1973). These techniques are most useful for the measuring of enterotoxin in purification assays. However, they are not applicable for the detection of enterotoxins in foods since a toxin control cannot be used in the test system because the band of precipitation cannot be related to a reference line of precipitation. One of the main features of radial diffusion systems is that the test line of precipitation can be related to a reference.

Microslide method. The microslide gel double diffusion test relies on the diffusion and migration through agar gel of the antibody, the reference toxin, and the material being tested. The radial system was first described by Ouchterlony (1949) and was later miniaturized on a microscope slide by Crowle (1958). This method was adapted for use in the detection of the staphylococcal enterotoxins (Casman and Bennett 1963) and has since been used by many laboratories.

The microslide technique is used for the detection of very small amounts of enterotoxin in concentrated food extracts and in bacterial culture filtrates (Casman and Bennett 1963; Hall et al. 1965). With this method, two layers of electrician's plastic tape are placed on a microscope slide, leaving an intervening 2-cm space between for the agar layer. A plastic template containing funnel-shaped holds for the reagents is placed on the agar layer. After preparing the gel diffusion assembly, specific antienterotoxin serum is placed in the center well and the known reference enterotoxin and test preparation are placed in peripheral wells. The slide is incubated 24–72 hr in a petri dish containing moist cotton or a synthetic sponge to prevent evaporation of the reagents. After incubation, the template is removed and the lines of precipitation are observed under oblique lighting. Faint lines of precipitation may be enhanced by staining. The main advantage of the microslide gel diffusion method is that it facilitates direct comparisons of the lines of precipitation formed by the interaction of antibody with toxin, in the sample under test and the line of precipitation formed by the antibody and the reference toxin. As little as 0.1–0.01 μg enterotoxin/mL has been detected by this method depending on the enterotoxin reference and antiserum concentrations. As little as 25 μL of reagents per well is required for the microslide technique. Hence it is possible to do 1000 or more tests with 1.0 mL of antiserum of sufficient titer. The method is most often applied in the detection and identification of two serological types of enterotoxin simultaneously and semiquantitatively. It has been described in detail (Bennett and McClure 1980; Bergdoll and Bennett 1984; Bennett 1984a) and seems to be the most often employed technique with good reliability between laboratories for detection and identification of enterotoxins in culture fluids (Bennett and McClure 1976) and in food extracts (Bennett and McClure 1980). This method is the official AOAC (1984) method and is recommended by APHA (Bergdoll and Bennett 1984) for the serological detection of the staphylococcal enterotoxins.

Optimum Sensitivity Plate (OSP). The Ouchterlony plate technique (Ouchterlony 1949) is also used for the detection of enterotoxins in unknown materials. There are a number of modifications of the original method, involving primarily the shape, size, and placement of the antigen and antibody wells in the agar. The wells are usually round and are normally placed in a circle around a center well with the edges of the outer wells 2–4 mm from the edge of the center well. The farther apart the wells, the longer the time it takes for precipitation to occur. Usually, good lines of identity can be obtained overnight at 25°C with 5–20 μg enterotoxin/mL when the wells are 2–3 mm apart. The detection of smaller amounts of toxin requires 2–3 days, but frequently the reagents disappear from the wells before the lines develop adequately. Generally, the antibody is placed in the center well, and the control toxin and unknown materials are placed in the outer wells. Although this method is not as sensitive as the microslide technique, it is adequate for detecting enterotoxin in concentrated culture fluids and appears to be easier than the slide test for personnel with limited manual dexterity.

Attempts have been made to make this method as sensitive as the microslide gel double diffusion test. A modification of this method, the optimum sensitivity plate, was reported by Robbins et al. (1974), which utilizes small petri dishes (50 x 12 mm). The primary modifications of the OSP method from those reported earlier (Bergdoll et al. 1965) by these investigators are less agar volume, well arrangement, well size, and distances of the wells from each other. Additional conditions such as plate incubation in a humidified environment at 37°C instead of at 25°C resulted in a test which could, generally, be read sooner (18 hr) with enterotoxin concentrations of 1–4 μg/ mL. These modifications of the OSP method, the sensitivity, enterotoxin volume requirements, and the necessity for large amounts of antiserum still do not make it equivalent to the microslide test. However, studies (Robbins et al. 1974) indicate that the OSP method is sufficiently sensitive for use when suspect enterotoxigenic *Staphylococcus aureus* are grown by the cellophane-over-agar and sac-culture toxin production methods. The OSP method is not recommended for the assay of food extracts suspected of containing enterotoxin because of its limited sensitivity (Bergdoll and Bennett 1984). A description for use of the OSP method for the serological determination of enterotoxigenicity of staphylococcal isolates from foods or other sources has been detailed by Bergdoll and Bennett (1984).

Single Radial Diffusion (SRD). A single radial immunodiffusion method was developed by Meyer and Palmieri (1980) to screen a large number of staphylococci in foods for enterotoxigenicity. The SRD method employs glass microscope slides layered with an agar gel coating containing an appropriate mixture of antisera to enterotoxins A, B, C, D, and E, thus establishing a polyvalent detection system. Staphylococcal isolates are cultured in a medium that supports toxin production. Cell-free culture supernatant fluids are added directly to wells bored in the agar layer on the slide. After incubation (24 hr, 35°C) in a moist chamber, a ring of precipitation around the well indicates presence of toxin in the test sample. Thus, a single slide can be used to screen 10 *S. aureus* isolates simultaneously. If polyvalent (serotypes A-E) antiserum has been used, the specific serotype will not be identified. However, the main objective is to determine if the suspect isolate is enterotoxigenic.

If the SRD method is used with the multiple culturing system (Meyer and Palmieri 1980), at least five isolates from the same sample can be grown on separate areas of a petri dish (150 × 15 mm) containing 40 mL of BHI semisolid (0.7%) agar, pH 5.3 (Casman and Bennett 1963; Bennett 1984a). The culture supernatant representing the five isolates is collected by centrifugation and a portion of the supernatant is tested in a single well. Thus, a single slide containing the agar immobilized antibodies can be used to screen up to 50 isolates for the five existing serotypes of enterotoxin. This method has potential in the quality control laboratory as a screening tool. Additionally, there are situations in which foods incriminated in food poisoning outbreaks may contain relatively few toxigenic *S. aureus* in the presence of high numbers of nontoxigenic staphylococci (Noleto and Bergdoll 1980). The method is reported by Meyer and Palmieri (1980) to have a sensitivity of 0.3 μg/mL and has been subjected to interlaboratory evaluation (Meyer et al. 1982).

Radioimmunoassay (RIA). Many studies have been conducted which apply various RIA systems for the detection and quantitation of the staphylococcal enterotoxins. The development of new and advanced technologies was the result of a need for faster results not afforded by some of the earlier methods.

Dickie (1970) suggested solid phase RIA as being potentially useful in meeting the requirements of a simple, rapid, and reasonably inexpensive approach in the quantitative determination of the staphylococcal enterotoxins. Johnson et al. (1971) and Collins et al. (1972) reported the use of solid phase radioimmunoassay for the detection of staphylococcal enterotoxin type B.

The solid phase radioimmunoassay system proposed by Johnson et al. (1971) employed partially purified antibody which was adsorbed onto the internal surface of polystyrene tubes. After adsorption of the antibody, protein adsorbing sites not covered by antibody were blocked by the addition of bovine serum albumin which is unrelated to the toxin-antienterotoxin system. The blocking of these unreacted sites was necessary in order to prevent nonspecific adsorption of radioactively labeled ^{125}I antigen to the walls of the polystyrene tubes. The extract from the test sample was added to the tubes. This provided an opportunity for adsorption of unknown enterotoxin. After an appropriate incubation period, labeled known enterotoxin was added. Again after an appropriate incubation period, the tubes were washed and their radioactivity was measured in a gamma counter. The higher the concentration of unlabeled enterotoxin, the lower the radioactive count. This procedure has been reported (Johnson et al. 1973; Park et al. 1973) to require 24–72 hr for completion with a minimum reproducible detection range of 0.0025–0.0015 μg of enterotoxin/g of food.

In the radioimmunoassay system proposed by Collins et al. (1972), the antibody was coupled to bromacetylcellulose and particles were suspended in a small amount (0.05 mL) of borate bovine serum albumin solution. The food extract or culture fluid (0.1 mL) for assay was added to the tubes followed by the addition of the ^{125}I labeled purified enterotoxin. The tubes were shaken vigorously for 15 min at room temperature and for 1-3/4 hr at 4°C. One and one-half milliliters of borate bovine serum albumin buffer were then added and the suspension was centrifuged. The radioactivity in 1.0 mL of the culture supernate or food extract was counted in a gamma counter in order to determine the amount of labeled antigen which was not bound and sedimented with the antibody. This procedure (Collins et al. 1973) required 3–4 hr for completion and was sensitive within the range 0.01–0.001 μg/mL for the detection of enterotoxin type A. Both tests are sufficiently sensitive for use in detecting enterotoxin in food extracts and were reported as being quantitative.

Comparative studies on the detection of enterotoxin in foods and culture media (Bennett et al. 1973) showed the RIA method employing bromace-tylcellulose particles (Collins et al. 1972) to be specific in distinguishing culture fluids which contained enterotoxins from those culture fluids not containing the enterotoxins (Table 16.4). Although radioimmunoassay systems offered economy in time with a high degree of sensitivity, certain meat products (e.g., salami) have been reported (Johnson et al. 1973) to cause as much as 50% or greater nonspecificity. However, much of the nonspecific inhibition caused with the salami extract was eliminated by dialysis against changes of phosphate buffered saline at 4°C. Other foods, such as ham salad, cheddar cheese, custard and condensed milk, produced nonspecific inhibitions of 15% or less. This assay was reported (Johnson et al. 1973) to be sensitive in a range 1–10 μg of toxin/g of food. The sensitivity of the RIA method of Collins et al. (1972) used in the study by Bennett et al. (1973) was approximately one-tenth that of the RIA method of Johnson et al. (1971). This can be attributed to the smaller volume of sample used (Bergdoll and Reiser 1980). Using RIA with polystyrene tubes as a solid phase support, Park et al. (1973) were able to detect as little as 1.25 ng enterotoxin type A/ g of cheddar cheese, while Bukovic and Johnson (1975) demonstrated the detection of enterotoxin type C at a level of 1.0 ng/g in a variety of foods. Other modifications of RIA employing polystyrene test tubes have been reported (Pober and Silverman 1977; Orth 1977; Miller et al. 1978; Areson et al. 1980). Pober and Silverman (1977) showed that the sensitivity of RIA for the detection of SEB in foods was decreased by food constituents that react with anti-SEB. They minimized this effect by a conditioning step involving overnight incubation (4°C) of the antibody coated tubes with food extracts not containing the toxin and by extraction of interfering constituents in the food samples. The assay was accomplished within 24 hr. The sensitivity was 1.0 ng/mL for milk and cheese and 1.3 ng/mL for chicken salad extract. Orth

(1977) demonstrated the reliability of RIA with a sensitivity of 1.0 ng/g with potato flakes.

Miller et al. (1978) developed a modification of RIA for the detection of staphylococcal enterotoxins A–E by employing inactivated *Staphylococcus aureus* cells containing protein A as an immunoadsorbent. A variety of food extracts were studied with this modified RIA which detected 1.0 ng or less toxin per gram of food. A similar approach to that of Miller et al. (1978) was utilized by Areson et al. (1980). They showed the applicability of using a single standard curve for the quantitation of toxin in foods as opposed to other RIA methods employing a standard curve for each material (sample) under test. They claimed the sensitivity of their assay to be 0.1 ng/mL for SEA and 0.5 ng/mL for SEB.

A third approach employing RIA, the double antibody RIA, was developed by using anti-rabbit gamma globulin from goats to separate the enterotoxin complex from the unreacted toxin (Robern et al. 1975). This method is reported to be highly sensitive and eliminates the need for purified antisera as required by other RIA methods. Robern et al. (1975), using a double antibody RIA, detected as little as 0.33 ng SEC_2/mL of reconstituted dehydrated soup. Robern et al. (1978) reported the applicability of this method to detect SEA and SEB in fermented sausage at a level of 5 ng/mL of extract. Using sheep anti-rabbit gamma globulin, Lindroth and Niskanen (1977) applied the double antibody RIA method and were able to detect as little as 2–5 ng of SEA/g of minced meat and sausage extracts with a reported method sensitivity of 200 pg of enterotoxin.

Still another approach employing RIA for the detection of the enterotoxins is the use of Sepharose 4B as the solid phase support instead of plastics or bromacetylcellulose particles. Niyomvit et al. (1978) covalently attached anti SEB to Sepharose 4B and passed the aqueous test sample through the Sepharose 4B column followed by labeled enterotoxin. They also reported that these columns could be used for over 100 determinations. This assay method could detect SEB at a level of 1.2 ng/mL in buffer, 2.2 ng/mL in nonfat dry milk, and 6.3 ng/g in hamburger.

A number of studies have been conducted in an attempt to resolve problems with RIA methodology regarding iodination techniques which might cause denaturation of the toxin, aggregation of the purified toxin, alteration of high specific gravity on the toxin during storage, and separation of labeled toxin from antibodies. These studies have been summarized by Bergdoll and Reiser (1980).

Although RIA methods appear to be useful in the detection of enterotoxins, only laboratories with gamma radiation counters can use them. However, RIA systems offer economy in assay time, especially in the examination of foods for toxins. General application of RIA is at present limited by the availability of large amounts of the various enterotoxin serotypes in the purified form and the requirement to be licensed to handle radioactive materials.

Enzyme-Linked Immunosorbent Assay (ELISA). A number of enzyme detection systems have been developed for the detection of staphylococcal enterotoxins. The principles of the ELISA assay are similar to those of the RIA. The primary difference is the substitution of an enzyme conjugate for radioactivated antigen in the ELISA assay. The enzyme detection systems can be divided into essentially two categories, competitive and noncompetitive. In competitive enzyme immunoassay (EIA), the antigen in the test sample (or unknown) competes with the antigen bound to a solid matrix for binding sites on the enzyme-labeled antibody (Swaminathan et al. 1985). Antibody binding to the immobilized antigen is decreased by the presence of antigen in the sample under test. Thus, the concentration of antigen in the test sample is inversely proportional to the concentration of product formed by enzyme action in the final reaction. EIAs are discussed more extensively in Chapter 12.

"Sandwich" type assays employing monoclonal antibodies may be less sensitive than those with polyclonal antibodies, since few antibody binding sites on the antigen molecules are being used. However, sandwich assays show a great deal of promise for testing food samples. The mechanics of some of these assays, choices of enzyme labels, assay preservation attempts, and limitations and precautions in the detection of staphylococcal enterotoxins in foods have been reviewed by Kuo and Silverman (1980).

Sanders and Bartlett (1977) employed double-antibody EIA to detect SEA in spiked foods. These investigators detected 0.4 ng SEA/mL in Vienna-type sausage extracts within 20 hr, 3.2 ng SEA/mL in milk within 1–3 hr, and 1.6 ng SEA/mL in a mayonnaise extract. Detection and quantitation of SEA from these spiked food products ranged from 72 to 98% of the added amount of SEA. The enzymes of choice are usually peroxidase or alkaline phosphatase, although Morita and Woodburn (1978) employed β-amylase coupled with SEB. Their reason for using this enzyme was that it is not produced by *S. aureus* and thus eliminates possible complication in assaying samples of culture media. They adapted the "homogeneous enzyme immune assay" for the detection of SEB in foods. In this technique, the free SEB in samples competed with the enzyme linked SEB for the homologous anti-SEB sites. Because the enzyme linked with SEB was rendered inactive with the attachment of anti SEB, the enzyme activity, which was measured photometrically, could be related directly to the concentration of free SEB in the samples under test. Morita and Woodburn (1978) were able to detect quantities of SEB as low as 5 ng/mL in food extracts with the homogeneous enzyme immune assay. The enzyme-multiplied immunoassay technique (Rubenstein et al. 1972) appears to be simpler than some others because it requires neither solid surfaces nor the separation of unbound from bound reactants.

Stiffler-Rosenberg and Fey (1978) described a competitive ELISA assay, the triple ball test, using polystyrene balls coated individually with antibody against SEA, SEB, and SEC in which they were able to detect 0.1 ng or less of enterotoxin/mL when 20 mL of food extract was incubated with three balls (anti SEA,SEB,SEC) followed by testing for uptake of the toxin serotypes. They were successful in detecting enterotoxins both in food extracts and in culture supernatants. With this assay, they observed no cross reactions nor nonspecific interference. An enzyme immunoassay procedure was proposed (Kauffman 1980), specifying alkaline phosphatase-labeled SEA to determine the presence of SEA in foods. In this assay, *Staphylococcus aureus* Cowan I cells were used to separate unbound from antibody-bound SEA. This method was sensitive to 2 ng SEA/mL of food extract. Kuo and Silverman (1980) have discussed the factors that ELISA and RIA share and also the advantages that ELISAs have over RIA. Among other common factors, such as specificity, sensitivity, rapidity, and nonspecific adsorption, the sensitivity of ELISA, as well as RIA is decreased by the presence of food components.

A number of investigators (Buning-Pfaue et al. 1980; Koper et al. 1980; Freed et al. 1982; Notermans et al. 1983) have also employed polyclonal antibodies in the detection of the enterotoxins by the "double-antibody sandwich" ELISA method. SEB was detected in vanilla custard at levels of 0.1 μg in 100 g of custard twice extracted and 20-fold concentrated (Buning-Pfaue et al. 1980). With the "sandwich" technique, Koper et al. (1980) studied nonspecific reactions which are caused by cross reacting antigens and protein A produced by some strains of *S. aureus*. In their studies, cross reacting antibodies were adsorbed from the antiserum using insolubilized culture filtrate of a nontoxigenic strain of *S. aureus*. In spite of this treatment, filtrates of nontoxin producing strains gave cross reactions with antiserum to SEB. In addition, extracts of food which had been inoculated with several different strains of *S. aureus* resulted in cross reactions. However, they were able to eliminate interference by protein A, which binds to the Fc fragments of the IgG antibodies, to SEB by using $F(ab')_2$ fragments of the IgG antibodies in their ELISA experiments. Freed et al. (1982) used the "double-antibody sandwich" ELISA to assay food extracts containing SEA, B, C, D, and E. In their studies, enterotoxin levels below 1.0 ng/g of food were consistently detectable by the ELISA in 8 hr. These studies confirm earlier studies (Koper et al. 1980) regarding the interference by protein A in "double-antibody sandwich" ELISAs and suggest screening samples, particularly culture supernates, for protein A interference with immunoglobulin G in sera from nonimmunized rabbits.

Notermans et al. (1983) employed the ELISA for the detection of SEA, B, C, and E in extracts of minced meat (beef and pork) at levels less than 0.5 μg of SE/100 g of product with neither false positive nor false negative results. Success was probably partially due to the utilization of IgG fractionated antisera.

Fey et al. (1984) made a comparative evaluation of four different ELISA systems for the detection of SEA, B, C, and D. Their general conclusions were that, although both the competitive and sandwich versions of the ELISA can measure 0.1–1.0 ng, the sandwich method proved to be the best in their study. According to them, the competitive method has the advantage of higher specificity because of lower nonspecific uptake. Additionally, it is not sensitive to staphylococcal protein A which interferes by binding to the Fc portion of the antibody. The primary disadvantages of the competitive method are that enterotoxins are difficult to produce and coating antibody and label concentrations are critical. Advantages of the sandwich method are: (1) higher sensitivity than the competitive ELISA; (2) extreme purity of enterotoxin is not necessary to produce specific antibody; (3) titration of reagents is not critical since they are used in excess; and (4) the system is suitable for the use of monoconal antibodies (Fey et al. 1984). Some disadvantages of the sandwich method are that antibody IgG cannot be purified by immunosorption for the conjugation because of the lack of available antigen; antibody reagents have a tendency for nonspecific absorption due to aggregate formation; and staphylococcal protein A removal from culture supernatants and foods may be necessary. Although protein A has not been demonstrated to be a problem in food extracts (Freed et al. 1982), an alternative to protein A interference is the use of sheep antibody (Notermans et al. 1982).

Meyer et al. (1984) developed a monoclonal antibody (McAb) capable of binding to determinants shared in common by staphylococcal enterotoxin serotypes A, B, C, D, and E. It has been proposed that these McAbs be used in the double-antibody sandwich method for the screening of foods for the presence of staphylococcal enterotoxin. Using sensitized spleen cells from mice immunized with SEA and fused with mouse myeloma cells, Edwin et al. (1984) developed clones for McAb production. When antibodies produced from SEA were tested by indirect ELISA, they showed reactivity with SEA and SEE, although the reactivity was higher with SEA than with SEE. Thompson et al. (1984) isolated McAbs reactive with SEB and SEC$_1$. These antibodies were employed to localize the specific and cross reacting epitopes on tryptic fragments of SEB and SEC_1. Progress in the application of monoclonal antibodies for detection of enterotoxins and the toxic shock syndrome antigen produced by *S. aureus* has been reviewed by Thompson et al. (1985).

REFERENCES

ABRAMSON, C. 1973. Hospital-acquired staphylococcal infections and the control programs. In *Proceedings of the Conference on Staphylococci in Foods*. Pennsylvania State University, University Park, PA.

AOAC. 1984. *Official Methods of Analysis*. 14th ed. Williams, S. (Ed.). Assoc. of Official Analytical Chemists, Arlington, VA.

ARESON, P. D. W., CHARM, S. E., and WONG, B. L. 1980. Determination of staphylococcal enterotoxins A and B in various food extracts, using staphylococcal cells containing protein A. *J. Food Sci.* 45: 400–401.

ARMIJO, R. D., HENDERSON, A., TIMOTHEE, R., and RABINSON, H. B. 1957. Food poisoning outbreaks associated with spray dried milk—an epidemiologic study. *Am. J. Public. Health* 47: 1093–1100.

ASHTON, D. H. and EVANCHO, G. M. 1973. Conditions necessary for survival, growth, and enterotoxin production by staphylococci. In *Proceedings of the Conference on Staphylococci in Foods*. Pennsylvania State University, University Park, PA.

ASSOC. FOOD DRUG OFFICIALS U.S. 1966. Microbiological examination of precooked frozen foods. Assoc. Food Drug Officials U.S. *Quart Bull.*

BAER, E. F., GRAY, R. J. H., and ORTH, D. S. 1976. Methods for the isolation and enumeration of *Staphylococcus aureus*. In *Compendium of Methods for the Microbiological Examination of Foods*. Speck, M. L. (Ed.). American Public Health Assoc., Washington, DC.

BAIRD-PARKER, A. C. 1965. The classification of staphylococci and micrococci from worldwide sources. *J. Gen. Microbiol.* 38: 363–387.

BARBER, L. E. and DEIBEL, R. H. 1972. Effect of pH and oxygen tension of staphylococcal growth and enterotoxin formation in fermented sausage. *Appl. Microbiol.* 24: 891–898.

BARBER, M. and KUPER, S. W. A. 1951. Identification of *Staphylococcus pyogenes* by the phosphatase reaction. *J. Pathol. Bacteriol.* 63: 65–68.

BARIZA, M. 1985. Listeriosis and milk. *N. Engl. J. Med.* 312: 438–440.

BENNETT, R. W. 1982. Staphylococcal foodborne illness. In *Microbiological Safety of Foods in Feeding Systems*. ABMPS Report #25. National Research Council, National Academy Press, Washington, DC.

BENNETT, R. W. 1984a. Staphylococcal enterotoxins. In *Bacteriological Analytical Manual*, 6th ed. Assoc. of Official Analytical Chemists, Arlington, VA.

BENNETT, R. W. 1984b. *Staphylococcus aureus*. In *Bacteriological Analytical Manual*. 6th ed. Assoc. of Official Analytical Chemists, Arlington, VA.

BENNETT, R. W. and AMOS, W. T. 1982. *Staphylococcus aureus* growth and toxin production in nitrogen - packed sandwiches. *J. Food Prot.* 45: 157–161.

BENNETT, R. and AMOS, W. T. 1983. *Staphylococcus aureus* growth and toxin production in imitation cheeses. *J. Food Sci.* 48: 1670–1673.

BENNETT, R. W., ARCHER, D. L., and LANCETTE, G. 1986a. Chromatographic selection of *Staphylococcus aureus* enterotoxin in food. *Appl. Environ. Microbiol.* (in press).

BENNETT, R. W., KEOSEYAN, S. A., TATINI, S. R., THOTA, H., and COLLINS, II, W. S. 1973. Staphylococcal enterotoxin: a comparative study of serological detection methods. *Can. Inst. Food Sci. Technol.* 6: 131–134.

BENNETT, R. W. and McCLURE, F. 1976. Collaborative study of the serological identification of staphylococcal enterotoxins by microslide gel double diffusion test. *J. Assoc. Off. Anal. Chem.* 59: 594–601.

BENNETT, R. W. and McCLURE, F. 1980. Extraction and separation of staphylococcal enterotoxin in foods. Collaborative study. *J. Assoc. Off. Anal. Chem.* 63: 1205–1210.

BENNETT, R. W., YETERIAN, M., SMITH, W., COLES, C. M., SASSAMAN, M., and McCLURE, F. D. 1986b. *Staphylococcus aureus* identification characteristics and enterotoxigenicity. *J. Food Sci.* (in press).

BERGDOLL, M. S. 1972. The enterotoxins. In *The Staphylococci*. Cohen, J. O. (Ed.). John Wiley and Sons, Inc. New York.

BERGDOLL, M. S. 1979. Staphylococcal intoxications. In *Foodborne Infections and Intoxications*. 2nd ed. Riemann, H. and Bryan, F. L. (Ed.). Academic Press, New York.

BERGDOLL, M. S. and BENNETT, R. W. 1976. Staphylococcal enterotoxins. In *Compendium of Methods for the Microbiological Examination of Foods*. Speck, M. L. (Ed.). American Public Health Assoc., Washington, DC.

BERGDOLL, M. S. and BENNETT, R. W. 1984. Staphylococcal enterotoxins. In *Compendium of Methods for the Microbiological Examination of Foods*. Speck, M. L. (Ed.). American Public Health Assoc., Washington, DC.

BERGDOLL, M. S., BORJA, C. R., and AVENA, R. M. 1965. Identification of a new enterotoxin as enterotoxin C. *J. Bacteriol.* 90: 1481–1485.

BERGDOLL, M. S. and REISER, R. 1980. Application of radioimmunoassay for detection of staphylococcal enterotoxins in foods. *J. Food Prot.* 43: 68–72.

BERGDOLL, M. S., REISER, R., and SPITZ, J. 1976. Staphylococcal enterotoxins—detection in food. *J. Food Technol.* 30: 80–84.

BOOTHBY, J., GENIGEORGIS, C., and FANELL, M. H. 1979. Tandem coagulase thermonuclease agar method for the detection of *Staphylococcus aureus. Appl. Environ. Microbiol.* 37: 298–302.

BRACHMAN, P. S., TAYLOR, A., GANGAROSA, E. J., MERSON, M. H., and BARKER, W. H. 1976. Food Poisoning in the U.S.A. In *The Microbiological Safety of Food.* Hobbs, B. C. and Christian, J. H. B. (Ed.). Academic Press, New York.

BRYAN, F. L. 1976. *Staphylococcus aureus.* In *Food Microbiology: Public Health and Spoilage Aspects.* de Figueiredo, M. P. and Splittstoesser, D. F. (Ed.). The Avi Publishing Co., Inc., Westport, CT.

BRYAN, F. L. 1978. Factors that contribute to outbreaks of foodborne disease. J. *Food Prot.* 41: 816–827.

BRYAN, F. L. 1979a. Prevention of foodborne disease in food service establishments. *J. Environ. Health* 41: 198–206.

BRYAN, F. L. 1979b. Infections and intoxications caused by other bacteria. In *Foodborne Infections and Intoxications.* 2nd ed. Riemann, H. and Bryan, F. L. (Ed.). Academic Press. New York.

BUKOVIC, J. A. and JOHNSON, H. M. 1975. Staphylococcal enterotoxin C: Solid-phase radioimmunoassay. *Appl. Microbiol.* 30: 700–701.

BUNING-PFAUE, H., TIMMERMANS, P., and NOTERMANS, S. 1980. Einfache Methods fur den Nachweis von Staphylokokken-Enteroxin-B in Vanillepudding mittels ELISA-Test. *Lebensm. Unters. Forsch.* 173: 351–355.

CASMAN, E. P. and BENNETT, R. W. 1963. Culture medium for the production of staphylococcal enterotoxin A. *J. Bacteriol.* 86: 18–23.

CASMAN, E. P. and BENNETT, R. W. 1965. Detection of staphylococcal enterotoxin in food. *Appl. Microbiol.* 13: 181–189.

CASMAN, E. P., BENNETT, R. W., DORSEY, A. E., and ISSA, J. A. 1967. Identification of a fourth staphylococcal enterotoxin, enterotoxin D. *J. Bacteriol* 94: 1875–1882.

CASMAN, E. P., BENNETT, R. W., DORSEY, E. E., and STONE, J. E. 1969. The micro-slide gel double diffusion test for the detection and assay of staphylococcal enterotoxins. *Health Lab. Sci.* 6: 185–198.

CENTERS FOR DISEASE CONTROL. 1976. Foodborne and Waterborne Disease Outbreaks. Annual Summary, 1975. CDC, Atlanta, GA.

CENTERS FOR DISEASE CONTROL. 1977. Foodborne and Waterborne Disease Outbreaks. Annual Summary, 1976. CDC, Atlanta, GA.

CENTERS FOR DISEASE CONTROL. 1979. Foodborne and Waterborne Disease Surveillance. Annual Summary, 1977. CDC, Atlanta, GA.

CENTERS FOR DISEASE CONTROL. 1981a. Foodborne and Waterborne Disease Surveillance. Annual Summary, 1978 (revised). CDC, Atlanta, GA.

CENTERS FOR DISEASE CONTROL. 1981b. Foodborne and Waterborne Disease Surveillance. Annual Summary, 1979. CDC, Atlanta, GA.

CENTERS FOR DISEASE CONTROL. 1983a. Foodborne Disease Surveillance. Annual Summary, 1980. CDC, Atlanta, GA.

CENTERS FOR DISEASE CONTROL. 1983b. Foodborne Disease Surveillance. Annual Summary, 1981. CDC, Atlanta, GA.

CLARK, B. R. and ENGVALL, E. 1980. Enzyme linked immunosorbent assay (ELISA): Theoretical and practical aspects. In *Enzyme Immunoassay*. Maggio, E. T. (Ed.). CRC Press. Boca Raton, FL.

COLLINS, W. S., JOHNSON, A. D., METZGER, J. F., and BENNETT, R. W. 1973. Rapid solid-phase radioimmunoassay for staphylococcal enterotoxin A. *Appl. Microbiol.* 25: 774–777.

COLLINS, W. S. II, METZGER, J. F., and JOHNSON, A. D. 1972. A rapid solid phase radioimmunoassay for staphylococcal B enterotoxin. *J. Immunol.* 108: 852–856.

COLLINS-THOMPSON, D. L., HURST, A., and ARIS, B. 1974. Comparison of selective media for the enumeration sublethally heated food-poisoning strains of *Staphylococcus aureus*. *Can. J. Microbiol.* 20: 1072–1075.

CRISLEY, F. D., ANGELOTTI, R., and FOSTER, M. J. 1964. Multiplication of *Staphylococcus aureus* in synthetic cream fillings and pies. *Public Health Rep.* 79: 369–376.

CRISLEY, F. D., PEELER, J. T., and ANGELOTTI, R. 1965. Comparative evaluation of five selective and differential media for the detection and enumeration of coagulase-positive staphylococci in foods. *Appl. Microbiol.* 13: 140–156.

CROWLE, A. J. 1958. A simplified micro double-diffusion agar precipitin technique. *J. Lab Clin. Med.* 52: 784–787.

CUNNINGHAM, L. B., CATLIN, W., and PRIVAT DE GARILHE, M. 1956. A deoxyribonuclease of *Micrococcus pyogenes*. *J. Am Chem. Soc.* 78: 4642–4645.

DACK, G. M. 1956. *Food Poisoning*. 3rd ed. University of Chicago Press, Chicago, IL.

DACK, G. M. 1963. Problems in foodborne diseases. In *Microbiological Quality of Foods*. Slanetz, L. W. et al., (Ed.). Academic Press, New York.

DANGERFIELD, H. G. 1973. Effects of enterotoxins after ingestion by humans. Paper presented at the 73rd Annual Meeting of the American Society for Microbiology, May 6–11, 1973, Miami Beach, FL.

De FIGUEIREDO, M. P. and JAY, J. M. 1976. Coliforms, enterotococci and other microbial indicators. In *Food Microbiology: Public Health and Spoilage Aspects*. de Figueiredo, M. P. and Splittstoesser, D. F. (Ed.). The Avi Publishing Co., Inc., Westport, CT.

DEIBEL, R. H. 1964. The group D streptococci. *Bacteriol. Rev.* 28: 330–366.

DEIBEL, R. H. and HARTMAN, P. A. 1984. The enterococci. In *Compendium of Methods for Microbiological Examination of Foods*. 2nd. ed. Speck, M. L. (Ed.). American Public Health Assoc., Washington, DC.

DEIBEL, R. H. and SILLIKER, J. H. 1963. Food poisoning potential of the enterococci. *J. Bacteriol.* 85: 827–832.

DENNY, C. B. and BOHRER, C. W. 1963. Improved cat test for enterotoxin. *J. Bacteriol.* 86: 347–348.

DENNY, C. B., TAN, P. L., and BOHRER, C. W. 1966. Heat inactivation of staphylococcal enterotoxin A. *J. Food Sci.* 31: 762–767.

DICKIE, N. 1970. Detection of staphylococcal enterotoxin. *Can. Inst. Food Sci. Technol. J.* 3: 143–144.

DOLMAN, C. E. and WILSON, R. J. 1940. The kitten test for staphylococcus enterotoxin. *Can. J. Public Health* 31: 68–71.

DONNELLY, C. B., LESLIE, J. E., BLACK, L. A., and LEWIS, K. H. 1967. Seriological identification of enterotoxigenic staphylococci from cheese. *Appl. Microbiol.* 15: 1382–1387.

DONNELLY, C. W. and BAIGENT, G. 1985. Use of flow cytometry for the selective identification of *Listeria monocytogenes*. *ASM Abstracts* 1985: 254 (P-18).

DONNELLY, L. S. and HARTMAN, P. A. 1978. Gentamicin-based medium for the isolation of group D streptococci and application of the medium to water analysis. *Appl. Environ. Microbiol.* 35: 576–581.

EDWIN, C., TATINI, S. R., STROBEL, R. S., and MAHESWARAN, S. K. 1984. Production of monoclonal antibodies to staphylococcal enterotoxin A. *Appl. Environ. Microbiol.* 48: 1171–1175.

ELEK, S. D. 1959. *Staphylococcus pyogenes and Its Relation to Disease*. E. S. Livingston, Ltd., Edinburg and London.

ELLIOTT, S. D., McCARTY, M., and LANCEFIELD, R. C. 1977. Teichoic acids of group D streptococci with special reference to strains from pig meningitis. *J. Exper. Med.* 145: 490–499.

FACKLAM, R. R. and MOODY, M. D. 1970. Presumptive identification of D streptococci: the bile-esculin test. *Appl. Microbiol.* 20: 245–250.

FEDERAL FOOD, DRUG, AND COSMETIC ACT, as Amended. January 1979. Code of Federal Regulations, Title 21. U.S. Government Printing Office, Washington, DC.

FELDMAN, H. A. 1946. Incidence of certain biological characteristics among food-poisoning staphylococci. *Am. J. Public Health* 36: 55–57.

FEY, H., PFISTER, H., and RUEGG, O. 1984. Comparative evaluation of different enzyme-linked assay systems for the detection of staphylococcal enterotoxins A,B,C and D. *J. Clin. Microbiol.* 19: 34–38.

FLEMING, D. W., COCHI, S. L., MacDONALD, K. L., BRONDUM, J., HAYES, P. S., PLIKAYTIS, B. D., HOLMES, M. B., ANDRIER, A., BROOME, V., and REINGOLD, A. L. 1985. Pasteurized milk as a vehicle of infection in an outbreak of listeriosis. *N. Engl. J. Med.* 312: 404–407.

FORSGREN, A. 1970. Significance of protein A production by staphylococci. *Infect. Immun.* 2: 672–673.

FOSTER, E. M. 1973. Food poisoning attributed to controversial agents: *B. cereus, Pseudomonas* sp. and fecal streptococci. In *Microbial Foodborne Infections and Intoxications.* Hurst, A. and de Man, J. M. (Ed.). 1972 Symposium Health Protection Branch, Dept. of National Health and Welfare, Ottawa, Canada.

FRANCIS, D. W., HUNT, J. M., PEELER, J., and LOVETT, J. 1984. Distribution of *Listeria monocytogenes* into fractions of whole milk during separation. *AOAC Abstracts.* 19: (# 147).

FREED, R. C., EVENSON, M. L., REISER, R. F., and BERGDOLL, M. S. 1982. Enzyme-linked immunosorbent assay for detection staphylococcal enterotoxins in foods. *Appl. Environ. Microbiol.* 44: 1349–1355.

FUNG, D. Y. C. 1973. Capillary agar tube system for the detection of staphylococcal enterotoxins in foods. In *Proceedings of the Conference on Staphylococci in Foods.* Pennsylvania State University, University Park, PA.

FUNG, D. Y. C. and WAGNER, J. 1971. Capillary tube assay for staphylococcal enterotoxin A, B, and C. *Appl. Microbiol.* 21: 559–561.

GANDHI, N. R. and RICHARDSON, G. H. 1971. Capillary tube immunological assay for staphylococcal enterotoxin. *Appl. Microbiol.* 21: 626–627.

GENIGEORGIS, C. and SADLER, W. W. 1966. Effect of sodium chloride and pH on enterotoxin B production by *Staphylococcus aureus*. *J. Bacteriol.* 92: 1383–1387.

GILBERT, R. J. and WIENEKE, A. A. 1973. Staphylococcal food poisoning with special reference to the detection of enterotoxin in food. In *The Microbiological Safety of Food*. Hobbs, B. C. and Christian, J. H. B. (Ed.). Academic Press, New York.

GILBERT, R. J., WIENEKE, A. A., LANSER, J., and SIMKOVICOVA, M. 1972. Serological detection of enterotoxin in foods implicated in staphylococcal food poisoning. *J. Hyg.* 70: 755–762.

GRAY, M. L. and KILLINGER, A. H. 1966. *Listeria monocytogenes* and listeric infections. *Bacteriol. Rev.* 30: 309–382.

HALL, H. E., ANGELOTTI, R., and LEWIS, K. H. 1965. Detection of staphylococcal enterotoxins in food. *Health Lab. Sci.* 2: 179–191.

HALLANDER, H. O. 1965. Production of large quantities of enterotoxin B and other staphylococcal toxins on solid media. *Acta Pathol. Microbiol. Scand.* 63: 299–305.

HAMMON, W. M. 1941. Staphylococcus enterotoxin: an improved cat test, chemical and immunological studies. *Am. J. Public Health* 31: 1191–1198.

HAUSCHILD, A. H. W., PARK, C. E., and HILHEIMER, R. 1979. A modified pork plasma agar for the enumeration of *Staphylococcus aureus* in foods. *Can. J. Microbiol.* 25: 1052–1057.

HEIDELBAUGH, N. D., ROWLEY, D. B., POWERS, E. M., BOURLAND, C. T., and McQUEEN, J. L. 1973. Microbiological testing of skylab foods. *Appl. Microbiol.* 25: 55–61.

HOBBS, B. C., KENDALL, M., and GILBERT, R. J. 1968. Use of phenolphthalein diphosphate agar with polymyxin as a selective medium for the isolation and enumeration of coagulase positive staphylococci from foods. *Appl. Microbiol.* 16: 535.

HOBBS, B. C., SMITH, M. E., OAKLEY, C. L., WARRACH, G. H., and CRUCKSHANK, J. C. 1953. *Clostridium welchii* food poisoning. *J. Hyg.* 51: 75–101.

ICMSF (International Commission on Microbiological Specifications for Foods of the International Assoc. of Microbiological Societies. 1978. *Microorganisms in Foods. I. Their Significance and Methods of Enumeration*. 2nd ed. University of Toronto Press, Canada.

JARVIS, A. W. and LAWRENCE, R. C. 1970. Production of high titers of enterotoxins for the routine testing of staphylococci. *Appl. Microbiol.* 19: 698–699.

JAY, J. M. 1978. *Modern Food Microbiology*. 2nd ed. D. Van Nostrand Co. New York.

JOHNSON, H. M., BUKOVIC, J. A., and KAUFFMAN, P. E. 1973. Staphylococcal enterotoxins A and B: Solid-phase radioimmunoassay in food. *Appl. Microbiol.* 26: 309–313.

JOHNSON, H. M., BUKOVIC, J. A., KAUFFMAN, P. E., and PEELER, J. T. 1971. Staphylococcal enterotoxin B: Solid phase radioimmunoassay. *Appl. Microbiol.* 22: 837–841.

JOHNSON, H. M., HALL, H. E., and SIMON, M. 1967. Enterotoxin B: serological assay in cultures by passive hemagglutination. *Appl. Microbiol.* 15: 815–818.

JULSETH, R. M. and DUDLEY, R. P. 1973. Improved methods for enumerating staphylococci and detecting staphylococcal enterotoxin in meat foods. 511–522. In *19th European Meeting of Meat Research Workers*, Vol. II. Centre Technique de la charcuterie, Paris, France.

KAUFFMAN, P. E. 1980. Enzyme immunoassay for staphylococcal enterotoxin A. *J. Assoc. Off. Anal. Chem.* 63: 1138–1143.

KENNER, B. A., CLARK, H. F., and SARAWALT, D. S. 1961. Fecal streptococci. I. Cultivation and enumeration of streptococci in surface waters. *Appl. Microbiol.* 9: 15–20.

KOPER, J. W., HAGENAARS, A. M., and NOTERMANS, S. 1980. Prevention of cross-reactions in the enzyme linked immunosorbent assay (ELISA) for the detection of *Staphylococcus aureus* enterotoxin type B in culture filtrates and foods. *J. Food Safety* 2: 35–45.

KUO, J. K. S. and SILVERMAN, G. J. 1980. Application of enzyme-linked immunosorbent assay for detection of staphylococcal enterotoxin in foods. *J. Food Prot.* 43: 404–407.

LACHICA, R. V. F., HOEPRICH, P. D., and GENIGEORGIS, C. 1971. Nuclease production and lysostaphin susceptibility of *Staphylococcus aureus* and other catalase-positive cocci. *Appl. Microbiol.* 21: 823–826.

LACHICA, R. V. F., HOEPRICH, P. D., and GENIGEORGIS, C. 1972. Metachromatic agar diffusion microslide technique for detecting staphylococcal nuclease in foods. *Appl. Microbiol.* 23: 168–169.

LANCETTE, G. 1985. Current resuscitation methods for recovery of stressed *Staphylococcus aureus* from foods. *J. Food Prot.* (in press).

LEE, W. S. 1972. Improved procedure for identification of group D enterococci with two new media. *Appl. Microbiol.* 24: 1–3.

LINDROTH, S. and NISKANEN, A. 1977. Double antibody solid-phase radioimmunoassay for staphylococcal enterotoxin A. *Eur. J. Appl. Microbiol.* 4: 137–143.

LITSKY, W., MALLMAN, W. L., and FIFFIELD, C. W. 1955. Comparison of the most probable numbers of *Escherichia coli* and enterococci in river water. *Am. J. Public Health* 45: 1049–1053.

LOVETT, J., FRANCIS, D. W., and HUNT, J. M. 1985. A method for isolating *Listeria monocytogenes* from milk. *ASM Abstracts* 1985: 253 (P 17).

MAHNKE, C., RATHMAN, K., and BERGDOLL, M. S. 1970. Food research institute technique for determination of staphylococcal enterotoxin in foods. (unpublished manuscript). Food Research Institute, University of Wisconsin, Madison, WI.

McBRIDE, M. E. 1960. A selective method for the isolation of *Listeria monocytogenes* from mixed bacterial populations. *J. Lab. Clin. Med.* 55: 153–157.

MEYER, R. F., BENNETT, R. W., MacMILLAN, J. D., and PALMIERI, M. J. 1982. Screening for enterotoxigenic staphylococci in foods. *FDA By-Lines* 12: 189–195.

MEYER, R. F., MILLER, L., BENNETT, R. W., and MacMILLAN, J. D. 1984. Development of a monoclonal antibody capable of interacting with five serotypes of *Staphylococcus aureus* enterotoxin. *Appl. Environ. Microbiol.* 47: 283–287.

MEYER, R. F. and PALMIERI, M. J. 1980. Single radial immunodiffusion method for screening staphylococcal isolates for enterotoxin. *Appl. Environ. Microbiol.* 40: 1080–1085.

MILLER, B. A., REISER, R. F. and BERGDOLL, M. S. 1978. Detection of staphylococcal enterotoxins A,B,C,D, and E in food by radioimmunoassay, using staphylococcal cells containing protein A as an immunoadsorbent. *Appl. Environ. Microbiol.* 36: 421–426.

MINOR, T. E. and MARTH, E. H. 1972. *Staphylococcus aureus* and staphylococcal food intoxication. A review. II. Enterotoxins and epidemiology. *J. Milk Food Technol.* 35: 21–29.

MORITA, T. N. and WOODBURN, M. J. 1978. Homogeneous enzyme immune assay for staphylococcal enterotoxin B. *Infect. Immun.* 21: 666–668.

MORSE, S. A. and MAH, R. A. 1967. Microtiter hemagglutination-inhibition assay for staphylococcal enterotoxin B. *Appl. Microbiol.* 15: 58–61.

NEFEDJEVA, M. P. 1964. Laboratovnaia diannostika infestsionnykh zabolevanii (*Laboratory Diagnosis of Infectious Diseases; methodological manual*). 2nd ed., p. 352. Beuro Nauchnoi. Informatsii, Moscow.

NIEMAN, R. E. and LOBER, B. 1980. Listeriosis in adults: a changing pattern: Report of eight cases and review of literature, 1968–1978. *Rev. Infect. Dis.* 2: 207–227.

NISKANEN, A. 1977. Staphylococcal enterotoxins and food poisoning. Production, properties and detection of enterotoxins. Pub. 19. Tech. Res. Centre Finland, Helsinki.

NIYOMIT, N., STEVENSON, K. E., and McFEETERS, R. F. 1978. Detection of staphyloccal enterotoxin B by affinity radioimmunoassay. *J. Food Sci.* 43: 735–739.

NOLETO, A. L. and BERGDOLL, M. S. 1980. Staphylococcal enterotoxin production in the presence of non-enterotoxigenic staphylococci. *Appl. Environ. Microbiol.* 39: 1167–1171.

NOTERMANS, S., BOOT, R., TIPS, P. D., and DENOOIJ, M. P. 1983. Extractions of staphylococcal enterotoxins (SE) from minced meat and subsequent detection of SE with enzyme linked immunosorbent assay (ELISA). *J. Food Prot.* 46: 238–241.

NYFELDT, A. 1929. Etiologie de la mononucleose infectieuse. C. P. *Soc. Biol*(Paris) 101: 590–592.

ORTH, D. S. 1977. Iodination of staphylococcal enterotoxin B by the use of chloramine-T. *Appl. Environ. Microbiol.* 33: 824–828.

OUCHTERLONY, O. 1949. Antigen antibody reactions in gels. *Acta Pathol. Microbiol. Scand.* 25: 507–515.

PARK, C. E., DICKIE, N., ROBERN, H., STAVRIC, S., and TODD, E. C. D. 1973. Comparison of solid-phase radioimmunoassay and slide gel double immunodiffusion methods for the detection of staphylococcal enterotoxins in foods. In *Proceedings of the Conference on Staphylococci in Foods* Pennsylvania State University, University Park, PA.

PAVLOVA, M. T., BREZENSKI, F. T., and LITSKY, W. 1972. Evaluation of various media for isolation, enumeration and identification of fecal streptocci from natural sources. *Health Lab. Sci.* 9: 289–298.

POBER, Z. and SILVERMAN, G. J. 1977. Modified radioimmunoassay determination for staphylococcal enterotoxin B in foods. *Appl. Environ. Microbiol.* 33: 620–625.

PUGSLEY, A. P. and EVISON, L. M. 1975. A fluorescent antibody technique for the enumeration of faecal streptococci in water. *J. Appl. Bacteriol.* 38: 63–65.

RALOVICH, B. 1984. *Listeriosis Research: Present Situation and Perspective.* Akademiai Kiado, Budapest, Hungary. Distributed by Heyden and Son, Philadelphia, PA.

RAY, B. 1979. Methods to detect stressed microorganisms. *J. Food Prot.* 42: 346–355.

RAYMAN, M. K., PARK, C. E., PHILPOTT, J., and TODD, E. C. D. 1975. Reassessment of the coagulase and thermostable nuclease test as a means of identifying *Staphylococcus aureus*. *Appl. Microbiol.* 29: 451–454.

READ, R. B. JR. and BRADSHAW, J. G. 1966. Thermal inactivation of staphylococcal enterotoxin B in Veronal buffer. *Appl. Microbiol.* 14: 130–132.

READ, R. B. JR., BRADSHAW, J., PRITCHARD, W. L., and BLACK, L. A. 1965b. Assay of staphylococcal enterotoxin from cheese. *J. Dairy Sci.* 48: 420–424.

READ, R. B. JR., PRITCHARD, W. L., BRADSHAW, J., and BLACK, L. A. 1965a. In vitro assay of staphylococcal enterotoxins A and B from milk. *J. Dairy Sci.* 48: 411–419.

REISER, R. F., CONAWAY, D., and BERGDOLL, M. S. 1974. Detection of staphylococcal enterotoxin in foods. *Appl. Microbiol.* 27: 83–85.

REISER, R. F. and WEISS, K. F. 1969. Production of staphylococcal enterotoxins A,B, and C in various media. *Appl. Microbiol.* 18: 1041–1043.

ROBBINS, R., GOULD, S., and BERGDOLL, M. S. 1974. Detecting the enterotoxigenicity of *Staphylococcus aureus* strains. *Appl. Microbiol.* 28: 946–950.

ROBERN, H., DIGHTON, M., YANO, Y., and DICKIE, N. 1975. Double-antibody radioimmunoassay for staphylococcal enterotoxin C_2. *Appl. Microbiol.* 30: 525–529.

ROBERN, H., GLEESON, T. M., and SZABO, R. A. 1978. Double-antibody radioimmunoassay for staphylococcal enterotoxins A and B. *Can. J. Microbiol.* 24: 436–439.

RUBENSTEIN, K. E., SCHNEIDER, R. S., and ULLMAN, E. F. 1972. "Homogeneous" enzyme immunoassay, a new immunochemical technique. *Biochem. Biophys. Res. Commun.* 47: 846–851.

SANDERS, G. C. and BARTLETT, M. L. 1977. Double-antibody solid-phase immunoassay for the detection of staphylococcal enterotoxin A. *Appl. Environ. Microbiol.* 34: 518–522.

SCHANTZ, E. J., ROESSLER, W. G., WAGMAN, J., SPERO, L., DUNNERY, D. A., and BERGDOLL, M. S. 1965. Purification of staphylococcal enterotoxin B. *Biochemistry* 4: 1011–1016.

SCHLECH, W. F. III, LAVIGNE, P. M., BORTOLUSSI, R. A., et al. 1983. Epidemic listerosis evidence for transmission by food. *N. Engl. J. Med.* 308: 203–206.

SHERMAN, J. M. 1937. The streptococci. *Bacteriol. Rev.* 1: 3–97.

SIEGEL, J. E. and NELSON, J. D. 1981. Listeriosis. In *Infectious Diseases* Sandford, J. P. and Luby, J. P. (Ed.). Grune and Stratton, New York.

SILVERMAN, S. J., KNOTT, A. R., and HOWARD, M. 1968. Rapid, sensitive assay for staphylococcal enterotoxin and a comparison of serological methods. *Appl. Microbiol.* 16: 1019–1023.

SIMKOVICOVA, M. and GILBERT, R. J. 1971. Serological detection of enterotoxin from food-poisoning strains of *Staphylococcus aureus*. *J. Med. Microbiol.* 4: 19–30.

SINELL, H. J. and BAUMGART, J. 1967. Selektivnahrboden mit Eigelbzur Isolierung von pathogenen staphylokokken aus Lebensmitteln. Zentralbl. Bakteriol. Parasitenk. Infektionskr. *Hyg. Abt. 1: Orig. Reihe B* 204: 248.

SMITH, J. L., BUCHANAN, R. L., and PALUMBO, S. A. 1983. Effect of food environment on staphylococcal enterotoxin synthesis: A review *J. Food Prot.* 46: 545–555.

SOMMERFELD, P. and TERPLAN, G. 1975. Methoden zum Nachweis von Staphylokokkenenterotoxinen. *Arch. Lebensmittel Hyg.* 26: 128–137.

SPERBER, W. H. 1976. The identification of staphylococci in clinical and food microbiology laboratories. *CRC Critical Reviews in Clinical Laboratory Science* 7: 121. CRC Press, Inc., Boca Raton, FL.

SPERBER, W. H. and TATINI, S. R. 1975. Interpretation of the tube for identification of *Staphylococcus aureus. Appl. Microbiol.* 29: 502–505.

STIFFLER-ROSENBERG, G. and FEY, H. 1978. Simple assay for staphyloccal enterotoxins A, B, and C: modification of enzyme-linked immunosorbent assay. *J. Clin. Microbiol.* 8: 473–479.

STOJANOW, I. M. and SCHENK, E. 1967. Verfahren zur preparativen Isolierung von Staphylokokken-enterotoxin in Fleischerzeugnisse. *XIII Kongr. Europae Fleisch Rotterdam Proceedings.*

STONE, R. V. SR. 1936. A cultural method for classifying staphylococci as of the food poisoning type. *Proc. Soc. Exp. Biol. Med.* 33: 185–187.

SURGALLA, M. J., BERGDOLL, M. S., and DACK, G. M. 1953. Some observations on the assay of staphylococcal enterotoxin by the monkey-feeding test. *J. Lab. Clin. Med.* 4: 782–788.

SWAMINATHAN, B., ALEIXO, J. A. G., and MINNICH, S. A. 1985. Enzyme immunoassay for *Salmonella*: one-day testing is now a reality. *Food Technol.* 39(3): 83–89.

TAGER, M. and DRUMMOND, M. C. 1965. Staphylocoagulase. *Ann. N.Y. Acad. Sci.* 128: 92–111.

TATINI, S. R. 1973. Influence of food environments on growth of *Staphylococcus aureus* and production of various enterotoxins. *J. Milk Food Technol.* 36: 559–563.

TATINI, S. 1976. Thermal stability of enterotoxins in food. *J. Milk Food Technol.* 39: 432–438.

TATINI, S. R., CORDS, B. R., and GRAMOLI, J. 1976. Screening for staphylococcal enterotoxins in food. *Food Technol.* 30(4): 64–74.

TATINI, S. R., HOOVER, D. G., and LACHICA, V. F. 1984. Methods for the isolation and enumeration of *Staphylococcus aureus*. In *Compendium of Methods for the Microbiological Examination of Foods*. Speck, M. L. (Ed.). American Public Health Assoc., Washington, DC.

THATCHER, F. S. and CLARK, D. S. (Ed.). 1968. *Microorganisms in Foods: Their Significance and Methods of Enumeration.* University of Toronto Press, Canada.

THIAN, T. S. and HARTMAN, P. A. 1981. Gentamicin-thallous-carbonate medium for isolation of fecal streptococci from foods. *Appl. Environ. Microbiol.* 41: 724–728.

THOMPSON, N. E., BERGDOLL, M. S., MEYER, R. F., BENNETT, R. W., MILLER, L., and MacMILLAN, J. D. 1985. Monoclonal antibodies to the enterotoxins and to the toxic shock syndrome toxin produced by *Staphylococcus aureus.* In *Monoclonal Antibodies.* Vol. II. Macario, A. J. L. and Macario, E. C. (Ed.). Academic Press, Inc., Orlando, FL (in press).

THOMPSON, N. E., KETTERHAGEN, M. J., and BERGDOLL, M. S. 1984. Monoclonal antibodies to staphylococcal enterotoxins B and C: cross-reactivity and localization of epitopes on tryptic fragments. *Infect. Immun.* 45: 281–285.

TOSHACH, S. and THORSTEINSON, S. 1972. Detection of staphylococcal enterotoxin by the gel diffusion test. *Can. J. Public Health* 63: 58–65.

TURNER, F. S. and SCHWARTZ, B. S. 1958. The use of lyophilized human plasma standardized for blood coagulation factors in the coagulase and fibrinolytic test. *J. Lab. Clin. Med.* 52: 888–894.

WATKINS, S. A., BALL, L. C., and FRASHER, C. A. 1980. Use of the API-ZYM system in rapid identification of B and non-hemolytic streptococci. *J. Clin. Pathol.* 33: 53–57.

YAMADA, S., IGARASHI, H., and TERAYAMA, T. 1977. Improved reversed passive hemagglutination for simple and rapid detection of staphylococcal enterotoxins A-E in food. *Microbiol. Immunol.* 21: 675–682.

ZEHREN, V. L. and ZEHREN, V. F. 1968. Examination of large quantities of cheese for staphylococcal enterotoxin A. *J. Dairy Sci.* 51: 635–644.

17

Detection and Quantitation of Sporeforming Pathogens and Their Toxins

Peggy M. Foegeding

North Carolina State University
Raleigh, North Carolina

This review will address methods to detect and/or quantitate *Clostridium perfringens, C. botulinum,* and *Bacillus cereus* organisms and their toxins. Both cultural and immunological methods will be reviewed, as prior chapters in this volume have reviewed details of immunological and other techniques.

CLOSTRIDIUM PERFRINGENS TYPE A

Five types of *Clostridium perfringens,* distinguished by the major exotoxins produced, have been identified to date. In addition to gas gangrene, septicemia, and other infections, *C. perfringens* type A causes foodborne illness and therefore will be the focus of this section.

Paper No. 9942 of the Journal Series of North Carolina Agricultural Research Service, Raleigh, NC 27695-7624. The use of trade names in this publication does not imply endorsement by the North Carolina Agricultural Research Service of the products named, nor criticism of similar ones not mentioned.

Hatheway and coworkers (1980) have published a review of epidemiological aspects of *C. perfringens* foodborne illness. Crowther and Baird-Parker (1984) and Craven (1980) briefly reviewed survival, growth, and sporulation of this organism in food. *C. perfringens* causes a generally mild gastroenteritis which typically follows ingestion of approximately 10^8 viable colony forming units. The vehicle of infection is frequently red meat or poultry. *C. perfringens* is capable of rapid growth to high numbers in these products, given a heating, cooling, and/or warming regime favorable for growth (Willardsen et al. 1979). The enterotoxin responsible for *C. perfringens* foodborne illness generally is produced in the intestine although sporulation and enterotoxin production may occur in foods (Craven 1980; Naik and Duncan 1977a).

Detection and Quantitation of *C. perfringens*

Foods in which *C. perfringens* detection and quantitation would be of interest include (a) foods in which the *C. perfringens* population is small and outnumbered by other microorganisms, as would be useful in quality control applications; and (b) foods in which *C. perfringens* populations are high, particularly food involved in a foodborne illness outbreak. In both instances, recovery of injured *C. perfringens* vegetative cells must be considered since injury of this organism may result from exposure to heat, cold, oxygen, and/or oxidized medium constituents (Shoemaker and Pierson 1976). Primarily vegetative cells rather than spores of *C. perfringens* are present in foods and of concern in recovery methodologies. In confirmation of a foodborne illness, *C. perfringens* may be isolated from the stools of patients. In this case, numbers of *C. perfringens* would be expected to be large in comparison to other microorganisms, and a significant spore population may be present (Hauschild et al. 1974, 1979).

In a recent overview of media for enumeration and confirmation of *C. perfringens*, Labbe (1983) noted that many media have evolved from a sulfate-glucose-iron-agar medium developed by Wilson and Blair (1924) for analysis of sulfite-reducing bacteria in water. In Wilson-Blair medium the clostridia reduce sulfite to sulfide, which is precipitated as ferrous sulfide in the presence of an iron salt, forming black colonies. This principle has proven useful for *C. perfringens* differentiation and still is employed. Other principles which have found some success in differential media used for recovery include incorporation of egg yolk for detection of lecithinase activity, use of blood agar for detection of hemolytic activity, use of milk-containing medium for detection of the typical *C. perfringens* stormy fermentation reaction, and incorporation of lactose for detection of abundant gas from fermentation of this sugar.

Selection of *C. perfringens* is by incorporation of one or more antibiotics in virtually all of the methodologies for isolation and enumeration. Alternatively, selection may employ incubation at approximately 46°C generally for ≤ 24 hr to take advantage of the rapid *C. perfringens* growth rate at this temperature. Antibiotics which have been incorporated alone or in combination into media for selection of *C. perfringens* with varying degrees of success include polymyxin B sulfate (10 mg/L; Mossel 1959), sulfadiazine (0.12 mg/mL; Angelotti et al. 1962), neomycin sulfate (50 mg/L; Marshall et al. 1965 or ca. 40 mg/L; Sutton and Hobbs 1968), D-cycloserine (800 mg/L; Fuzi and Csudas 1969 or 400 mg/L; Harmon et al. 1971), kanamycin (12 mg/L; Shahidi and Ferguson 1971), and oleandomycin phosphate (0.5 mg/L; Hanford and Cavett 1973; Hanford 1974).

Media currently in common use for isolation and enumeration of *C. perfringens* include Tryptose Sulfite Cycloserine agar (TSC; Harmon et al. 1971), egg yolk-free TSC (Hauschild and Hilsheimer 1974a), oleandomycin-polymyxin-sulphadiazine perfringens medium (OPSP; Hanford 1974), neomycin blood agar (Sutton and Hobbs 1968), and Shahidi-Ferguson-perfringens agar (SFP; Shahidi and Ferguson 1971). Formulations for these media are shown in Table 17.1 .

For specificity and high recovery, TSC and egg yolk-free TSC are superior to SFP and neomycin blood agar (Hauschild et al. 1977, 1979). Since not all enterotoxin-producing *C. perfringens* are lecithinase producers, and because of the added complexity of preparing medium with egg yolk, many laboratories prefer egg yolk-free TSC (Hauschild and Hilsheimer 1974; Hauschild et al. 1977). OPSP medium is widely used in the United Kingdom. Adams and Mead (1980) compared media for *C. perfringens* enumeration and reported that OPSP medium compared favorably with egg yolk-free TSC medium. OPSP medium suppresses *C. bifermentans* colony formation more effectively than does TSC medium; however, it permits the growth of some fecal streptococci which form small white or cream-colored colonies since they do not reduce sulfite. The United States Food and Drug Administration (Harmon and Duncan 1978) uses TSC with or without egg yolk for presumptive enumeration of *C. perfringens* in foods, and TSC with or without egg yolk has been adopted as official first action for this purpose by the Association of Official Analytical Chemists (Anonymous, 1980). Confirmation of typical colonies is required.

A need to detect small numbers of *C. perfringens* has led to the development of enrichment media and other recovery systems. Debevere (1979) enriched low populations using fluid thioglycollate medium without glucose and with 0.4 mg D-cycloserine/mL incubated at 46°C. This was followed by isolation on iron plus sulfite agar followed by confirmation. Others have enriched small populations using cooked meat medium or incubation in meat foods

Table 17.1. Media Currently in Common Use for Selective Enumeration of *Clostridium perfringens*

	SFP[a]	Egg Yolk-Free TSC[b]	OPSP[c]	Neomycin Blood-Agar[d]
	Amount per 100 mL medium			
Tryptose	1.5 g	1.5 g	1.5 g	—
Soytone	0.5 g	0.5 g	0.5 g	—
Yeast extract	0.5 g*	0.5 g	0.5 g	—
Sodium metabisulfite	0.1 g	0.1 g	0.1 g	—
Ferric ammonium citrate	0.1 g	0.1 g	0.1 g	—
Agar	2.0 g	2.0 g	2.0 g	—
Blood agar	—	—	—	(base plus blood)[e]
D-cycloserine	—	40 mg	—	—
Sodium sulfadiazine	12 mg	—	1.0 mg	—
Polymyxin B sulfate	3000 units	—	1000 i.u.	—
Kanamycin sulfate	1.2 mg	—	—	—
Oleandomycin phosphate	—	—	0.05 mg	—
Neomycin sulfate	—	—	—	ca. 4 mg[f]
Egg Yolk emulsion (50% in saline)	10 mL	(8 mL)[g]	—	—
pH (pre-autoclave)	7.6	7.6	7.6	7.2

[a]Shahidi and Ferguson (1971).
[b]Hauschild and Hilsheimer (1974a).
[c]Hanford (1974).
[d]Sutton and Hobbs (1968).
[e]Blood agar plates are prepared using a standard basal medium plus blood (5 g/100 mL).
[f]Approximately 0.06 mL of a 1.0% solution spread evenly over the surface of a plate.
[g]TSC is made according to the formula for egg yolk-free TSC to which 8 mL of egg yolk emulsion is added per 100 mL medium. Egg yolk emulsion is omitted from the overlay medium. Harmon et al. (1971).

(Hobbs and Cross 1984). Enrichment for *C. perfringens* is not routinely incorporated in methodologies (Harmon and Duncan 1978; Mead et al. 1982; Duncan and Harmon 1976).

A most probable number (MPN) method for estimating *C. perfringens* was proposed by Erickson and Diebel (1978). They employed Rapid Perfringens Medium (RPM), a fortified mixture of litmus milk plus fluid thioglycollate with polymyxin and neomycin for selection. Organisms causing the characteristic stormy fermentation were isolated and confirmed. This procedure is laborious but effectively recovers small populations. A similar MPN method utilizes iron milk medium (St. John et al. 1982). Recovery by this procedure was similar to SFP recovery, and false-positive results from clostridial strains with biochemical characteristics similar to *C. perfringens* appear unlikely. The procedure has the advantages of rapid positive responses (< 3 hr) from inocula with $\geq 10^7$ CFU/mL *C. perfringens* and apparently good recovery and specificity (Abeyta et al. 1985).

Beerens et al. (1982) used the MPN procedure with a lactose plus sulfite broth (LS) medium incubated at 46°C for *C. perfringens* enumeration. Dilutions were made with cysteine-Ringer solution and confirmation of positive tubes (black from FeS and gassy) was not required. Of 43 clostridia species and species from 10 other genera tested (100 strains total, including 24 *C. perfringens* strains), only *C. barati (C. paraperfringens)* may be confused with *C. perfringens* and the authors noted that this organism rarely is associated with foods. Recovery of *C. perfringens* from food and feces was comparable for the LS medium-MPN procedure and egg yolk-free TSC without cycloserine enumeration. Since confirmation of positive LS cultures is not required, results can be obtained in ≤ 24 hr and small *C. perfringens* populations (5–10 cells/tube) in inoculated samples can be detected.

The formula for RPM, iron milk medium, and LS medium and suggested incubation for MPN enumeration of *C. perfringens* are shown in Table 17.2 for comparison.

Successful *C. perfringens* enumeration requires adequate anaerobiosis which can be achieved by N_2 (Harmon et al. 1971), H_2 plus 5% CO_2 (Hanford 1974), or N_2, H_2 and CO_2 in varying proportions (Willardsen et al. 1979; Labbe 1983; Labbe and Norris 1982). Mead (1969) has indicated that reducing conditions in the recovery medium are more critical for consistent blackening of colonies (due to FeS) than for *C. perfringens* colony formation *per se*. Colony count procedures for *C. perfringens* (pour and spread plating procedures) incorporate an agar medium overlay to assure blackening and consistent colony formation. Smith (1972) recommends anaerobically diluting samples for quantitative recovery of *C. perfringens* regardless of the enumeration medium to protect vegetative cells from organic peroxides which may form in medium due to air exposure. Alternatively, incorporation of catalase

Table 17.2. Formulations of Media for *C. perfringens* MPN Enumeration and Suggested Incubation Conditions

	Iron milk medium[a]	LS medium[b]	RPM[c]
	Amount per 100 mL medium		
Whole milk	(10 mL/tube)[d]	—	—
Litmus milk powder[e]	—	—	7.0 g
Fluid thioglycolate medium	—	—	3.0 g
Trypsin-digested peptone from casein	—	0.5 g	—
Yeast Extract	—	0.25 g	0.3 g
Gelatin	—	—	6.0 g
Peptone	—	—	0.5 g
Glucose	—	—	0.5 g
Lactose	—	1.0 g	—
NaCl	—	0.25 g	0.15 g
K_2HPO_4	—	—	0.5 g
L-cysteine-HCl	—	0.03 g	—
Na-metabisulphite	—	67 mg	—
Ferric ammonium citrate	—	56 mg	—
Ferrous sulfate	—	—	0.05 g
Iron (elemental)	2 g	—	—
Neomycin sulfate	—	—	7.5 g
Polymyxin B sulfate	—	—	1.25 mg
pH (pre-autoclave)	nd[f]	7.1	nd
Incubation time	16–18 hr	18–24 hr	24 hr
Incubation temperature	46°C	46°C	46–48°C

[a]St. John et al. (1982).
[b]Beerens et al. (1982).
[c]Erickson and Diebel (1978).
[d]Information for this ingredient is not per 100 mL. Milk (whole, pasteurized, homogenized) is placed in test tubes and 0.2 g iron is added per tube.
[e]The authors used Difco Laboratories (Detroit, MI) products.
[f]Not defined.

into medium to degrade peroxide may be effective (Harmon and Kautter 1976).

Incubation for *C. perfringens* colony counts is generally at 35–37°C for 18–24 hr. For enumeration of heat-damaged *C. perfringens* spores, prolonged incubation may be required (Labbe 1983). Excessive blackening may occur in sulfite plus iron-containing media incubated >20 hr (Harmon 1976; Orth 1977). In some instances ca. 46°C incubation is used for selection (Marshall et al. 1965). Hanford (1974) indicated incubation at 35°C was more favorable than 46°C for recovery of *C. perfringens* on tryptone sulfite-neomycin medium (Marshall et al. 1965). Most probable number procedures using iron milk medium or other liquid recovery media successfully employ 46°C incubation.

Confirmatory procedures are required to exclude physiologically similar species of clostridia which form black colonies on the sulfite plus iron-containing media. Confirmation typically includes testing for nitrate reduction, lack of motility, lactose fermentation, and/or gelatin liquification. The CAMP (authors' initials) test has been suggested for presumptive identification of lecithinase-positive *C. perfringens*. This procedure depends upon the synergistic hemolysis pattern (arrowhead shape) of *Streptococcus agalactiae* and *C. perfringens* when streaked at right angles on blood-agar plates (Hansen and Elliot 1980). Confirmation procedures have been discussed by Walker (1975) and Harmon and Kautter (1978) and are detailed by Mead et al. (1982), Duncan and Harmon (1976), and the Food and Drug Administration (Harmon and Duncan 1978). Serological identification of cultures is used to confirm diagnoses, where the goal is to isolate organisms of the same serotype from the epidemiologically incriminated food and stools of patients or to isolate the same serotypes from the stools of most patients but not from controls. Serotyping procedures have been detailed by Stringer et al. (1982). Watson (1985) typed 802 isolates of *Clostridium perfringens* from food poisoning outbreaks and other sources using 50 bacteriocins. Isolates of the same serotype generally had a similar pattern of sensitivity to bacteriocins. Some isolates could be typed using bacteriocins but not serologically. Bacteriocin typing appears useful for identifying *C. perfringens* isolates from foodborne illness outbreaks.

In contrast to vegetative cells, recovery of *C. perfringens* spores has received little attention. The subject has been reviewed briefly by Labbe (1983). Labbe and Norris (1982) reported that tryptone-sulfite-neomycin medium (TSN) (Marshall et al. 1965) and sulfite-polymyxin-sulfadiazine medium (SPS) (Angelotti et al. 1962) were preferable to nonselective media for enumeration of heat-activated spores. Barach et al. (1974) reported that enumeration of *C. perfringens* spores was essentially equal using SPS, TSN, SFP, TSC, and TSC without antibiotics. However, TSC and SFP were superior for recovery of spores surviving high (105–120°C) temperature heating. Incorporation of lysozyme into the plating medium may improve recovery of heat-injured spores (for discussion, see Labbe 1983).

Vegetative cells of *C. perfringens* are sensitive to refrigeration or frozen storage, causing populations to decrease 3–4 log cycles after a few days' storage at low temperatures (Canada et al. 1964; Harmon and Kautter 1974). Since confirmation of *C. perfringens* foodborne illness outbreaks depends on detection of large numbers of the organism in the suspect food, cold storage of samples may result in false-negative confirmation of *C. perfringens*. To minimize loss of viability of *C. perfringens* vegetative cells prior to micro-biological examination, Hauschild and Hilsheimer (1974a) suggested, and a collaborative study confirmed (Harmon and Placencia 1978), that samples be mixed (1:1 w/v) with 20% glycerol and stored in dry ice or frozen at $-60°C$. The potential for falsely low numbers of *C. perfringens* being recovered from foods stored at cold temperatures led Harmon and Kautter (1970, 1974) to propose lecithinase (phospholipase C, alpha toxin) as an indicator of the prior presence of high *C. perfringens* populations. Using hemolysin indicator plates, the titer of lecithinase is determined and used to estimate the previous *C. perfringens* population from a standard table. A population of at least ca. 4×10^5 is required to produce detectable levels of lecithinase. Shortcomings of the test are numerous, including variability in the amount of lecithinase produced depending upon the food substrate, time and temperature of growth (Park and Mikolajcik 1979), and the strain (Foegeding and Busta 1980a). Furthermore, the lecithinase activity may peak and decline at temperatures above about 51°C, paralleling the population changes during cooking or reheating (Foegeding and Busta 1980b). Generally, presence of detectable lecithinase activity would indicate the *C. perfringens* population was $\geq 10^5$ CFU/g food at one time. This is significant since this population level is used by the Centers for Disease Control for confirmation of a foodborne illness outbreak (Anonymous 1981). However, absence of detectable leci-thinase does not exclude prior presence of a high titer and therefore prior presence of significant numbers of *C. perfringens*.

Detection and Quantitation of *C. perfringens* Enterotoxin

It is well established that an enterotoxin is responsible for the typical symp-toms of *C. perfringens* foodborne illness. The relationship between sporulation and enterotoxin production by *C. perfringens* has been reviewed by Labbe (1980) and the mechanism of action of enterotoxin was reviewed by McDonel (1980). Methodologies to detect *C. perfringens* enterotoxin have been reviewed recently by Stringer et al. (1982) and will be briefly treated in this manuscript.

As for any enterotoxin, the methods available for toxin detection and quantitation can be classified as biological tests involving animals or human volunteers and serological tests which utilize specific antisera prepared against purified enterotoxin. The convenience, sensitivity, reproducibility, and brevity of most serological procedures make them preferable to the bioassays if they accurately reflect biologically active enterotoxin and are acceptably sensitive. The procedure used by the U.S. Food and Drug Administration (Harmon and Duncan 1978) is the erythemal assay using the guinea pig, although new serological procedures with apparent promise are being developed (Stelma et al. 1985; Naik and Duncan 1977b; Stelma et al. 1983).

Preparation of purified enterotoxin and antitoxin has been reviewed by Stringer et al. (1982). Antisera to *C. perfringens* enterotoxin currently is not available commercially.

Symptoms of *C. perfringens* foodborne illness have been produced in mammals by feeding cells, spores, culture filtrates, and purified enterotoxin (Duncan and Strong 1969, 1971; Bartlett et al. 1972; Skjelkvale and Uemura 1977). The ligated ileal loop test, generally carried out in rabbits, has been described by Duncan et al. (1968) and demonstrates fluid accumulation in the intestine by enterotoxin. Hauschild (1970) showed that extracts which caused fluid accumulation in ligated ileal loops also caused erythema when injected intradermally into guinea pigs and rabbits. Where diameters of erythema are between 0.5 and 1.2 cm, the area of erythema is proportional to the concentration of enterotoxin injected. Increased capillary permeability results from the action of *C. perfringens* enterotoxin injected intradermally into guinea pigs (Stark and Duncan 1972). The increased capillary permeability can be detected if the intradermal enterotoxin injection is followed by an intravenous injection of Evans blue dye. Higher concentrations of enterotoxin result in more intense blue areas surrounding the enterotoxin injection site.

Several serological detection methods have been developed. Applications of the double gel diffusion procedure similar to that used for staphylococcal enterotoxin detection, electroimmunodiffusion (Duncan and Somers 1972), counterimmunoelectrophoresis (Naik and Duncan 1977b), single gel diffusion (Genigeorgis et al. 1973), reversed passive hemagglutination (Uemura et al. 1973), and fluorescent antibody (Niilo 1977) procedures for *C. perfringens* type A enterotoxin detection and quantitation have been reviewed clearly and succinctly by Genigeorgis et al. (1973) and Stringer et al. (1982).

The counterimmunoelectrophoresis procedure of Naik and Duncan (1977b) or other immunoprecipitation methods are used most commonly to confirm the enterotoxigenicity of isolates. A more sensitive radioimmunoassay recently has been developed by Stelma and coworkers (1983). Stelma and others (1985) also have developed a sensitive enzyme-linked immunosorbent assay

(ELISA) for detection of enterotoxin directly from the surface of an agar medium. *C. perfringens* are allowed to grow and sporulate on the surface of agar medium, after which the colonies are blotted from the agar surface with Whatman filter paper. This step is necessary to remove cellular components, most likely the spore coat protein (Labbe 1980), which nonspecifically bind the rabbit IgG. The enterotoxin which remains at the sites of the colonies is adsorbed to nitrocellulose filter paper and a standard ELISA assay is performed. Stelma et al. (1985) obtained positive ELISA results for 11 of 12 enterotoxigenic strains (positive rabbit ileal loop or radioimmunoassay) in each of 43 total replicates with these strains. The strain which did not initially yield a positive ELISA did produce positive results if grown with starch in the medium (presumably to stimulate sporulation and enterotoxin production). No false positives were obtained. This procedure requires 48 hr for completion. More discouraging is the requirement for an as yet undefined medium component (fecal extract) to assure sporulation and enterotoxin production. Nonetheless, the ELISA procedure appears to have great promise for simple, sensitive, and efficient screening of a large number of *C. perfringens* isolates for enterotoxin production. Stelma et al. (1985) predicted that this assay could be used instead of the confirmatory procedures currently used to identify *C. perfringens* colonies.

CLOSTRIDIUM BOTULINUM

Clostridium botulinum is a metabolically diverse species of anaerobic, spore-forming, rod-shaped microorganism having in common the production of one or more pharmacologically similar but serologically distinct protein neurotoxins. Although rare, foodborne botulism has a high fatality rate and results from consumption of foods which contain botulinum toxin produced during growth of *C. botulinum* in the food. A recent collection of papers has reviewed chemical, immunological, and biomedical aspects of the botulinum neurotoxin (Lewis 1981).

   C. botulinum spores are found in soil, freshwater sediments, and marine environments throughout the world (Huss 1980; Smith 1977). *C. botulinum* types A, B, C_1, C_2, D, E, and F occur widely throughout the world while type G has been isolated only from soil in Argentina (Gimenez and Ciccarelli 1970). Because of their ubiquitous nature, *C. botulinum* spores are contaminants of a wide variety of raw foods. Botulism results when a contaminated food is processed inadequately for *C. botulinum* spore inactivation or the product becomes contaminated after processing, the food supports growth and toxin production of *C. botulinum*, and the toxic food is ingested (Eklund 1982). Foods typically associated with foodborne botulism include canned vegetables and meats, fish and meats preserved by smoking, salting, or curing and other low-acid products. Several reviews are available which address the potential for *C. botulinum* growth and toxin production in a variety of foods (Hauschild 1982; Eklund 1982; Sugiyama 1982; Hobbs 1976; Simunovic et al. 1985). The requirements of *C. botulinum* for growth and toxin production were reviewed recently by Sperber (1982) and Crowther and Baird-Parker (1984).

Smith (1977), following classifications in the 8th edition of *Bergy's Manual of Determinative Bacteriology* (Buchanan and Gibbons 1974), divided the species into four groups based upon metabolic and serological similarities. Characteristics of these groups are identified in Table 17.3. This grouping is supported by the morphology of inducible temperate phages (Dolman and Chang 1972), the distinct activity spectra of boticins (Lau et al. 1974), and the distinct host ranges of wild-type phages (Sugiyama and King 1972). This categorization and other reports (Dowell and Dezfulian 1981; Hobbs and Cross 1984; Lynt et al. 1982) illustrate the metabolic diversity of this species. Furthermore, several biochemically indistinguishable species which do not produce toxin may be isolated from food, feces, or other materials (Kiritani et al. 1973; Gutteridge et al. 1980; Hobbs and Cross 1984). Lysogenic phages have been found in *C. botulinum* types A, B, D, E, and F (Eklund and Poysky 1974; Dolman and Chang 1972; Sugiyama and King 1972). Studies by Eklund, Poysky, and others (Eklund et al. 1971, 1972, 1974; Eklund and Poysky 1974; Inoue and Iida 1970) have shown that the syntheses of C_1 and D toxins are controlled by the presence of a specific phage. The work of Eklund and Poysky shows that a nontoxic clostridial strain can give rise to either *C. botulinum* type C or D or *C. novyi*, depending on the infecting phage. The role of bacteriophage in toxigenicity has been summarized succinctly by Eklund and Poysky (1981).

Table 17.3. Characteristics of *C. botulinum* Groups

Group	Characteristics
I	Type A and proteolytic strains of types B and F
II	Type E and nonproteolytic strains of types B and F
III	Types C and D (all are nonproteolytic)
IV	Type G (all are proteolytic but nonsaccharolytic)

(*From Smith 1977*)

There are two possible approaches for laboratory detection of *C. botulinum*. One may look for the presence of toxins by biological or serological procedures, or one may look for the presence of cells or spores by microscopic or cultural procedures. Detection of toxin is more critical when a suspected botulinal outbreak is being investigated. Toxin may be present in the feces of humans several weeks after ingestion. Therefore, toxin assays routinely are used to analyze epidemiologically implicated foods as well as feces, serum, and other clinical specimens of patients (Kautter and Lynt 1978). Microscopic or cultural methods for isolation of the organism are useful for quality control purposes, to provide cultures for taxonomic identification of the causative organism, and to supplement epidemiological investigations. In foods, detection of viable *C. botulinum* without detection of toxin is not proof that the suspect food caused botulism and in clinical specimens does not mean that the patient had botulism.

Detection of C. botulinum

Due to the species diversity, no single method or protocol is equally successful for isolation of all types of this organism. *C. botulinum* is an obligate anaerobe, therefore successful isolation of the vegetative cells dictates careful anaerobic technique. Numerous methods have been published for the detection of *C. botulinum* from foods, clinical specimens, soil, and other samples. Most procedures are not designed to quantitate *C. botulinum*, rather they are enrichment procedures so that small populations can be detected. Procedures and media which have found use for detection of *C. botulinum* are listed in Table 17.4 and discussed below.

If the sample is capable of supporting growth it can be vacuum packed and incubated for enrichment of the microorganism. Enrichment media which have been used include Robertson's Cooked Meat Broth with or without added carbohydrate (1% w/v) (Hobbs et al. 1982), cooked meat medium (Kautter and Lynt 1978) peptone-glucose broth, glucose-peptone broth, fish infusion broth, reinforced clostridial medium, brain-heart infusion broth (Bott et al. 1968), papain broth (Rymkiewicz 1968), corn extract medium (Tsarapkin 1971), and others (Hobbs et al. 1982). Incubation generally is between 26 and 35°C for 5 to 10 days.

Lilly et al. (1971) developed an enrichment medium designated TPGYT which contains trypticase, peptone, glucose, yeast extract, and trypsin (1 mg/mL) for detection of *C. botulinum* type E. TPGYT was designed to potentiate the toxin of this nonproteolytic strain as it is produced and to render the boticins of competing strains inactive. The TPGYT medium and cooked

Table 17.4. Steps in Determination of C. *botulinum* as a Causative Agent of a Foodborne Illness Outbreak and Media or Procedures Which May be Used to Accomplish Each Step

Step	Media or procedure[a,b]
Enrichment[c]	Food or other specimen, Robertson's cooked meat broth ± 1% carbohydrate, cooked meat medium, peptone-glucose broth, glucose-peptone broth, fish-infusion broth, reinforced clostridial medium, brain-heart infusion broth, papain broth, corn extract medium, TPGYT medium, botulinal enrichment medium.
Isolation, selection, and/or differention of C. *botulinum*[c]	Horse blood agar ± antibiotics, egg yolk agar ± antibiotics, CB1 medium, TPGY with added antitoxin.
Confirmation of cultures	Toxin test (mouse bioassay or other), none necessary for colonies with zones of Ag-Ab precipitation on TPGY with added antitoxin. (Pyrolysis-gas chromatography, anaerobic growth on blood agar, casein hydrolysis, lecithinase, catalase, lipase and protease activities, end-product analysis from growth on glucose or with phenylalanine and indole production[d]

[a]For references, see text.
[b]The listing is not comprehensive.
[c]These steps are not included in many instances.
[d]Tests in parentheses are supplemental to confirmation by demonstrating toxin production or presence.

meat medium are officially recommended by the U.S. Food and Drug Administration for isolation of *C. botulinum* from foods (Kautter and Lynt 1978). Holdeman and coworkers (1977) developed botulinum enrichment medium which incorporated trypsin and lysozyme in a medium designed to recover fastidious anaerobes. This medium appears to enhance recovery of *C. botulinum* from naturally contaminated materials compared to reinforced clostridial medium (Hobbs et al. 1982).

Crowther and Baird-Parker (1984) have observed that *C. botulinum* recovery may be improved if attention is paid to promoting germination of spores by adding compounds known to stimulate germination, such as lysozyme, lactate plus L-alanine, or bicarbonate. Indeed, they reported observations (unpublished) that these compounds improve recovery when added to TPGYT medium.

Many studies have used a heat treatment to select for *C. botulinum* spores against competing microflora. Heat treatments of 80°C for 10 min or 70°C for 30 min to 2 hr have commonly been used. It is now understood that the less heat-resistant strains of *C. botulinum*, in particular the nonproteolytic strains of types B, E, and F, would be inactivated by these treatments. Several alternative procedures have been developed to reduce the number of competitors. For example, samples may be treated with ethanol to inactivate vegetative cells (equal volumes of enrichment culture and ethanol held ca. 1 hr at 25°C prior to incubation), a milder heat treatment may be employed prior to enrichment (for example 60°C, 30 min), or incorporation of antibiotics into the enrichment broth for selection may be used (Hobbs et al. 1982; Mossel and DeWaart 1968). To be certain that vegetative cells of *C. botulinum* are recovered in the absence of spores, an untreated sample always should be included.

Isolation of *C. botulinum* is achieved by subculturing an enrichment culture using suitable agar media. Seldom is direct plating successful since *C. botulinum* is normally outnumbered by other anaerobic or facultatively anaerobic microorganisms. Horse blood agar and egg yolk agar commonly are used for isolation. Neither medium is selective but the differential reactions of slight hemolysis and egg yolk lipolysis can be observed. Selection can be accomplished by addition of antibiotics or other inhibitors to the media, although many *C. botulinum* strains may be inhibited by antibiotics. Hence, selection generally is not incorporated at this stage. Useful basal media for egg yolk agar are freshly prepared meat infusion or chopped-liver broth, or commercially dehydrated brain-heart infusion agar or liver-veal-egg yolk agar.

Recently, a selective agar medium for isolation of *C. botulinum* from human feces has been developed (Dowell and Dezfulian 1981). The medium, CB1 agar, contains cycloserine (250 mg/L), sulfamethoxazole (76 mg/L), and trimethoprim (4 mg/L) in a base of modified McClung-Toabe egg yolk agar. Some type E strains were inhibited by this medium and type G strains were more difficult to recognize than other colonies due to absence of the lipolytic reaction. Several other clostridia will grow on CB1, but few are lipase positive and most anaerobic or facultative species tested were inhibited on CB1 medium (Dowell and Dezfulian 1981). This medium may be used to obtain isolates within 1 or 2 days.

Typically, enriched cultures are confirmed to contain *C. botulinum* by testing the toxicity of the cultures by the mouse bioassay or another procedure. Since toxicity is a requirement for speciation and since metabolically similar strains otherwise can not be differentiated from *C. botulinum*, a toxicity test is mandatory for speciation and identification of the toxin type. Many nontoxic isolates otherwise cannot be differentiated from *C. botulinum*.

Extending the procedure of Ferreira et al. (1981), Lilly et al. (1984) recently published an immunodiffusion procedure for detection of *C. botulinum* types A, B, E, and F colonies. *C. botulinum* cultures were streaked for isolation on TPGY agar (TPGYT without trypsin) with added specific antitoxin and incubated anaerobically. Thiazine red R stain was used to highlight the zones of toxin-antitoxin precipitate around each *C. botulinum* colony. Among the advantages of this procedure is that individual toxic colonies of *C. botulinum* can be selected from nontoxic isolates without further in vivo toxin assays. Procedures such as this could reduce the time and difficulty for determining the presence of known botulinal toxin types.

Other procedures are being developed and show promise for confirmation and identification of *C. botulinum* and related organisms. For example, Gutteridge et al. (1980) could differentiate types A and B *C. botulinum* from types E and F and from types C and D using low resolution pyrolysis gas-liquid chromatography. This technique thermally degrades small samples of whole cells to generate a series of low molecular weight fragments, which are separated and detected to produce a complex analog trace known as a pyrogram. Using pyrolysis gas-chromatography, *C. sporogenes* could not be distinguished from types A, B, and F *C. botulinum*. Dowell and Dezfulian (1981) suggested confirmation of isolates from CB1 medium using blood agar incubated aerobically and anaerobically, glucose fermentation, casein hydrolysis, lecithinase, lipase and proteolytic activity tests, measurement of volatile and nonvolatile acids from peptone-yeast extract-glucose medium with added phenylalanine, and testing for catalase and indole production in addition to toxin production.

The gas chromatographic endproduct analysis of Holdeman et al. (1977) is used successfully to identify many anaerobes and facultative anaerobes, yet it cannot differentiate types of *C. botulinum* and *C. sporogenes*. In related work, headspace gas chromatographic analysis of food samples may be useful to separate botulinum-positive and -negative samples (Snygg et al. 1979). Although the chromatograms were complex and no single peak was unique to toxic samples, the procedure does show promise. Procedures such as this would be useful as rapid screening tests but false-positive samples may result.

A fluorescent antibody procedure has been developed which may be useful as a screening or backup diagnostic test to detect *C. botulinum* cells or spores in samples (Aalvik et al. 1973). Antisera prepared against one toxin type cross react with other toxin types and with *C. sporogenes* so the results are not conclusive.

Detection and Quantitation of *C. botulinum* Toxin

The standard procedure for detection of *C. botulinum* toxin from food, feces, other clinical specimens, or enriched cultures is the mouse bioassay. This procedure is detailed in the *Bacteriological Analytical Manual* (Kautter and Lynt 1978), by Hobbs et al. (1982), Kautter and Solomon (1977), and others. Briefly, it entails injecting mice intraperitoneally with unheated, heated (100°C, 5 min), and trypsinized sample extracts and observing the mice over a 3-day period for typical botulism symptoms and death. Botulinum toxin is readily inactivated by heat, and trypsin treatment will activate the toxin of nonproteolytic strains. Following demonstration of toxin, protection with monovalent antitoxin is used to identify the serological toxin type. The amount of toxin can be determined by injecting dilutions of the sample and reporting the reciprocal of the highest dilution giving typical symptoms and death (minimum lethal dose).

One drawback of the mouse bioassay is the long time period required (3 days) for death with samples containing small amounts of toxin. Furthermore, determination of the presence or absence of botulinum toxin sometimes is difficult due to nonspecific deaths. That is, antitoxin-protected mice and other mice die without typical *C. botulinum* symptoms. Nonspecific deaths may result from an infection (Segner and Schmidt 1968), from heat-stable endotoxins of Gram-negative organisms (Solberg et al. 1985), or by other means. Nonspecific deaths may be reduced by treatment of assay samples with bovine serum albumin (bovine serum albumin added to assay sample and held 1 hr at 37°C prior to injection of mice). Solberg et al. (1985) identified immunoglobulin M as the active fraction of bovine serum albumin. Immunoglobulin M eliminated nonspecific deaths due to endotoxin.

Several in vitro serological methods have been considered as possible replacements for the conventional mouse toxicity test. None of the tests developed to date has the sensitivity and specificity of the mouse bioassay.

The mouse bioassay is the only procedure which can detect as yet unidentified toxins. In vitro methods developed for detection of *C. botulinum* toxin have been reviewed by Crowther and Holbrook (1976) and include electroimmunodiffusion (Miller and Anderson 1971), reversed passive hemagglutination (Evancho et al. 1973), capillary tube diffusion (Mestrandrea 1974), radioimmunoassay (Boroff and Shu-Chen 1973), and an enzyme-linked immunosorbent assay (ELISA) (Notermans et al. 1979; Notermans and Kozaki 1981).

The ELISA procedure appears to be promising since it is simple, rapid to perform, does not require experimental animals or special laboratory provisions, and approaches the sensitivity of the mouse bioassay. Notermans et al. (1979), using formalinized type E toxin for production of antiserum and the "double-sandwich" ELISA procedure, were able to detect about 80 mouse intraperitoneal 50% lethal doses of toxin. Some cross reaction was observed with types A and B toxins, but not with type C or other *Clostridium* species. Similar results have been obtained with other toxin types. Use of monoclonal antibodies selected for their high activity may increase the sensitivity of the ELISA procedure.

BACILLUS CEREUS

Two types of *Bacillus cereus* foodborne illness are recognized. The emetic and diarrheal responses are caused by two distinct enterotoxins produced by this organism (Melling et al. 1976). Presently, it is unclear whether the toxin produced in an outbreak is strain specific, food specific, or dependent upon other environmental factors (Johnson 1984). A scheme for serotyping *B. cereus* isolates from foodborne illness outbreaks using their flagellar antigens has been developed by Taylor and Gilbert (1975). Serotyping indicates that the type of illness may be a function of the strain (Crowther and Baird-Parker 1984; Gilbert 1979), although some serotypes have been associated with both illness types. A wide variety of foods, including vegetables, salads, and meat-based foods, have been implicated in the diarrheal-type outbreaks. The emetic-type outbreaks have been almost exclusively related to rice products. Occasionally other starchy foods (macaroni and cheese, etc.) have been involved. Several excellent reviews of *B. cereus* foodborne illness are available (Johnson 1984; Gilbert 1979; Terranova and Blake 1978; Gilbert and Taylor 1976; Goepfert et al. 1972).

Detection and Quantitation of *B. cereus*

B. cereus spores are distributed widely in nature, and *B. cereus* is recovered commonly from a variety of foods. Indeed, the incidental finding of this organism in many food products should be expected. Therefore, detection of *B. cereus* in foods does not justify implication of the food in an outbreak, making enrichment procedures of little or no value for determination of *B. cereus* in foods. However, finding large populations ($>10^5$ colony forming units/g) of *B. cereus* in a food is indicative of active growth and multiplication of the organism in the food and is consistent with a potential hazard. Therefore, methods for evaluation of *B. cereus* in foods are based upon quantitation of the organism. Generally, confirming *B. cereus* as the cause of a foodborne outbreak requires either (1) isolation of strains of the same serotype from the suspect food and feces or vomitus of the patient, (2) isolation of significant numbers ($>10^5$ colony forming units/g) of a *B. cereus* serotype known to cause foodborne illness from the suspect food or from the feces or vomitus of the patient, or (3) isolation of significant numbers ($>10^5$ colony forming units/ g) of *B. cereus* from the suspect food and from the feces or vomitus of the patient (Kramer et al. 1982).

   B. cereus is a Gram-positive, facultatively aerobic sporeformer which does not ferment mannitol, xylose, or arabinose, ferments glucose anaerobically, reduces nitrate to nitrite, and is lecithinase positive. Cells are large rods and the spores do not swell the sporangium. These and other characteristics have been used to differentiate and confirm *B. cereus* although these characteristics are shared by *B. cereus*, *B. cereus* var. *mycoides*, *B. thuringiensis*, and *B. anthracis*. Differentiation of these organisms depends upon determination of motility (most *B. cereus* are motile), presence of crystals of protein toxin (*B. thuringiensis* is positive), hemolytic activity (*B. cereus* and others are beta hemolytic while *B. anthracis* usually is nonhemolytic), and rhizoid growth which is characteristic of *B. cereus* var. *mycoides*. It is not always possible to distinguish *B. cereus* from these culturally similar organisms (Harmon 1980). However, one generally would not expect to find *B. cereus* var. *mycoides* or *B. anthracis* in foods.

   Several media for the isolation and identification of *B. cereus* in foods have been described. Donovan (1958) recommended a medium containing lithium chloride and polymyxin B as selective agents. This medium is similar to the mannitol-egg yolk-polymyxin agar (MYP) medium developed by Mossel et al. (1967) currently in common use. MYP medium contains mannitol plus phenol red and egg yolk for differentiation and polymyxin (100 units/mL) for selection.

   Kim and Goepfert (1971) developed KG medium as a rapid presumptive enumeration medium for *B. cereus*. KG medium also uses polymyxin for selection. The lecithinase reaction on egg yolk and sporulation due to low levels of peptone and absence of carbohydrate and meat extract provide differentiation properties.

Holbrook and Anderson (1980) proposed polymyxin-pyruvate-egg yolk-mannitol-bromothymol blue agar (PEMBA, also referred to as *Bacillus cereus* Selective Medium) for enumeration of *B. cereus*. Again, selection is by polymyxin and egg yolk aids in differentiation. Low levels of peptone promote sporulation and pyruvate reduces the colony size. Holbrook and Anderson (1980) claim that the medium is superior in detecting lecithinase-negative *B. cereus*. Szabo et al. (1984) modified this medium, replacing bromocresol purple for bromothymol blue and calling the modified medium PEMPA. Using PEMPA, Szabo et al. (1984) claimed incubation could be reduced from 48 to 22 hr and recognition of presumptive isolates was enhanced. Performance of PEMPA compared favorably to the medium with bromothymol blue and to MYP when recovering *B. cereus* from naturally contaminated food samples or inoculated samples.

The U.S. Food and Drug Administration (Harmon 1980) recommends an MPN procedure using trypticase-soy-polymyxin (89 units/mL) broth for enumeration of *B. cereus* in foods that are expected to contain fewer than 10^3 *B. cereus*/g or to examine dehydrated or starchy foods. Tubes with growth are streaked onto MYP medium for confirmation of typical colonies. Others (Kramer et al. 1982) have proposed use of blood agar plates for isolation of *B. cereus* from clinical and food samples associated with a foodborne illness outbreak, but selective media are required to recover *B. cereus* in the presence of other organisms. The formula of the commonly used selective media, including MYP, KG, PEMBA, PEMPA, and trypticase-soy-polymyxin broth, are listed in Table 17.5.

Stec and Burzynska (1980) compared MYP medium, KG agar, egg yolk medium, and blood agar medium for enumeration of *B. cereus*. Egg yolk medium and MYP medium were superior for numbers recovered and required the shortest recovery time. MYP medium currently is recommended by the U.S. Food and Drug Administration (Harmon 1980). Several combinations of confirmatory tests have been recommended by various groups. The U.S. Food and Drug Administration (Harmon 1980) confirms presumptive *B. cereus* colonies from MYP medium (large Gram-positive rods with spores which do not swell the sporangium and are lecithinase positive and mannitol negative) using anaerobic production of acid from glucose, reduction of nitrate to nitrite, production of acetylmethylcarbinol, decomposition of L-tyrosine, and growth in the presence of 0.001% lysozyme. Bouwer-Hertzberger and Mossel (1982) reported that more than 95% of the typical colonies on MYP medium are indeed *B. cereus* so that confirmation is not necessary in most instances.

Table 17.5. Media Currently in Common Use or Recommended for Selective Enumeration of *Bacillus cereus*

	MYP[a]	KG[b]	PEMBA[c]	PEMPA[d]	Trypticase-Soy-Polymyxin Broth[c,f]
			Amount per 100 mL medium		
Meat extract	0.1 g	—	—	—	—
Peptone	1.0 g	0.1 g	0.1 g	—	0.3 g
Phytone peptone	—	—	—	0.1 g	—
Tryptone	—	—	—	—	1.7 g
Trypticase peptone	—	—	—	—	—
Yeast extract	—	—	—	—	0.25 g
Glucose	—	—	—	—	0.25 g
D-mannitol	1.0 g	—	0.9 g	0.9 g	—
Agar	1.5 g	1.8 g	1.6 g	1.6 g	—
$MgSO_4 \cdot 7H_2O$	—	—	0.01 g	0.01 g	—
Na_2HPO_4	—	—	0.23 g	0.23 g	—
KH_2PO_4	—	—	0.023 g	0.023 g	—
K_2HPO_4	—	—	—	—	0.25 g
NaCl	1.0 g	—	0.2 g	0.2 g	0.5 g
Sodium pyruvate	—	—	1 g	1 g	—
Polymyxin B sulfate	1.0 mg	1.0 mg	10^4 units	8260 USP units	8900 units
Phenol red	2.5 mg	2.5 mg	—	—	—
Bromocresol purple	—	—	—	6 mg	—
Bromothymol blue	—	—	0.01 g	—	—
Egg yolk emulsion (20%)	10 ml	10 ml	5 ml	5 ml	—
pH (pre-autoclave)	7.1 g	6.8	7.4	6.9	7.3

[a] Mossel et al. (1967).
[b] Kim and Goepfert (1971).
[c] Holbrook and Anderson (1980).
[d] Szabo et al. (1984).
[e] Harmon (1980).
[f] Used as an MPN procedure.

Aerobic incubation at 30–35°C for 24–48 hr is advised for most enumeration and confirmation procedures. *B. cereus* is not reported to be sensitive to cold or frozen storage, although freezing of samples prior to examination is not recommended. MYP medium will recover thermally injured *B. cereus* (Johnson et al. 1982; Rappaport and Goepfert 1978).

Procedures for serotyping of cultures are available and may be useful for confirmation of foodborne illness outbreaks. H-specific antisera used for serotyping are not available commercially and cultures for serotyping typically are sent to established laboratories for this purpose (Kramer et al. 1982).

Detection and Quantitation of *B. cereus* Enterotoxins

Because practical tests for detection of *B. cereus* enterotoxins presently are not available, the U.S. Food and Drug Administration uses cultural procedures to confirm isolates as *B. cereus* and confirmation does not include reference to toxin production. Tests for enterotoxin are used to evaluate isolates of particular interest, to monitor toxin purification procedures, and for other limited research purposes. Currently, established tests for enterotoxin are in vivo tests, although in vitro serological procedures for detection of the toxins are being developed and may prove widely applicable.

Tests applicable for enterotoxin detection and/or quantitation include the vascular permeability reaction test using guinea pigs or rabbits for the diarrheal toxin (Glatz and Goepfert 1973), the ligated ileal loop test for the diarrheal toxin (Spira and Goepfert 1972), and the rhesus monkey feeding test for diarrheal or emetic toxins (observe for diarrhea or vomiting response). The ligated ileal loop and vascular permeability tests are essentially identical to the tests used for detection of *C. perfringens* enterotoxin. A positive vascular permeability test may be elicited by other cellular metabolites so that the test may not be specific for *B. cereus* enterotoxin (Glatz et al. 1974).

Purification of the enterotoxins for production of specific antisera is the main obstacle to development of useful in vitro immunological procedures for assay of the *B. cereus* enterotoxins.

FUTURE DIRECTION

Methodologies for each of the toxigenic sporeformers will evolve rapidly with the development of effective toxin purification schemes and specific, sensitive antibodies. Undoubtedly, monoclonal antibody production will further these goals. Development of phage and bacteriocin typing schemes and DNA or phage probes also will simplify detection and identification of these organisms. However, cultural procedures for recovery of *C. perfringens* and *B. cereus* will continue to be important. Simplified systems for isolation and confirmation of toxigenic species such as the procedures introduced by Stelma et al. (1983) [ELISA to detect *C. perfringens* enterotoxin directly from the surface of agar medium] and Ferreira, Lilly, and coworkers (Ferreira et al. 1981; Lilly et al. 1984) [incorporation of *C. botulinum* antitoxin in recovery medium and identification of toxigenic isolates by Ag-Ab precipitation zone] will advance the methods. Success of procedures to simplify cultural isolation and identification methods is dependent on assuring quantitative recovery (including injured organisms) and dependable toxin production by the isolates (and sporulation of *C. perfringens*) in many cases. Finally, bioassays cannot be replaced for detection of as yet unidentified serological toxin types.

REFERENCES

AALVIK, B., SAKAGUCHI, G., and RIEMANN, H. 1973. Detection of type E botulinal toxin in cultures by fluorescent-antibody microscopy. *Appl. Microbiol.* 25: 153.

ABEYTA, C. JR., MICHALOVSKIS, A., and WEKELL, M. M. 1985. Differentiation of *Clostridium perfringens* from related clostridia in iron milk medium. *J. Food Prot.* 48: 130.

ADAMS, B. W. and MEAD, G. C. 1980. Comparison of media and methods for counting *Clostridium perfringens* in poultry meat and further-processed products. *J. Hyg. Camb.* 84: 151.

ANGELOTTI, R., HALL, H. E., FOTER, M. J., and LEWIS, K. H. 1962. Quantitation of *Clostridium perfringens* in foods. *Appl. Microbiol.* 10: 193.

AOAC. 1980. *Official Methods of Analysis.* 13th ed., p. 829. Assoc. of Official Analytical Chemists, Washington, DC.

ANONYMOUS. 1981. Food-borne disease surveillance, annual summary for 1979. Centers for Disease Control, U.S. Department of Health and Human Services, Atlanta, GA.

BARACH, J. T., ADAMS, D. M., and SPECK, M. L. 1974. Recovery of heated *Clostridium perfringens* type A spores on selective media. *Appl. Microbiol.* 28: 793.

BARTLETT, M. L., WALDER, H. W., and ZIPRIN, R. 1972. Use of dogs as an assay for *C. perfringens* enterotoxin. *Appl. Microbiol.* 23: 196.

BEERENS, H., ROMOND, C., LEPAGE, C., and CRIQUELION, J. 1982. A liquid medium for the enumeration of *Clostridium perfringens* in food and faeces. In *Isolation and Identification Methods for Food Poisoning Organisms.* Corry, J. E. L., Roberts, D., and Skinner, F. A. (Ed.), p. 217. Academic Press, London.

BOROFF, D. A. and SHU-CHEN, G. 1973. Radioimmunoassay for type A toxin of *Clostridium botulinum. Appl. Microbiol.* 25: 545.

BOTT, T. L., JOHNSON, J., FOSTER, E. M., and SUGIYAMA, H. 1968. Possible origin of the high incidence of *Clostridium botulinum* type E in an inland bay (Green Bay of Lake Michigan). *J. Bacteriol.* 95: 1542.

BOUWER-HERTZBERGER, S. A. and MOSSEL, D. A. A. 1982. Quantitative isolation and identification of *Bacillus cereus.* In *Isolation and Identification Methods for Food Poisoning Organisms.* Corry, J. E. L., Roberts, D., and Skinner, F. A. (Ed.), p. 255. Academic Press, London.

BUCHANAN, R. E. and GIBBONS, N. E. (Ed.). 1974. *Bergey's Manual of Determinative Bacteriology.* 8th ed. The William and Wilkins Co., Baltimore.

CANADA, J. C., STRONG, D. H., and SCOTT, L. G. 1964. Response of *Clostridium perfringens* spores and vegetative cells to temperature variation. *Appl. Microbiol.* 12: 273.

CRAVEN, S. E. 1980. Growth and sporulation of *Clostridium perfringens* in foods. *Food Technol.* 34(4): 80.

CROWTHER, J. S. and BAIRD-PARKER, A. C. 1984. The pathogenic and toxigenic spore-forming bacteria. Ch. 8. In *The Bacterial Spore* Vol. 2, Hurst, A. and Gould, G. W. (Ed.), p. 275. Academic Press, London.

CROWTHER, J. S. and HOLBROOK, R. 1976. Trends in methods for detecting food-poisoning toxins produced by *Clostridium botulinum* and *Staphylococcus aureus.* In *Microbiology in Agriculture, Fisheries and Food.* Skinner, F. A. and Carr, J. G. (Ed.), p. 215. Academic Press, London.

DEBEVERE, J. M. 1979. A simple method for the isolation and determination of *Clostridium perfringens. Eur. J. Appl. Microbiol. Biotechnol.* 6: 409.

DOLMAN, C. E. and CHANG, E. 1972. Bacteriophages of *Clostridium botulinum. Can. J. Microbiol.* 18: 67.

DONOVAN, K. O. 1958. A selective medium for *Bacillus cereus* in milk. *J. Appl. Bacteriol.* 21: 100.

DOWELL, V. R. JR. and DEZFULIAN, M. 1981. Physiological characterization of *Clostridium botulinum* and development of practical isolation and identification procedures. In *Biomedical Aspects of Botulism.* Lewis, G. E. Jr. (Ed.), p. 205. Academic Press, New York.

DUNCAN, C. L. and HARMON, S. M. 1976. *Clostridium perfringens.* Ch. 35. In *Compendium of Methods for the Microbiological Examination of Foods.* Speck, M. (Ed.), p. 437. American Public Health Assoc., Washington, DC.

DUNCAN, C. L. and SOMERS, E. B. 1972. Quantitation of *Clostridium perfringens* type A enterotoxin by electroimmunodiffusion. *Appl. Microbiol.* 24: 801.

DUNCAN, C. L. and STRONG, D. H. 1969. Experimental production of diarrhoea in rabbits with *C. perfringens*. *Can. J. Microbiol.* 15: 765.

DUNCAN, C. L. and STRONG, D. H. 1971. *Clostridium perfringens* type A food poisoning. I. Response of the rabbit ileum as an indication of enteropathogenicity of strains of *Clostridium perfringens* in monkeys. *Inf. Immun.* 3: 167.

DUNCAN, C. L., SUGIYAMA, H., and STRONG, D. H. 1968. Rabbit ileal loop response to strains of *C. perfringens*. *J. Bacteriol.* 95: 1560.

EKLUND, M. W. 1982. Significance of *Clostridium botulinum* in fishery products preserved short of sterilization. *Food Technol.* 36(12): 107.

EKLUND, M. W. and POYSKY, F. T. 1974. Interconversion of type C and D strains of *Clostridium botulinum* by specific bacteriophages. *Appl. Microbiol.* 27: 251.

EKLUND, M. W. and POYSKY, F. T. 1981. Relationship of bacteriophages to the toxigenicity of *Clostridium botulinum* and closely related organisms. In *Biomedical Aspects of Botulism*. Lewis, G. E. Jr. (Ed.), p. 93. Academic Press, New York.

EKLUND, M. W., POYSKY, F. T., MEYERS, J. A., and PELROY, G. A. 1974. Interspecies conversion of *Clostridium botulinum* type C to *Clostridium novyi* type A by bacteriophage. *Science* 186: 456.

EKLUND, M. W., POYSKY, F., and REED, S. M. 1972. Bacteriophage and toxigenicity of *Clostridium botulinum* type D. *Nature* 235: 16.

EKLUND, M. W., POYSKY, F. T., REED, S. M., and SMITH, C. A. 1971. Bacteriophage and toxigenicity of *Clostridium botulinum* type C. *Science* 172: 480.

ERICKSON, J. E. and DEIBEL, R. H. 1978. New medium for rapid screening and enumeration of *Clostridium perfringens* in foods. *Appl. Environ. Microbiol.* 36: 567.

EVANCHO, G. M., ASHTON, D. H., BRISKEY, E. J., and SCHANTZ, E. J. 1973. A standardized reverse passive haemagglutination technique for the determination of botulinum toxin. *J. Food Sci.* 38: 764.

FERREIRA, J. L., HAMDY, M. K., ZAPATKA, F. A., and HEBERT, W. O. 1981. Immunodiffusion method for detection of type A *Clostridium botulinum*. *Appl. Environ. Microbiol.* 42: 1057.

FOEGEDING, P. M. and BUSTA, F. F. 1980a. Production of phospholipase C by nine strains of *Clostridium perfringens* at 37°C and at a constantly rising temperature. *J. Food Prot.* 43: 15.

FOEGEDING, P. M. and BUSTA, F. F. 1980b. *Clostridium perfringens* cells and phospholipase C activity at constant and linearly rising temperatures. *J. Food Sci.* 45: 918.

FUZI, M. and CSUKAS, Z. 1969. New selective medium for the isolation of *Clostridium perfringens*. *Acta Microbiol. Acad. Sci. Hungary* 16: 273.

GENIGEORGIS, C., SAKAGUCHI, G., and RIEMANN, H. 1973. Assay methods for *Clostridium perfringens* type A enterotoxin. *Appl. Microbiol.* 26: 111.

GILBERT, R. J. 1979. *Bacillus cereus* gastroenteritis, Ch. X. In *Food-borne Infections and Intoxications*. 2nd ed. Riemann, H. and Bryan, F. L. (Ed.), p. 495. Academic Press, New York.

GILBERT, R. J. and TAYLOR, A. J. 1976. *Bacillus cereus* food poisoning. In *Microbiology in Agriculture, Fisheries and Food*. Skinner, F. A. and Carr, J. G. (Ed.), p. 197. Academic Press, London.

GIMINEZ, D. F. and CICCARELLI, A. S. 1970. Another type of *Clostridium botulinum*. *Zentrabl. Bakteriol. Phrasitenk. Infektionski. Hyg. Abt. I. Orig.* 215: 212.

GLATZ, B. A. and GOEPFERT, J. M. 1973. Extracellular factor synthesized by *Bacillus cereus* which evokes a dermal reaction in guinea pigs. *Infect. Immun.* 8: 25.

GLATZ, B. A., SPIRA, W. M., and GOEPFERT, J. M. 1974. Alteration of vascular permeability in rabbits by culture filtrates of *Bacillus cereus* and related species. *Infect. Immun.* 10: 299.

GOEPFERT, J. M., SPIRA, W. M., and KIM, H. U. 1972. *Bacillus cereus*: food poisoning organism. A review. *J. Milk Food Technol.* 35: 213.

GUTTERIDGE, C. S., MACKEY, B. M., and NORRIS, J. R. 1980. A pyrolysis gas-liquid chromatography study of *Clostridium botulinum* and related organisms. *J. Appl. Bacteriol.* 49: 165.

HANFORD, P. M. 1974. A new medium for the detection and enumeration of *Clostridium perfringens* in foods. *J. Appl. Bacteriol.* 37: 559.

HANFORD, P. M. and CAVETT, J. J. 1973. A medium for the detection and enumeration of *Clostridium perfringens* (*welchii*) in foods. *J. Sci. Food Agric.* 24: 487.

HANSEN, M. W. and ELLIOT, L. P. 1980. New presumptive identification test for *Clostridium perfringens*: reverse CAMP test. *J. Clin. Microbiol.* 12: 617.

HARMON, S. M. 1976. Collaborative study of an improved method for the enumeration and confirmation of *Clostridium perfringens* in foods. *J. Assoc. Off. Anal. Chem.* 59: 606.

HARMON, S. M. 1980. *Bacillus cereus*, Ch. XVI. In *Bacteriological Analytical Manual* 5th ed. (1978, rev. 1980). Food and Drug Administration (Ed.), p. XVI-1. Association of Official Analytical Chemists, Washington, DC.

HARMON, S. M. and DUNCAN, C. L. 1978. *Clostridium perfringens:* enumeration, identification, and enterotoxin detection. Ch. XV. In *Bacteriological Analytical Manual*, 5th ed. Food and Drug Administration (Ed.), p. XV-1. Association of Official Analytical Chemists, Washington, DC.

HARMON, S. M. and KAUTTER, D. A. 1970. Method for estimating the presence of *Clostridium perfringens* in food. *Appl. Microbiol.* 20: 913.

HARMON, S. M. and KAUTTER, D. A. 1974. Collaborative study of the α-toxin method for estimating population levels of *Clostridium perfringens* in food. *J. Assoc. Offic. Anal. Chem.* 57: 91.

HARMON, S. M. and KAUTTER, D. A. 1976. Beneficial effect of catalase treatment on growth of *Clostridium perfringens*. *Appl. Environ. Microbiol.* 32: 409.

HARMON, S. L. and KAUTTER, D. A. 1978. Media for confirming *Clostridium perfringens* from food and feces. *J. Food Prot.* 41: 626.

HARMON, S. M., KAUTTER, D. A., and PEELER, J. T. 1971. Improved medium for enumeration of *Clostridium perfringens*. *Appl. Microbiol.* 22: 688.

HARMON, S. M. and PLACENCIA, A. M. 1978. Methods for maintaining viability of *Clostridium perfringens* in foods during shipment and storage: collaborative study. *J. Assoc. Off. Anal. Chem.* 61: 785.

HATHEWAY, C. L., WHALEY, D. N., and DOWELL, V. R. JR. 1980. Epidemiological aspects of *Clostridium perfringens* foodborne illness. *Food Technol.* 34(4): 77.

HAUSCHILD, A. H. W. 1970. Erythemal activity of the cellular enteropathogenic factor of *Clostridium perfringens* type A. *Can. J. Microbiol.* 16: 651.

HAUSCHILD, A. H. W. 1982. Assessment of botulism hazards from cured meat products. *Food Technol.* 36(12): 95.

HAUSCHILD, A. H., DESMARCHELIER, P., GILBERT, R. J., HARMON, S. M., and VAHLEFELD, R. 1979. ICMSF methods studies. XII. Comparative study for the enumeration of *Clostridium perfringens* in feces. *Can. J. Microbiol.* 25: 953.

HAUSCHILD, A. H., GILBERT, R. J., HARMON, S. J., O'KEEFFE, M. F., and VAHLEFELD, R. 1977. ICMSF methods studies. VII. Comparative study for the enumeration of *Clostridium perfringens* in foods. *Can. J. Microbiol.* 23: 884.

HAUSCHILD, A. H. and HILSHEIMER, R. 1974a. Evaluation and modifications of media for enumeration of *Clostridium perfringens*. *Appl. Microbiol.* 27: 78.

HAUSCHILD, A. H. and HILSHEIMER, R. 1974b. Enumeration of food-borne *Clostridium perfringens* in egg yolk-free tryptose-sulfite-cycloserine agar. *Appl. Microbiol.* 27: 521.

HAUSCHILD, A. H., HILSHEIMER, R., and GRIFFITH, D. W. 1974. Enumeration of fecal *Clostridium perfringens* spores in egg yolk-free tryptose-sulfite-cycloserine agar. *Appl. Microbiol.* 27: 527.

HOBBS, G. 1976. *Clostridium botulinum* and its importance in fishery products. *Adv. Food Res.* 22: 135.

HOBBS, G. and CROSS, T. 1984. Identification of endospore-forming bacteria. Ch. 2. In *The Bacterial Spore.* Vol. 2. Hurst, A. and Gould, G. W. (Ed.), p. 49. Academic Press, London.

HOBBS, G., CROWTHER, J. S., NEAVES, P., GIBBS, P. A., and JARVIS, B. 1982. Detection and isolation of *Clostridium botulinum*. In *Isolation and Identification Methods for Food Poisoning Organisms.* Corry, J. E. L., Roberts, D., and Skinner, F. A. (Ed.), p. 151. Academic Press, London.

HOLDEMAN, L. V., CATO, E. P., and MOORE, W. E. C. (Ed.). 1977. *Anaerobe Laboratory Manual.* 4th ed. Virginia Polytechnic Institute and State University, Blacksburg, VA.

HOLBROOK, R. and ANDERSON, J. M. 1980. An improved selective and diagnostic medium for the isolation and enumeration of *Bacillus cereus* in foods. *Can. J. Microbiol.* 26: 753.

HUSS, H. H. 1980. Distribution of *Clostridium botulinum*. *Appl. Environ. Microbiol.* 39: 764.

INOUE, K. and IIDA, H. 1970. Conversion of toxigenicity in *Clostridium botulinum* type C. *Jpn. J. Microbiol.* 14: 87.

JOHNSON, K. M. 1984. *Bacillus cereus* foodborne illness—an update. *J. Food Prot.* 47: 145.

JOHNSON, K. M., NELSON, C. L., and BUSTA, F. F. 1982. Germination and heat resistance of *Bacillus cereus* spores from strains associated with diarrheal and emetic food-borne illnesses. *J. Food Sci.* 47: 1268.

KAUTTER, D. A. and LYNT, R. K. 1978. *Clostridium botulinum*, Ch. XIV. In *Bacteriological Analytical Manual.* 5th ed., p. XIV-1. Food and Drug Administration (Ed.). Association of Official Analytical Chemists, Washington, DC.

KAUTTER, D. A. and SOLOMON, H. M. 1977. Collaborative study of a method for the detection of *Clostridium botulinum* and its toxins in foods. *J. Assoc. Off. Anal. Chem.* 60: 541.

KIM, H. U. and GOEPFERT, J. M. 1971. Enumeration and identification of *Bacillus cereus* in foods. I. 24-Hour presumptive test medium. *Appl. Microbiol.* 22: 581.

KIRITINI, K., MITSUI, N., NAKAMURA, S., and NISHIDA, S. 1973. Numerical taxonomy of *Clostridium botulinum* and *Clostridium sporogenes* strains and their susceptibility to induced lysins and to mitomycin C. *Jpn. J. Microbiol.* 17: 361.

KRAMER, J. M., TURNBULL, P. C. B., MUNSHI, G., and GILBERT, R. J. 1982. Identification and characterization of *Bacillus cereus* and other *Bacillus* species associated with foods and food poisoning. In *Isolation and Identification Methods for Food Poisoning Organisms.* Corry, J. E. L., Roberts, D., and Skinner, F. A. (Ed.), p. 261. Academic Press, London.

LABBE, R. G. 1980. Relationship between sporulation and enterotoxin production in *Clostridium perfringens* type A. *Food Technol.* 34(4): 88.

LABBE, R. G. 1983. Enumeration and confirmation of *Clostridium perfringens*. *J. Food Prot.* 46: 68.

LABBE, R. G. and NORRIS, K. E. 1982. Evaluation of plating media for recovery of heated *Clostridium perfringens* spores. *J. Food Prot.* 45: 686.

LAU, A. H. S., HAWIRKO, R. Z., and CHOW, C. T. 1974. Purification and properties of boticin P produced by *Clostridium botulinum*. *Can. J. Microbiol.* 20: 385.

LEWIS, G. E. JR. (Ed.). 1981. *Biomedical Aspects of Botulism.* Academic Press, New York.

LILLY, T. JR., HARMON, S. M., KAUTTER, D. A., SOLOMON, H. M., and LYNT, R. K. JR. 1971. An improved medium for detection of *Clostridium botulinum* type E. *J. Milk Food Technol.* 34: 492.

LILLY, T. JR., KAUTTER, D. A., LYNT, R. K., and SOLOMON, H. M. 1984. Immunodiffusion detection of *Clostridium botulinum* colonies. *J. Food Protect.* 47: 868.

LYNT, R. K., KAUTTER, D. A., and SOLOMON, H. M. 1982. Differences and similarities among proteolytic and nonproteolytic strains of *Clostridium botulinum* types A, B, E and F: a review. *J. Food Prot.* 45: 466.

MARSHALL, R. S., STEENBERGEN, J. F., and McCLUNG, L. 1965. Rapid technique for the enumeration of *Clostridium perfringens*. *Appl. Microbiol.* 13: 559.

McDONEL, J. L. 1980. Mechanism of action of *Clostridium perfringens* enterotoxin. *Food Technol.* 34(4): 91.

MEAD, C. G. 1969. The use of sulfite-containing media in the isolation of *Clostridium welchii*. *J. Appl. Bacteriol.* 32: 358.

MEAD, G. C., ADAMS, B. W., ROBERTS, T. A., and SMART, J. L. 1982. Isolation and enumeration of *Clostridium perfringens*. In *Isolation and Identification Methods for Food Poisoning Organisms.* Corry, J. E. L., Roberts, D., and Skinner, F. A. (Ed.), p. 99. Academic Press, London.

MELLING, J., CAPEL, B. J., TURNBULL, P. C. B., and GILBERT, R. J. 1976. Identification of a novel enterotoxigenic activity associated with *Bacillus cereus. J. Clin. Pathol.* 29: 938.

MESTRANDREA, L. W. 1974. Rapid detection of *Clostridium botulinum* toxin by capillary tube diffusion. *Appl. Microbiol.* 27: 1017.

MILLER, C. A. and ANDERSON, A. W. 1971. Rapid detection and quantitative estimation of type A botulism toxin by electroimmunodiffusion. *Infect. Immun.* 4: 126.

MOSSEL, D. A. A. 1959. Enumeration of sulfite-reducing clostridia occurring in foods. *J. Sci. Food Agric.* 19: 662.

MOSSEL, D. A. A. and DeWAART, J. 1968. The enumeration of clostridia in foods and feeds. *Ann. Inst. Pasteur, Lille* 19: 13.

MOSSEL, D. A. A., KOOPMAN, M. J., and JONGERIUS, E. 1967. Enumeration of *Bacillus cereus* in foods. *Appl. Microbiol.* 15: 650.

NAIK, H. S. and DUNCAN, C. L. 1977a. Enterotoxin formation in foods by *Clostridium perfringens* type A. *J. Food Safety* 1: 7.

NAIK, H. S. and DUNCAN, C. L. 1977b. Rapid detection and quantitation of *Clostridium perfringens* enterotoxin by counterimmunoelectrophoresis. *Appl. Environ. Microbiol.* 34: 125.

NIILO, L. 1977. Enterotoxin formation by *Clostridium perfringens* type A studied by the use of fluorescent antibody. *Can. J. Microbiol.* 23: 908.

NOTERMANS, S., DUFRENNE, J., and KOZAKI, S. 1979. Enzyme-linked immunosorbent assay for detection of *Clostridium botulinum* type E toxin. *Appl. Environ. Microbiol.* 37: 1173.

NOTERMANS, S. and KOZAKI, S. 1981. Isolation and identification of botulinum toxins using the ELISA. In *Biomedical Aspects of Botulism.* Lewis, G. E. (Ed.), p. 181. Academic Press, New York.

ORTH, D. S. 1977. Comparison of sulfite-polymyxin-sulfadiazine medium and tryptose-sulfite-cycloserine medium without egg yolk for recovering *Clostridium perfringens. Appl. Environ. Microbiol.* 33: 986.

PARK, Y. and MIKOLAJCIK, E. M. 1979. Effect of temperature on growth and alpha toxin production by *Clostridium perfringens. J. Food Prot.* 42: 848.

RAPPORT, H. and GOEPFERT, J. M. 1978. Thermal injury and recovery of *Bacillus cereus. J. Food Prot.* 41: 533.

RYMKIEWICZ, D. 1968. Studies on type F *Clostridium botulinum.* II. Isolation and properties of highly active toxin. *Medycyna Doswiadczalna Mikrobiol.* 20: 288.

ST. JOHN, W. D., MATCHES, J. R., and WEKELL, M. M. 1982. Use of iron milk medium for enumeration of *Clostridium perfringens. J. Assoc. Off. Anal. Chem.* 65: 1129.

SEGNER, W. P. and SCHMIDT, C. F. 1968. Nonspecific toxicities in the mouse assay test for botulinum toxin. *Appl. Microbiol.* 16: 1105.

SHAHIDI, S. A. and FERGUSON, A. R. 1971. New quantitative, qualitative, and confirmatory media for rapid analysis of food for *Clostridium perfringens*. *Appl. Microbiol.* 21: 500.

SHOEMAKER, S. P. and PIERSON, M. D. 1976. "Phoenix phenomenon" in the growth of *C. perfringens*. *Appl. Environ. Microbiol.* 32: 803.

SIMUNOVIC, J., OBLINGER, J. L., and ADAMS, J. P. 1985. Potential for growth of nonproteolytic types of *Clostridium botulinum* in pasteurized restructured meat products: a review. *J. Food Prot.* 48: 265.

SKJELKVALE, R. and UEMURA, T. 1977. Experimental diarrhoea in human volunteers following oral administration of *C. perfringens* enterotoxin. *J. Appl. Bacteriol.* 43: 281.

SMITH, L. DS. 1972. Factors involved in the isolation of *Clostridium perfringens*. *J. Milk Food Technol.* 35: 71.

SMITH, L. DS. 1977. *Botulism: The Organism, its Toxins, and the Disease*, p. 15. Charles C. Thomas, Springfield, IL.

SNYGG, B. G., ANDERSSON, J. E., KRALL, C. A., STÖLLMAN, U. M., and AKESSON, C. A. 1979. Separation of botulinum-positive and -negative fish samples by means of a pattern recognition method applied to headspace gas chromatograms. *Appl. Microbiol.* 38: 1081.

SOLBERG, M., POST, L. S., FURGANG, D., and GRAHAM, C. 1985. Bovine serum eliminates rapid nonspecific toxic reactions during bioassay of stored fish for *Clostridium botulinum* toxin. *Appl. Environ. Microbiol.* 49: 644.

SPERBER, W. H. 1982. Requirements of *Clostridium botulinum* for growth and toxin production. *Food Technol.* 36(12): 89.

SPIRA, W. M. and GOEPFERT, J. M. 1972. *Bacillus cereus*-induced fluid accumulation in rabbit ileal loops. *Appl. Microbiol.* 24: 341.

STARK, R. L. and DUNCAN, C. L. 1972. Transient increase in capillary permeability induced by *Clostridium perfringens* type A enterotoxin. *Inf. Immun.* 5: 147.

STEC, E. and BURZYNSKA, K. 1980. Comparison of media for quantitative determination of *Bacillus cereus* in certain food products. *Roczn. Panstwowego Zakladu Higien.* 31: 407. (in Russian, English summary).

STELMA, G. N. JR., JOHNSON, C. H., and SHAH, D. B. 1985. Detection of enterotoxin in colonies of *Clostridium perfringens* by a solid phase enzyme-linked immunosorbent assay. *J. Food Prot.* 48: 227.

STELMA, G. N., WIMSATT, J. C., KAUFFMAN, P. E., and SHAH, D. G. 1983. A radioimmunoassay for *Clostridium perfringens* enterotoxin and its use in screening isolates implicated in food-poisoning outbreaks. *J. Food Prot.* 46: 1069.

STRINGER, M. F., WATSON, G. N., and GILBERT, R. J. 1982. *Clostridium perfringens* type A: serological typing and methods for the detection of enterotoxin. In *Isolation and Identification Methods for Food Poisoning Organisms.* Corry, J. E. L., Roberts, D., and Skinner, F. A., (Ed.), p. 111. Academic Press, London.

SUGIYAMA, M. W. 1982. Botulism hazards from nonprocessed foods. *Food Technol.* 36(12): 113.

SUGIYAMA, H. and KING, G. J. 1972. Isolation and taxonomic significance of bacteriophages for non-proteolytic *Clostridium botulinum. J. Gen. Microbiol.* 70: 517.

SUTTON, R. G. A. and HOBBS, B. C. 1968. Food poisoning caused by heat-sensitive *Clostridium welchii.* A report of five recent outbreaks. *J. Hyg. Camb.* 66: 135.

SZABO, R. A., TODD, E. C. D., and RAYMAN, M. K. 1984. Twenty-four hour isolation and confirmation of *Bacillus cereus* in foods. *J. Food Prot.* 47: 856.

TAYLOR, A. J. and GILBERT, R. J. 1975. *Bacillus cereus* food poisoning: a provisional serotyping scheme. *J. Med. Microbiol.* 8: 543.

TERRANOVA, W. and BLAKE, P. A. 1978. Current concepts: *Bacillus cereus* food poisoning. *New Engl. J. Med.* 298: 143.

TSARAPKIN, V. P. 1971. Preparation of sorbed botulinum toxoid type F. Comparative assessment of various nutrient media to obtain active botulinum toxin type F. *Zhurnal Microbiol. Epidemiol. Immunobiol.* 48: 28.

UEMURA, T., SAKAGUCHI, G., and RIEMANN, H. P. 1973. *In vitro* production of *Clostridium perfringens* enterotoxin and its detection by reversed passive haemagglutination. *Appl. Microbiol.* 26: 381.

WALKER, H. W. 1975. Food borne illness from *Clostridium perfringens. Crit. Rev. Food Sci. Nutr.* 7: 71.

WATSON, G. N. 1985. The assessment and application of a bacteriocin typing scheme for *Clostridium perfringens. J. Hyg., Camb.* 94: 69.

WILLARDSEN, R. R., BUSTA, F. F., and ALLEN, C. E. 1979. Growth of *Clostridium perfringens* in three beef media and fluid thioglycollate medium at static and constantly rising temperatures. *J. Food Prot.* 42: 144.

WILSON, W. J. and BLAIR, E. M. 1924. The application of a sulphite-glucose-iron-agar medium to the quantitative estimation of *Bacillus welchii* and other reducing bacteria in water supplies. *J. Path. Bacteriol.* 27: 11.

18

Official Methods of Analysis of Foods for Mycotoxins

Douglas L. Park and Albert E. Pohland

Food and Drug Administration
Washington, D.C.

INTRODUCTION

Mycotoxins are toxic secondary metabolites produced by fungi. The growth of molds on foods results frequently in their contamination by mycotoxins. Ingestion of contaminated foods can, if the level of toxin is sufficiently high, lead to illness and even death in man and animals (Goldblatt 1977; Stoloff 1977). Such illnesses are termed mycotoxicoses and have been known for many years. The earliest human mycotoxicoses were probably a result of eating toxic mushrooms. The frequent, widespread occurrence during the Middle Ages of ergotism, resulting from ingestion of rye contaminated by the fungus *Claviceps purpurea*, has been well documented. More recent outbreaks of ergotism have occurred in Russia (1926), England (1928), France, and India (1951). Immediately following World War II, severe mycotoxicoses in man and animals were reported in the Eastern European countries, apparently caused by contamination of overwintered grain by Fusarium species leading to a condition referred to as alimentary toxic aleukia (ATA).

In Japan (1945) a human mycotoxicosis resulting from eating "yellowed" rice (probably contaminated with *Pencillium citreoviridin*) was reported. More recently, a severe acute human mycotoxicosis resulting from ingestion of aflatoxin-contaminated corn was reported in India, resulting in over 200 deaths. These examples, as well as an extensive body of scientific literature describing mycotoxicoses in animals, have prompted public health officials to make a concerted, continuing effort to understand and control exposure to mycotoxins. This effort was spurred by the findings in the early 1960s that aflatoxin was a potent liver carcinogen in every animal species tested.

Health officials are constantly faced with the challenge of assessing the risks associated with man's exposure to mycotoxins. However, every assessment dealing with food contamination contains the same basic elements, i.e., the toxicological nature of the contaminant and the degree of human exposure to the toxicant. In making such an assessment, an in-depth review of the toxicological properties of the substance is performed. The toxicological analysis takes into account data on pathology, metabolism, species/strain susceptibility, no observable effect concentration, and epidemiology.

The exposure assessment requires information on natural occurrence of the substance—incidence/levels and commodities affected—and the potential for human exposure, either directly or indirectly. Other information required in the assessment includes an inventory of all sources of exposure—human food, human foods from animal sources (milk, eggs), and edible animal tissues (liver, kidney, muscle)—identification of subpopulations at risk (age, sex, ethnic group, physical status, etc.), and consumption patterns for each population group identified. Although not part of the exposure assessment per se, information on chemical and physical properties such as structural formulae, substance stability, analytical method capabilities and limitations, and availability of decontamination methods is also necessary.

Once the potential for mycotoxin contamination has been identified, it is necessary to develop suitable analytical methods for the detection and quantitation of the toxin(s). These methods could be based either on the biological responses or on the chemical characteristics of the toxin(s). Analytical methods for use under a variety of applications, i.e., screening, survey, regulatory control, etc., need to be developed and, where applicable, validated by an interlaboratory collaborative study. Organizations such as the Association of Official Analytical Chemists (AOAC), American Oil Chemists' Society (AOCS), American Association of Cereal Chemists' (AACC), and International Union of Pure and Applied Chemistry (IUPAC) have method validation programs. Table 18.1 lists several mycotoxin methods adopted by these organizations. A committee composed of representatives from these organizations was formed to establish priorities for methods development programs and to exchange information on many aspects of mycotoxin research.

Table 18.1. Mycotoxin Methods Approved by AOAC, IUPAC, AACC, and AOCS[a]

Analyte	Commodity	AOAC	IUPAC	AACC	AOCS
Total aflatoxins	almonds, white & yellow corn, peanut & cottonseed meals, peanuts, peanut butter, pistachio nuts, mixed feeds	26.014–26.019	—	45–10:1–4 (1975)	—
Total aflatoxins	corn, raw peanuts	26.020–26.025	—	45–14:1–9 (1980)	—
Aflatoxin B_1, B_2, G_1, G_2	peanut & peanut products	26.026–26.031	IB-31 (1968)	—	—
Aflatoxin B_1, B_2, G_1, G_2	peanuts & peanut products	26.032–26.036	—	—	Ab6–68 (1973)
Aflatoxin B_1, B_2, G_1, G_2	cocoa beans	26.037–26.043	IB–8 (1973)	—	—
Aflatoxin B_1, B_2, G_1, G_2	coconut, copra, & copra meal	26.044–26.048	IB-9 (1974)	—	Ah1–72
Aflatoxin B_1, B_2, G_1, G_2	corn	26.049–26.051	—	45–05:1–9 (1972)	—
Aflatoxin B_1, B_2, G_1, G_2	cottonseed products	26.052–26.060	—	—	Aa8–83
Aflatoxin B_1, G_1	confirmation	26.076–26.082	—	45–30:1–8 (1977)	—
Aflatoxin B_1, G_1	confirmation	26.083	—	45–25:1–5 (1977)	—
Aflatoxin M_1	milk, cheese	26.095–26.100	—	—	—
Aflatoxin B_1, M_1	animal tissues	26.101–26.106	—	—	—
Ochratoxin A, B	barley, green coffee	26.111–26.117 26.119–26.124	IB–14 (1976)	—	—
Sterigma-tocystin	barley, wheat	26.132–26.137	—	—	—
Patulin	apple juice	26.126–26.131	—	—	—
Zearalenone	corn	26.139–16.147	—	45–20:1–6 (1976)	—

[a]AOAC—Association of Official Analytical Chemists; IUPAC—International Union of Pure and Applied Chemistry; AACC—American Association of Cereal Chemists; AOCS—American Oil Chemists' Society.

An annual report of this committee is published in the *Journal of the AOAC*. Park and Yess (1983) have identified scientific organizations that sponsor programs aiding in the development and validation of analytical methods for mycotoxins. These programs provide a forum for the exchange of ideas and dissemination of information in all aspects of mycotoxin research and in the development of programs for natural resource utilization.

Method validation studies are designed to demonstrate that a given method will provide reliable results within the limits of variation of the method in the hands of competent analysts. Check sample programs enable individual laboratories to critically judge the analytical performance of its analysts. To analyze the check samples, laboratories may use any method they desire (in contrast to a collaborative study in which a specific set of directions is to be followed). The purpose of a collaborative study, on the other hand, is to evaluate the performance of a method rather than that of a laboratory or an analyst. The International Agency for Research on Cancer (IARC), IUPAC, Association of American Feed Control Officials (AAFCO), and AOCS routinely organize check sample series for mycotoxins.

Validated Mycotoxin Methods

The observation by Platt et al. (1962) that the "groundnut toxin" caused deaths when injected into the yolk of 5-day-old chicken embryos led to increased investigation of the feasibility of using the chicken embryo as a bioassay for aflatoxin (Verrett et al. 1964). The test was routinely used for the detection of aflatoxin B_1 for many years and in 1970 was collaboratively studied and adopted by AOAC as Official First Action (Verrett et al. 1973). Regulatory scientists, however, quickly realized that a more rapid analytical method was needed. Nesheim and co-workers (1964) and Nesheim (1964) published a rapid thin-layer chromatographic (TLC) procedure applicable to the analysis of aflatoxins in peanut products. This method was later collaboratively studied (Campbell and Funkhouser 1966) and adopted Official First Action by AOAC (commonly called the BF Method). Several other researchers followed up these efforts, resulting in the development of another AOAC approved TLC method (Eppley 1966; Eppley et al. 1968; Stack 1974). This method (CB Method) showed a little more versatility and included a step for confirmation of aflatoxin identity. The basis for these methods was subsequently applied and/or modified for the analysis of aflatoxins in other food commodities and feeds, i.e., cottonseed products (Pons 1969), green coffee beans (Levi 1969), cocoa beans (Scott 1969; Scott and Przybylski

1971), coconut, copra, and copra meal (Baur and Armstrong 1971), corn
and soybeans (Shotwell and Stubblefield 1972), pistachio nuts (DiProssimo
1974), dairy products (Pons et al. 1973; Stubblefield and Shannon 1974a,
b), eggs (Trucksess et al. 1969), and liver (Stubblefield and Shotwell 1981;
Stubblefield et al. 1982). In 1980 (Pons et al.) a high performance liquid
chromatographic (HPLC) and TLC method was adopted for aflatoxins in
cottonseed products. A complete listing of aflatoxin methods validated by
AOAC is included in Table 18.2.

As the significance and incidence of aflatoxin contamination became better
understood, the need for qualitative screening methods became apparent for
use in feed and food processing plants. Several minicolumn methods were
developed (Velasco 1972; Velasco and Whitten 1973, Shotwell and Stubblefield 1973; Romer 1975) and eventually collaboratively studied for mixed
feeds, white and yellow corn, peanut and cottonseed meals, peanuts, peanut
butter, and pistachio nuts (Romer and Campbell 1976), almonds (Stanley
et al. 1979), corn (Shannon and Shotwell 1979), and raw peanuts (Shotwell
and Holaday 1981).

Several methods have been adopted by AOAC for mycotoxins other than
aflatoxin, including ochratoxins A and B and their esters (Nesheim et al.
1973; Neshein 1973; Levi 1975); sterigmatocystin (Stack and Rodricks 1971,
1973), patulin (Scott 1974), zearalenone (Shotwell et al. 1976), and zearalenone and α-zearalenol (Bennett et al. 1985). These methods employ primarily TLC techniques; however, the method for zearlenone and α-zearalenol
(Bennett et al. 1985) is based on reverse phase liquid chromatography (HPLC)
with fluorescence detection. These methods are listed in Table 18.3.

Confirmation of Identity Methods—Mycotoxins

Early in the research it was observed that substances other than the analyte
under study could interfere with positive identification, i.e., have similar
chromatographic and fluorescence properties. Therefore, other techniques
were employed in establishing chemical confirmation of the identity of the
mycotoxin detected. Although used for many years for confirmation of identity of aflatoxin B_1, the chicken embryo assay was not collaboratively studied
until 1970 and not adopted by AOAC until 1973 (Verrett et al. 1973).
Although the BF method (Campbell and Funkhouser 1966) contained a
section for the confirmation of aflatoxin G_1 and G_2 using two alternative
TLC development systems, the first chemical confirmation method for aflatoxin B_1 involved the preparation of a water adduct (aflatoxin B_{2a}) by treatment with either formic acid-thionyl chloride or trifluoroacetic acid (TFA)

Table 18.2. Aflatoxin Methods Adopted by the Association of Official Analytical Chemists (AOAC)

Section No.	Analyte	Technique	Determination level (ng/g)	Commodity
26.014– 26.019	total aflatoxins (B_1, B_2, G_1, G_2)	minicolumn (Romer)	> 5 > 10	almonds white & yellow corn, peanut & cottonseed meals, peanuts,
			> 15	peanut butter, pistachio nuts mixed feeds
26.020– 26.025	total aflatoxins (B_1, B_2, G_1, G_2)	minicolumn (Holaday-Velasco)	> 10	white & yellow corn, raw, shelled peanuts
26.026– 26.031	aflatoxin B_1, B_2, G_1, G_2	TLC (CB method)	2.5	peanuts, peanut products
26.032– 26.036	aflatoxin B_1, B_2, G_1, G_2	TLC (BF method)	10	peanuts, peanut products
26.037– 26.043	aflatoxin B_1, B_2, G_1, G_2	TLC (modified CB method)	10	cocoa beans
26.044– 26.048	aflatoxin B_1, B_2, G_1, G_2	TLC	50	coconut, copra, copra meal
26.049– 26.051	aflatoxin B_1, B_2, G_1, G_2	TLC	10	corn
26.052– 26.060	aflatoxin B_1, B_2, G_1, G_2	TLC/HPLC	20	cottonseed products
26.061– 26.066	aflatoxin, B_1, B_2, G_1, G_2	TLC	25	green coffee
26.067	aflatoxin B_1, B_2, G_1, G_2	TLC (Method I)	15	pistachio nuts
26.068	aflatoxin B_1, B_2, G_1, G_2	TLC (Method II)	10	pistachio nuts
26.069	aflatoxin B_1, B_2, G_1, G_2	TLC	10	soybeans
26.070– 26.075	aflatoxin B_1	TLC	1	whole egg, egg white & yolk, dried whole egg, egg yolk & white

(Continued)

Table 18.2 (*Continued*).

Section No.	Analyte	Technique	Determination level (ng/g)	Commodity
26.090– 26.094	aflatoxin M_1	TLC	0.1 ($\mu g/L$, milk) 0.2 (cheese) 0.1 (milk powder)	fluid, powdered milk, blue, ricotta, cheddar cheese, butter
26.095– 26.100	aflatoxin M_1	TLC	0.1	milk and cheese
26.101– 26.106	aflatoxin B_1, M_1	TLC	2.5– 6.0(B_1) 6.4–32 (M_1)	liver

and the preparation of a mixture of epimeric acetates by reaction with acetic acid-thionyl chloride (AOAC 1967). Pohland et al. (1970) and Stoloff (1970) developed and collaboratively studied a rapid chemical confirmatory method based on the acid-catalyzed hydration of aflatoxin B_1 to yield aflatoxin B_{2a} or on the reaction with acetic anhydride to yield two acetates.

Przybylski (1975) outlined two confirmatory techniques using the TLC plate directly. The first involved the conversion of aflatoxin B_1 and G_1 to B_{2a} and G_{2a}, respectively, by applying TFA directly to the unknown and aflatoxin standards spots and developing with acetone-chloroform ($15 + 85$). The B_{2a} and G_{2a} derivatives appear at an R_f about one-fourth that of aflatoxin B_1 and G_1, respectively. The second technique, performed after TLC development, showed a change in fluorescence from blue to yellow after spraying with 25% sulfuric acid. These methods were collaboratively studied and adopted by AOAC (Stack and Pohland 1975).

For samples contaminated with low levels of aflatoxin B_1 or M_1, where interfering fluorescent substances may be present, a two-dimensional technique utilizing water adduct formation was developed and approved (van Egmond et al. 1978; Stubblefield 1979; van Egmond and Stubblefield 1981). A confirmatory method for sterigmatocystin was adopted in 1973 (Stack and

Table 18.3. Mycotoxin Methods Other than Aflatoxin Adopted by the Association of Official Analytical Chemists (AOAC)

Section No.	Analyte	Technique	Determination level (ng/g)	Commodity
26.111– 26.117	ochratoxin A, B & esters of ochratoxin A, B	TLC	45	barley
26.119– 26.124	ochratoxin A	TLC	50	green coffee
26.126– 26.131	patulin	TLC	20 μg/L	apple juice
26.132– 26.137	sterigma- tocystin	TLC	75 (barley) 100 (wheat)	barley, wheat
26.139– 26.147	zearalenone	TLC	300	corn
26.A09– 26.A16	zearalenone, α-zearalenol	LC	50 50	corn

Rodricks) where an acetate derivative is formed which fluoresces blue (instead of brick red) and has an R_f about one-half that of sterigmatocystin. A separate reaction with acid forms a derivative which fluoresces yellow after spraying with potassium hydroxide and has an R_f about one-fourth that of sterigmatocystin. Ochratoxins are confirmed by formation of derivatives directly on the TLC plate by spraying with either an alkaline sodium bicarbonate or an aluminum chloride solution or exposure to ammonia vapor (Nesheim et al. 1973; Nesheim 1973). Ochratoxin fluorescence changes to bright blue and increases in intensity.

All confirmation of identity procedures discussed thus far are based on either physical or chemical properties or biological activity and are often nonspecific. To adhere to a high degree of specificity in confirmation of aflatoxin identity, mass spectrometric (MS) techniques were investigated and one procedure based on negative ion chemical ionization (NICI) was collaboratively studied (Park et al. 1985). Partially purified extracts are subjected to additional cleanup by two-dimensional TLC before MS analysis. Table 18.4 summarizes the methods for confirmation of identity.

Table 18.4. Mycotoxin Methods of Confirmation of Identity Adopted by the Association of Official Analytical Chemists (AOAC)

Section No.	Analyte	Technique	Result
26.076– 26.083	aflatoxin B_1, G_1	derivative formation with TFA, TLC	change in R_f
		derivative formation with H_2SO_4, TLC	change in fluorescent color
26.084– 26.089	aflatoxin B_1	chicken embryo	mortality
26.A01– 26.A08	aflatoxin B_1	MS/NICI	MS spectrum of B_1 fragmentation
26.100	aflatoxin M_1	derivative formation with TFA, TLC	change in R_f
26.107– 26.109	aflatoxin M_1 (liver)	derivative formation with TFA, TLC	change in R_f
26.118	ochratoxin A, B	formation of ethyl esters, TLC	change in R_f
26.125	ochratoxin A	derivative formation	change in fluorescence color and intensity
26.131(d)	patulin	different developing solvents, TLC	change in R_f
26.138	sterigmatocystin	derivative formation, TLC	change in R_f and fluorescence color

SUMMARY

Method validation is a continuing process. Currently two methods for deoxynivalenol, one a TLC method (Eppley et al. 1984) and one a gas chromatographic method (Ware et al. 1984), have been submitted to the AOAC for approval for official status. As better methods become available these also will be submitted to collaborative study for validation. The process, admittedly time-consuming and expensive, is still the best way to evaluate methods before they can be considered for "official" status. The AOAC, in conjunction with many other organizations, has recently put a great deal of effort into developing standard procedures for conducting collaborative studies.

REFERENCES

AOAC. 1967. Changes in Methods, 25. Nuts and Nut Products. *J. Assoc. off. Anal. Chem.* 50: 214–216.

BAUR, F. J. and ARMSTRONG, J. C. 1971. Collaborative study of a modified method for the determination of aflatoxins in copra, copra meal, and coconut. *J. Assoc. Off. Anal. Chem.* 54: 874–878.

BENNETT, G. A., SHOTWELL, O. L., and KWOLEK, W. F. 1985. Liquid chromatographic determination of α-zearalenol and zearalenone in corn: Collaborative study. *J. Assoc. Off. Anal. Chem.* 68: 958–961.

CAMPBELL A. D. and FUNKHOUSER, J. T. 1966. Collaborative study on the analysis of aflatoxins in peanut butter. *J. Assoc. Off. Anal. Chem.* 49: 730–739.

DiPROSSIMO, V. 1974. Collaborative study comparing two methods for the determination of aflatoxins in pistachio nuts. *J. Assoc. Off. Anal. Chem.* 67: 1114–1120.

EPPLEY, R. M. 1966. A versatile procedure for the assay and preparatory separation of aflatoxins from peanut products. *J. Assoc. Off. Anal. Chem.* 49: 1218–1223.

EPPLEY, R. M., STOLOFF, L., and CAMPBELL, A. D. 1968. Collaborative study of "a versatile procedure for assay of aflatoxins in peanut products," including preparatory separation and confirmation of identity. *J. Assoc. Off. Anal. Chem.* 51: 67–73.

EPPLEY, R. M., TRUCKSESS, M. W., NESHEIM, S., THORPE, C. W., and POHLAND, A. E. 1984. Collaborative study of a thin-layer chromatographic method for the determination of deoxynivalenol in wheat. *J. Assoc. Off. Anal. Chem.* 69:37–40.

GOLDBLATT, L. A. 1977. Mycotoxins—past, present and future. *J. Am. Oil Chem. Soc.* 54: 302A–309A.

LEVI. C. P. 1969. Collaborative study on a method for detection of aflatoxin B_1 in green coffee beans. *J. Assoc. Off. Anal. Chem.* 52: 1300–1303.

LEVI, C. P. 1975. Collaborative study of a method for the determination of ochratoxin A in green coffee. *J. Assoc. Off. Anal. Chem.* 58: 258–262.

NESHEIM, S. 1964. Mycotoxins: Studies of the rapid procedure for aflatoxins in peanuts, peanut meal, and peanut butter. *J. Assoc. Off. Agric. Chem.* 47: 1010–1017.

NESHEIM, S. 1973. Analysis of ochratoxin A and B and their esters in barley, using partition and thin-layer chromatography. II. Collaborative study. *J. Assoc. Off. Anal. Chem.* 56: 822–826.

NESHEIM, S., BANES, D., STOLOFF, L., and CAMPBELL, A. D. 1964. Note on aflatoxin analysis in peanuts and peanut products. *J. Assoc. Off. Agric. Chem.* 47: 586.

NESHEIM, S., HARDIN, N. F., FRANCIS, O. J. JR., and LANGHAM, W. S. 1973. Analysis of ochratoxin A and B and their esters in barley, using partition and thin layer chromatography. I. Development of the method. *J. Assoc. Off. Anal. Chem.* 56: 817–821.

PARK, D. L., DiPROSSIMO, V., ABDEL-MALEK, E., TRUCKSESS, M. W., NESHEIM, S., BRUMLEY, W. C., SPHON, J. A., BARRY, T. L., and PETZINGER, G. 1985. Negative ion chemical ionization mass spectrometric method for confirmation of identity of aflatoxin B_1: Collaborative study. *J. Assoc Off. Anal. Chem.* 68: 636–640.

PARK, D. L. and YESS, N. 1983. Scientific societies sponsoring mycotoxin programs. In *Mycotoxin Symposium.* Naguib, K., Naguib, M. M., Park, D. L., and Pohland, A. E. (Ed.). National Research Centre, Dokki, Cairo, Egypt.

PLATT, B. S., STEWART, R. J. C., and GUPTA, R. 1962. *Proc. Nutr. Soc.* 30: 21.

POHLAND, A. E., YIN, L., and DANTZMAN, J. G. 1970. Rapid chemical confirmatory method for aflatoxin B_1. Development of the method. *J. Assoc. Off. Anal. Chem.* 53: 101–102.

PONS, W. A. JR. 1969. Collaborative study on the determination of aflatoxin in cottonseed products. *J. Assoc. Off. Anal. Chem.* 52: 61–72.

PONS, W. A. JR., CUCULLU, A. F., and LEE, L. S. 1973. Method for the determination of aflatoxin M_1 in fluid milk and milk products. *J. Assoc. Off. Anal. Chem.* 56: 1431–1436.

PONS, W. A. JR., LEE, L. S., and STOLOFF, L. 1980. Revised method for aflatoxins in cottonseed products, and comparison of thin layer and high performance liquid chromatography determinative steps: Collaborative study. *J. Assoc. Off. Anal. Chem.* 63: 899–906.

PRZYBYLSKI, W. 1975. Formation of aflatoxin derivatives on thin layer chromatographic plates. *J. Assoc. Off. Anal. Chem.* 58: 163–164.

ROMER, T. R. 1975. Screening method for the detection of aflatoxins in mixed feeds and other agricultural commodities with subsequent confirmation and quantitative measurement of aflatoxins in positive samples. *J. Assoc. Off. Anal. Chem.* 58: 500–506.

ROMER, T. R. and CAMPBELL, A. D. 1976. Collaborative study of a screening method for the detection of aflatoxins in mixed feeds, other agricultural products and foods. *J. Assoc. Off. Anal. Chem.* 59: 110–117.

SCOTT, P. M. 1969. Analysis of cocoa beans for aflatoxins. *J. Assoc. Off. Anal. Chem.* 52: 72–74.

SCOTT, P. M. 1974. Collaborative study of a chromatographic method for determination of patulin in apple juice. *J. Assoc. Off. Anal. Chem.* 57: 621–625.

SCOTT, P. M. and PRZYBYLSKI, W. 1971. Collaborative study of a method for the analysis of cocoa beans for aflatoxins. *J. Assoc. Off. Anal. Chem.* 54: 540–544.

SHANNON, G. M. and SHOTWELL, O. L. 1979. Minicolumn detection methods for aflatoxin in yellow corn: Collaborative study. *J. Assoc. Off. Anal. Chem.* 62: 1070–1075.

SHOTWELL, O. L., GOULDEN, M. L., and BENNETT, G. A. 1976. Determination of zearalenone in corn: Collaborative study. *J. Assoc. Off. Anal. Chem.* 59: 666–670.

SHOTWELL, O. L. and HOLADAY, C. E. 1981. Minicolumn detection methods for aflatoxin in raw peanuts: Collaborative study. *J. Assoc. Off. Anal. Chem.* 64: 674–677.

SHOTWELL, O. L. and STUBBLEFIELD, R. D. 1972. Collaborative study of the determination of aflatoxin in corn and soybeans. *J. Assoc. Off. Anal. Chem.* 55: 781–788.

SHOTWELL, O. L. and STUBBLEFIELD, R. D. 1973. Collaborative study of three screening methods for aflatoxin in corn. *J. Assoc. Off. Anal. Chem.* 56: 808–812.

STACK, M. E. 1974. Collaborative study of AOAC methods I and III for the determination of aflatoxins in peanut butter. *J. Assoc. Off. Anal. Chem.* 57: 871–874.

STACK, M. E. and POHLAND, A. E. 1975. Collaborative study of a method for chemical confirmation of the identity of aflatoxin. *J. Assoc. Off. Anal. Chem.* 58: 110–113.

STACK, M. E. and RODRICKS, J. V. 1971. Method for analysis and chemical confirmation of sterigmatocystin. *J. Assoc. Off. Anal. Chem.* 54: 86–90.

STACK, M. E. and RODRICKS, J. V. 1973. Collaborative study of the qualitative determination and chemical confirmation of sterigmatocystin in grains. *J. Assoc. Off. Anal. Chem.* 56: 1123–1125.

STANLEY, G. I., DiPROSSIMO, V. P., and KOONTZ, A. C. 1979. Minicolumn detection method applied to almonds: Collaborative study. *J. Assoc. Off. Anal. Chem.* 62: 136–140.

STOLOFF, L. 1970. Rapid chemical confirmatory method for aflatoxin B_1. II. Collaborative study. *J. Assoc. Off. Anal. Chem.* 53: 102–104.

STOLOFF, L. 1977. Aflatoxins—an overview. In *Mycotoxins in Human and Animal Health.* Rodricks, J. V., Hesseltine, C. W., and Mehlman, M. A. (Ed.). p. 7–28. Pathotox Publishers Inc., Park Forest South, IL.

STUBBLEFIELD, R. D. 1979. The rapid determination of aflatoxin M_1 in dairy products. *J. Am. Oil Chem. Soc.* 56: 800–802.

STUBBLEFIELD, R. D., KWOLEK, W. F., and STOLOFF, L. 1982. Determination and thin layer chromatographic confirmation of identity of aflatoxins B_1 and M_1 in artificially contaminated beef livers: Collaborative study. *J. Assoc. Off. Anal. Chem.* 65: 1435–1444.

STUBBLEFIELD, R. D. and SHANNON, G. M. 1974a. Aflatoxin M_1: Analysis in dairy products and distribution in dairy foods made from artificially contaminated milk. *J. Assoc. Off. Anal. Chem.* 57: 847–851.

STUBBLEFIELD, R. D. and SHANNON, G. M. 1974b. Collaborative study of methods for the determination and chemical confirmation of aflatoxin M_1 in dairy products. *J. Assoc. Off. Anal. Chem.* 57: 852–857.

STUBBLEFIELD, R. D. and SHOTWELL, O. L. 1981. Determination of aflatoxins in animal tissues. *J. Assoc. Off. Anal. Chem.* 64: 964–968.

TRUCKSESS, M. W., STOLOFF, L., PONS, W. A. JR., CUCULLU, A. F., LEE, L. S., and FRANZ, A. O. JR. 1969. Thin layer chromatographic determination of aflatoxin B_1 in eggs. *J. Assoc. Off. Anal. Chem.* 60: 795–798.

VAN EGMOND, H. P., PAULSCH, W. E., and SCHULLER, P. L. 1978. Confirmatory test for aflatoxin M_1 on a thin-layer plate. *J. Assoc. Off. Anal. Chem.* 61: 809–812.

VAN EGMOND, H. P. and STUBBLEFIELD, R. D. 1981. Improved method for confirmation of identity of aflatoxin B_1 and M_1 in dairy products and animal tissue extracts. *J. Assoc. Off. Anal. Chem.* 65: 152–155.

VELASCO, J. 1972. Modified ferric gel method for determining aflatoxin in cottonseed meals. *J. Assoc. Off. Anal. Chem.* 55: 1359–1360.

VELASCO, J. and WHITTEN, M. E. 1973. Evaluation of florisil tubes in detection of aflatoxin. *J. Am. Oil Chem. Soc.* 50: 120–121.

VERRETT, M. J., MARLIAC, J. P., and McLAUGHLIN, J. JR. 1964. Use of the chicken embryo in the assay of aflatoxin toxicity. *J. Assoc. Off. Anal. Chem.* 47: 1003–1006.

VERRETT, M. J., WINBUSH, J., REYNALDO, E. F., and SCOTT, W. F. 1973. Collaborative study of the chicken embryo bioassay for aflatoxin B_1. *J. Assoc. Off. Anal. Chem.* 56: 901–904.

WARE, G. M., CARMAN, A., FRANCIS, O., and KHAN, S. 1984. Gas chromatographic determination of deoxynivalenol in wheat with electron capture detection. *J. Assoc. Off. Anal. Chem.* 67: 731–734.

19

Detection, Quantitation, and Public Health Significance of Foodborne Viruses

Edward P. Larkin

Food and Drug Administration
Cincinnati, Ohio

INTRODUCTION

The virus disease historically associated with food and water is infectious hepatitis (hepatitis A). This agent has been responsible for most life-threatening outbreaks of foodborne virus disease and has been shown to be transmitted via the fecal-oral route. About 4,000 cases were reported in the United States between 1944 and 1982 (Table 19.1). As with most diseases, the number of hepatitis A cases is underestimated (Cliver 1983). Many infections of children are mild and easily misdiagnosed. Probably only 5–10% of the cases are reported.

Consumption of raw and undercooked shellfish has resulted in a variety of foodborne disease outbreaks in the United States (Table 19.2). Between 1900 and 1984 more than 11,000 cases were reported (Verber 1984). A number of studies on pollution of shellfish harvesting waters resulted in much better control over the sanitary harvesting and shipment of shellfish.

Table 19.1. Food-Associated Hepatitis in the United States, 1944–1982

	1944–49	1950–59	1960–69	1970–79	1980–82	Total
Number of cases associated with shellfish			1,047[a]	343	8	1,398
Number of cases associated with other foods	38	257	733	1,346	479	2,853

[a]Cliver (1983).

Such activity should have reduced the number of cases of shellfish-associated disease outbreaks. However, this has not been the case, chiefly because of widespread transport and distribution of the product and the increase in the number of shellfish consumers. This increase in consumption and overfishing produced a shortage of native shellfish used in the raw clam and oyster trade. As a result, foreign shippers attempted to penetrate the American market, and four English companies were quite successful in the early 1980s. However, between March and June 1982 more than 1,800 cases of gastrointestinal disease occurred in consumers of raw clams (Verber 1984). In one instance, more than 50% of the 3,000 individuals at a picnic became ill (Fig. 19.1). Shellfish importation ceased as a result of joint agreement between the responsible agencies in the United States and England. Later investigations showed that the shellfish had been harvested from polluted waters and relayed in waters having similar levels of contamination.

DETECTION AND QUANTITATION OF FOODBORNE VIRUSES

In recent years viruses have been incriminated in only two types of foodborne disease: hepatitis A virus in a number of foods that were consumed raw or undercooked and the Norwalk agent that was identified in the feces of consumers of contaminated foods by immune electron microscopy (IEM) or radioimmunoassay (RIA). A large outbreak occurred in 1978 in Australia when shellfish harvested from sewage-contaminated waters were eaten over a period of weeks by thousands of consumers (Christopher et al. 1982; Murphy et al. 1979; Cross et al. 1979). Two different-sized virus particles

Table 19.2. Shellfish-Associated Disease in the United States

Disease agent or symptomatology	1900–09	1910–19	1920–29	1930–39	1940–49	1950–59	1960–69	1970–79	1980–84	Total cases
Typhoid	310[a]	129	2,130	471	224	4	—	—	—	3,268
Gastroenteritis	—[b]	—	—	70	1,316	88	261	6	4,355	6,096
Hepatitis A	—	—	—	—	—	—	1,051	342	11	1,404
Norwalk agent	—	—	—	—	—	—	—	—	6	6
Vibrio	—	—	—	—	—	—	71	34	37	142
Unspecified	52	79	31	26	300	12	—	328	—	828
Total cases	362	208	2,161	567	1,840	104	1,383	710	4,409	11,744

[a]Verber (1984).
[b]Data not available or not known.

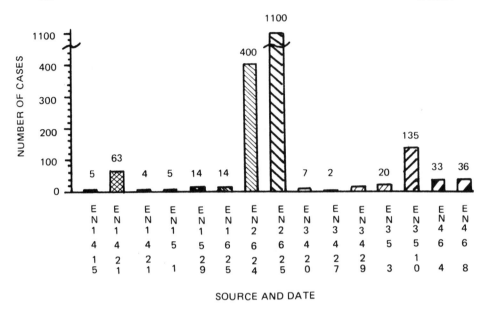

FIG. 19.1   Foodborne disease outbreaks associated with consumption of clams imported from four English sources (En-1, 2, 3, and 4) between 4/15 and 6/25, 1983.

were found in feces obtained from ill consumers: a 27–30 nm particle that reacted with Norwalk antiserum and a 22–25 nm particle. The Norwalk-like agent was believed to be disease-related but the role of the smaller particle in the disease process was unknown. It was interesting that a number of secondary infections developed in family members who were in contact with sick consumers of shellfish. Several enteroviruses and reoviruses have been isolated from foods but have not been incriminated in disease outbreaks because similar contact infections that continuously occur in the population masked the infection source.

Each year a number of gastroenteritis cases of unknown origin are reported. Scientists in different parts of the world have been screening feces recovered from both ill and well patients and have observed a variety of virus-like particles (Middleton et al. 1977). The structure of the particles has been used to attempt to classify them into groups with known viruses (Caul and Appleton 1982; Flewett and Boxall 1976; Flewett et al. 1974). This system has allowed for an orderly description of the agents, and comparisons could be made with agents in other disease outbreaks. The morphological characteristics plus the presence of specific antibody confirmed by IEM in the diseased individual effectively showed the association of the particle with the specific disease.

Viruses and virus-like particles have been found in fecal preparations. A number of agents such as adenoviruses, enteroviruses, reoviruses, and rotaviruses are identifiable and usually can be grown in an animal or cell culture system. A number of surveys have been made of human populations in different areas of the world, and the presence of serum antibody has been used to indicate past infections with viral agents. The volume of information available is dependent on the interests of the scientists and the availability of serum from the various age groups (Table 19.3). The intestinal adenoviruses, astroviruses, caliciviruses, and rotaviruses are the chief agents producing gastrointestinal disease in young children and infants, while the Norwalk-type viruses usually infect older children and adults (Kapikian et al. 1972). Any of these agents can produce infections in any age group, however.

Rotaviruses and Norwalk-type viruses usually elicit detectable antibody, which does not necessarily protect the individual from a second infection. This is especially evident in the case of rotavirus infections in which passive immunity, i.e., antibody in mother's milk, results in greater protection than serum antibody in the child. However, the presence of serum antibody usually results in a more rapid recovery from a rotavirus infection (Cukor and Blacklow 1984).

The great variety and chemical complexity of foods present a number of problems to the investigator attempting to determine if viruses are present in/on the food. The selection process is reduced to foods subjected to limited or no thermal contact, for viruses are inactivated by the high processing temperatures used in many food products. The past experience of the consumer with the food and its history in viral foodborne disease outbreaks present the investigator with a choice of foods that have a higher potential for contamination. A number of these foods have been investigated using procedures outlined in Fig. 19.2 (Larkin 1982a).

Most of the methods utilized to examine foods for viruses use pH adjustments to detach the virus from the food particles or adsorb it to them. This technique has been shown to be very efficient when testing foods for picornaviruses, and low level virus contaminants can be extracted. However, the same procedure had little success in extracting parvoviruses and rotaviruses; only a small fraction of the viruses known to be present in the food has been recovered. We are investigating other procedures in an attempt to enhance recovery of such viruses.

A number of viruses do not grow or are not able to be detected by the cell cultures now in use in virus laboratories. Many viruses that infect humans will grow only in human or primate cells. Logistical restrictions and costs limit the use of many such cells, especially when routine surveys are made to compare methods for recovering viruses from commercial products.

The same cell cultures propagated in different laboratories over a period of time change in their sensitivity to virus growth. Thus, comparisons made

Table 19.3. Characteristics of Gastrointestinal Disease Caused by Viruses

Virus	Clinical disease and antibody production
Adenoviruses 70–90 nm[a] DS–DNA[b]	Clinical intestinal infections occur chiefly in patients less than 3 years of age; percentage of adults with antibody not known.
Astroviruses 20–29 nm Not known	Clinical infection occurs between 3 and 4 years of age, ~70% of older children and adults have antibody (England); high percentage of children over 4 years of age have antibody (U.S.).
Caliciviruses 20–25 nm Not known	Clinical infection occurs between 6 and 24 months of age, ~ 95% of older Japanese children and adults have antibody; incidence in the U.S. not known.
Coronaviruses 80–180 nm SS–RNA[c]	Viruses detected in both ill and well children and adults; causative agent of gastroenteritis not proven.
Norwalk virus ~ 27 nm Not known	Clinical infection occurs in late adolescence; ~ 70% of adults have antibody.
Rotaviruses ~ 70 nm DS–RNA	Clinical infection occurs between 6 and 24 months of age; great majority of children over 2 years of age possess antibody; highest percentage of hospital gastrointestinal illness in age group 6 months to 2 years due to these viruses.
Small round viruses	~ 5 other virus-like agents detected in feces by electron microscopy: 1. Parvovirus-like agent (22–25 nm). 2. Minireoviruses (35–40 nm).

[a]Size.
[b]Double-stranded DNA.
[c]Single-stranded RNA.

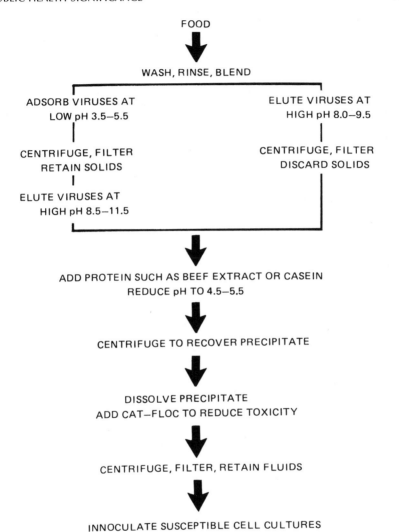

FIG. 19.2   Summary of procedures used to enhance virus recovery from foods.

of the same food in different laboratories may vary extensively. When different methods are examined, such cells may give results that differ significantly and the method may be thought to be ineffective, when actually the cell cultures were at fault.

An interesting study was reported in which the infectious dose of virus was compared on two occasions several years apart. Echovirus 12 was passed twice in primary monkey kidney cells after isolation from an 8-year-old girl. A number of studies with this virus, after it was originally isolated, had shown it to be a very mild pathogen, and owing to this attenuation it was approved for human infectivity studies (Ward and Akin 1984). The virus was suspended in distilled water and consumed by human subjects in 100-mL portions. Doses in pfu were 0, 10, 30, 100, and 300, and the % infectivities were 0, 30, 45, 73, and 100. The virus titers were all calculated by growth in monkey kidney culture (LLC-MK). The human infectious dose ($HID/_{50}$) was determined to be 30 pfu, and it was estimated that about 2% of the subjects would be infected with approximately 1 pfu.

A few years later, using the identical inocula, another cell line and another plaque assay procedure, it was determined that the $HID/_{50}$ was 919 and that about 2% of the subjects would have been infected with approximately 17 pfu. The variation in infectivity was reported to be due to the increased sensitivity of the new cell line and plaque assay. In this study the inocula from the earlier study were available for comparison, an unusual circumstance, for in most similar cases inocula were used in other studies or discarded. It is apparent that interpretations made in any such study are affected by the sensitivity of the culture systems used to measure both the dose and virus shedding data. Similar information could be obtained from other studies in which virus recovery data had been reported.

A number of methods are used to detect and quantify viruses. Some of the procedures, like plaque assay and detection by CPE, are inexpensive and require little or no equipment or special laboratory facilities. However, the use of electron microscopy and some other procedures requires the availability of expensive and complicated microscopes and radioisotope measurement systems (Table 19.4). Some of the methods used in virus quantitative studies are:

1. Cytopathic effect—visible destruction of the cell sheet, tube cultures, and most probable number (MPN).

2. Electron microscopy—visualization of the particles by direct EM with or without specific antibody.

3. Plaque formation—visual observation of areas in cell sheets destroyed by virus growth—live cells stained with vital dye.

Table 19.4. Growth and Identification Characteristics of Possible Foodborne Viruses

Virus (human)	Grown in culture	Method of detection and identification
Adenoviruses (intestinal)	Yes	CPE, plaques
Astroviruses	No	EM immunological methods
Caliciviruses (Norwalk)	No	EM immunological methods
Enteroviruses Polioviruses Coxsackieviruses A and B Echoviruses	Yes; variety of cultures and lab animals needed	Variety of methods
Hepatitis A (Enterovirus 72)	Yes; slow, cell associated, direct isolation quantitation is questionable	EM immunological methods, gene probes
Parvoviruses	Yes and No	EM, hemagglutination, gene probes
Papovaviruses	Yes; culture requirements difficult	Immunological methods
Reoviruses	Yes; variety of cultures	Variety of methods
Rotaviruses	Yes; direct isolation is slow, quantitation is not presently available	EM immunological methods, gene probes

4. Immunofluorescence—addition of fluoroescent specific antibody to virus infected cells, antibody-antigen complex fluorescent in UV light.

5. Radioimmunoassy—specific antibody tagged with radioactive ^{125}I, level of viral antigen detected by amount of bound radioactivity.

6. ELISA (enzyme-linked-immunoabsorbent assay) horseradish peroxidase or alkaline phosphatase-enzyme conjugated to antigen, levels bound to antibody measured by intensity of color reaction.

7. Radioimmuno-focus assay—fixation of infected cells with acetone and reaction with ^{125}I labeled antibody. The antibody which binds to infected

cells is visualized by autoradiography as individual foci are produced on the photographic plate.

Susceptible culture systems provide the most effective way to grow and quantitate viruses. As can be seen in Table 19.4, many viruses associated with human gastroenteritis either have not been cultured, grow slowly, or produce little or no CPE in cell cultures (Birch et al. 1983; Wyatt et al. 1983). It is only recently that the intestinal adenoviruses, the rotaviruses, and hepatitis A virus have been propagated directly from feces obtained from patients with the infection (Binn et al. 1984). "Wild" rotaviruses and hepatitis A virus are detectable only after 2–4 weeks in culture, while the intestinal adenoviruses have been propagated in transformed human cultures and were detectable within a few days (Wigand et al. 1983; de Jong et al. 1983). The Norwalk viruses, the astroviruses, and some parvoviruses may grow in some cell cultures without cell destruction, and thus were discarded as useful means of propagation. In some cases a large number of viruses inoculated onto the cultures will produce sufficient antigen to be detected, as was the case with rotaviruses where CPE appeared in rotary cell cultures several weeks after inoculation with heavily contaminated feces. A number of laboratories have been investigating cultures and procedures for growing the Norwalk virus but have been unsuccessful (Caul et al. 1979; Cukor and Blacklow 1984). Possibly the low virus concentration in the feces may be responsible for the poor results. It is anticipated that a breakthrough in this quest will soon be achieved.

PUBLIC HEALTH SIGNIFICANCE

On a worldwide basis a number of viruses have been isolated from foods (Larkin 1981, 1982b). Most of these viruses were enteroviruses: polioviruses, coxsackieviruses, and echoviruses. A number of foods were incriminated, including lettuce, tomatoes, beets, carrots, potatoes, cucumbers, parsley, dill, cherries, and rhubarb. Animal products such as eggs, chicken, fish fillets, beef, lamb, milk, and butter have been shown on occasion to be contaminated by animal or human viruses. Shellfish are foods of concern in the U.S. because they are one of the few foods consumed raw, and viruses have been recovered from market samples of raw oysters and mussels and from oysters and clams harvested from approved waters (Larkin and Hunt 1982). None of the enteroviruses recovered was shown to be agents of disease in shellfish consumers. Recently we have grown parvoviruses in cell culture inoculated with feces obtained from ill consumers of raw shellfish and from other ill and well patients. Whether these agents are associated with foodborne disease is not known at the present time. Until recently, methods for detecting hepatitis A and rotaviruses were not available. It is anticipated that such studies will be initiated in the near future as these methods are adapted to food virology.

Viruses and bacteria associated with foodborne disease are transmitted to the consumer via the fecal-oral route. Viruses require living cells in order to propagate, and unless a living food animal is infected the viruses will usually persist for only a short time. This phenomenon is different from that of bacteria, which may increase in numbers in the food. Viruses may be concentrated in shellfish by a filter-feeding process in which viruses are removed from the ingested water along with food particulates. Virus concentrations inside the shellfish have been reported to be equivalent to the virus concentration in the surrounding water. Removal of the shellfish to clean waters should result in a reduction in virus numbers. If the contamination level is too high, the viruses may persist for longer than the time usually allocated for virus reduction. If such shellfish are sent to market, there is a high potential for foodborne disease outbreaks. In some instances, the level of indicator bacteria used to monitor the microbiological quality of the product may be low while viruses are still present in the shellfish.

Protecting the food supply from virus contamination may be accomplished by procedures used to prevent contamination by other organisms. Good sanitary practices and personal hygiene along with control of the environment will reduce the potential for contamination. Where prevention measures are not possible, processing the food at temperatures of $> 90°C$ should ensure inactivation of any viruses present in or on the food (Larkin 1983).

REFERENCES

BINN, L. N., LEMON, S. M., MARCHWICKI, R. M., REDFIELD, R. R., GATES, N. L., and BANCROFT, W. H. 1984. Primary isolation and serial passage of hepatitis A virus strains in primate cell cultures. *J. Clin. Microbiol.* 20(1): 28–33.

BIRCH, C. J., RODGER, S. M., MARSHALL, J. A., and GUST, I. D. 1983. Replication of human rotavirus in cell culture. *J. Med. Virol.* 11: 241–250.

CAUL, E. O. and APPLETON, H. 1982. The electron microscopical and physical characteristics of small round human fecal viruses: An interim scheme for classification. *J. Med. Virol.* 9: 257–265.

CAUL, E. O., ASHLEY, C. R., and PETHER, J. V. S. 1979. 'Norwalk'-Like particles in epidemic gastroenteritis in the UK. *Lancet* ii: 1292.

CHRISTOPHER, P. J., GROHMANN, G. S., MILLSON, R. H., and MURPHY, A. M. 1982. Parvovirus gastroenteritis. A new entity for Australia. *Med. J. Aust.* 1: 121–124.

CLIVER, D. O. 1983. *Manual on Food Virology*. VPH83.46. WHO, Geneva, Switzerland.

CROSS, G., FORSYTH, J., GREENBERG, H., HARRISON, J., IRVING, L., LUKE, R., MOORE, B., and SCHNAGL, R. 1979. Oyster-associated gastroenteritis. *Med. J. Aust.* 1: 56–57.

CUKOR, G. and BLACKLOW, N. R. 1984. Human viral gastroenteritis. *Microbiol. Rev.* 48: 157–179.

DE JONG, J. C., WIGAND, R., KIDD, A. H., WADELL, G., KAPSENBERG, J. G., MUZERIE, C. J., WERMENBOL, A. G., and FIRTZLAFF, R. -G. 1983. Candidate adenoviruses 40 and 41: Fastidious adenoviruses from human infant stool. *J. Med. Virol.* 11: 215–231.

FLEWETT. T. H., BRYDEN, A. S., and DAVIES, H. A. 1974. Diagnostic electron microscopy of the faeces. I. The viral flora of the faeces as seen by electron microscopy. *J. Clin. Pathol.* 27: 603–608.

FLEWETT, T. H. and BOXALL, E. 1976. The hunt for viruses in infections of the alimentary system. *Clin. Gastroenterol.* 5: 359–385.

KAPIKIAN, A. Z., WYATT, R. G., DOLIN, R., THORNHILL, T. S., KALICA, A. R., and CHANOCK, R. M. 1972. Visualization by immune electron microscopy of a 27 nm particle associated with acute infectious non-bacterial gastroenteritis. *J. Virol.* 10: 1075–1081.

LARKIN, E. P. 1981. Food contaminants—viruses. *J. Food Protect.* 44: 320–325.

LARKIN, E. P. and HUNT, D. A. 1982. Bivalve mollusks: Control of microbiological contaminants. *BioScience* 32(3): 193–197.

LARKIN, E. P. 1982a. Detection of viruses in foods. In *Methods in Environmental Virology*. Gerba, C. and Goyal, S. (Ed.) p. 221–241. Marcel Dekker, Inc., New York.

LARKIN, E. P. 1982b. Viruses in wastewater sludges and effluents used for irrigation. *Environm. Int.* 7: 29–33.

LARKIN, E. P. 1983. Viruses of vertebrates: Thermal resistance. In CRC Handbook of Foodborne Diseases of Biological Origin. Rechcigl, M. Jr. (Ed.), p. 3–24. CRC Press, Inc., Boca Raton, FL.

MIDDLETON, P. J., SZYMANSKI, T., and PETRIC, M. 1977. Viruses associated with acute gastroenteritis in young children. *Am. J. Dis. Child.* 131: 733–737.

MURPHY, A. M., GROHMANN, S. S., CHRISTOPHER, P. J., LOPEZ, W. A., DAVEY, G. R., and MILLSOM, R. H. 1979. An Australia-wide outbreak of gastroenteritis from oysters caused by Norwalk virus. *Med. J. Aust.* 2: 329–333.

VERBER, J. L. 1984. *Shellfish borne disease outbreaks.* p. 2–36. USPHS, FDA, Shellfish Sanitation Branch, Northeast Technical Services Unit, Davisville, RI.

WARD, R. L. and AKIN, E. W. 1984. Minimum infective dose of animal viruses. In CRC *Critical Review and Environmental Control* 14: 297–310. CRC Press, Inc., Boca Raton, FL.

WIGAND, R., BAUMEISTER, H. G., MAASS, G., KÜHN, J., and HAMMER, H. J. 1983. Isolation and identification of enteric adenoviruses. *J. Med. Virol.* 11: 233–240.

WYATT, R. G., JAMES, H. D., JR., PITTMAN, A. L., HOSHINO, Y., GREENBERG, H. B., KALICA, A. R., FLORES, J., and KAPIKIAN, A. Z. 1983. Direct isolation in cell culture of human rotaviruses and their characterization into four serotypes. *J. Clin. Microbiol.* 18(2): 310–317.

20

Detection of Foodborne Microorganisms and Their Toxins: The Future

Anthony N. Sharpe

Health & Welfare Canada
Ottawa, Ontario, Canada

MIRACLES AND MILLSTONES

However touching the true story of its introduction, agar fulfilled the perceived needs of early microbiologists so consummately, it channelled future developments into a monotony almost unparalleled in science, and with a rigidity belying its clammy fragility.

For almost a century thereafter, analytical microbiology—and particularly food microbiology—became the science of agar jelly. To be sure, tube counts and other deviations might grudgingly be made at the dictates of gas production and other clues, but only the rarest of analyses totally avoided agar. Microbiological specifications (whenever not calling for apparent absence) became, in the main, counts of colony-forming units (CFU) or their equivalent. Food microbiologists seemed eternally damned to doing counts, and media room technicians became resigned to their personal foretaste of the Inferno. Such, just a few years ago, was the gloomy outlook.

SPIRALS AND SQUARES

The intractability of the problem of automating counts, from the engineering feasibility and cost/effectiveness angles, gave little hope until recently that the outlook might change. In recent years, two approaches, both based on ingeniously avoiding the knotty problem of how to make dilutions automatically, aseptically and reliably, have appeared. The Spiral Plater™ (AOAC 1981) and Iso-Grid™ membrane filters both—in their own ways—lend some hope that, even if the count does remain with us for another century, at least a portion of the tedium will eventually wither away.

Both systems also feature electronic colony counters which, though still leaving something to be desired, promise through continued development a chance of softening the second dismal reality of counts. The Iso-Grid system also offers attractions in microbial identification and is rapidly being steered in this direction. Both systems have generated much interest and official methodology, and both enjoy an acceptability heightened by their resemblance to traditional ways of doing things. These are definitely systems for the immediate future. Although some reductions in analysis times are possible, for example, in *Escherichia coli* and *Salmonella* determinations by Iso-Grid (AOAC 1984, 1985), neither system undercuts what is currently perceived as a third major drawback of agar microbiology—the analysis time imposed by a need for microbial multiplication in order to get a result.

NEW LAMPS

Very recently, one senses a quickening mood of expectancy and optimism among food microbiologists. Agar methodology has been taken about as far as it can go, and fresh motivation could only come from other directions. Several developments from other sciences are poised to infiltrate food microbiology. Certainly they will modify the ways we detect microbial contamination; perhaps ultimately our very perceptions of spoilage and hazard. The three fields with most immediate impact are: (1) hybridoma, (2) DNA probe, and (3) electronic technologies. Of these, the last is likely to have the most far-reaching and unpredictable consequences.

I shall not spend much time discussing DNA probes and monoclonal antibodies; previous chapters cover these areas capably. There is likely to be considerable overlap between these two fields for many years. Immunological methods of all types are currently engulfing microbiological analysis and monoclonals—if only because of their potential specificity—should enjoy an assured future in identification systems and the determination of toxins in foods. Whether they will completely supercede polyclonal preparations remains to be seen. For detection of preformed toxins in foods, much applicability depends on development of preparations specific against common sites or pooled preparations able to react reliably and specifically across groups of related toxins. For microbial identification, much depends on developing reagents of adequate sensitivity and even more on development of preparations specific to reliably expressed antigenic sites.

It seems likely that, even though some pause in progress is currently evident, DNA probes must eventually overtake totally immunochemically based methods for microbial identification. The early hope for systems capable of detecting any or all organisms without need for incubation steps is, for many species, still very much an early hope. Much remains to be done in the way of developing satisfactory labeling systems. However, the potential seems to be there and we can be confident that the performance of gene probes will improve steadily.

Except perhaps for dilutors, readers, and other equipment for ELISA, neither the immunological nor DNA probe identification procedures are available as automated methods, and here may be a major impediment to widescale use. My impression is that few of the techniques yet described would drastically reduce manipulative time. Whilst there is a general clamor for faster methods, only in a few situations can earlier results be justified at the expense of increased labor requirement or disruptions to laboratory organization. Currently, I think, only a minority of laboratories—those with unusual demands for rapidity—would jump at these techniques. However, development of more streamlined or automated procedures will make them much more universally appreciated. A few years from now simplified, automated, nonradiological EIA and DNA hybridization tests, also combining speed and sensitivity with selectivity, should be very powerful and popular tools.

Neither of these approaches will cause a major shift in attitudes to microbiological contamination. They are basically more effective ways of getting the same information that we look for today. The present "Electronics Age" and the encroaching "Information Age" will produce much more fundamental changes of concept. Those concerned with long range forecasting of or investment in food microbiological methods might well find themselves caught on the horns of a dilemma. For electronics could lead us in two very different directions—approaches with very different outcomes in respect to the need for and types of microbiological analyses we do.

END OF AN ERA

For years agar reigned supreme among the microbiological analyses, because the noise-free amplification made available through colony growth overwhelms most other sources of interference. Physical methods of detecting microorganisms suffered too badly from poor signal to noise problems, and the techniques that were available demanded too much effort for the information they yielded. Techniques such as the determination of microbial numbers through analysis of various metabolic products or adenosinetriphosphate were usually confounded by the existence in foods of large and variable quantities of the analyte. Even when intrinsic analyte could be removed, it was found that correlations between such determinations and plate counts were less than satisfactory. In the climate of yesteryear, nonconformance was too easily blamed on failure of the upstart technique and confirmed the general consensus that only plate counts yielded plate counts as convincingly as plate counts, which was a quite valid opinion, though it sidestepped the question of whether plate counts are convincing determinants of food quality.

There is no doubt that, wherever comparison studies were committed (by the pre-existence of statutory or other regulatory standards couched in terms of microbial numbers) to evaluating alternative techniques for their ability to predict plate counts, then the nonmultiplicative methods had little to attract to them. They did not yield *counts*. Even more important, neither the manipulations involved in them nor the type of data produced engendered the same feeling of closeness to the product or the organisms within it that the count produces.

Electronics—in particular, the computer—is ushering in a wave of new approaches to food microbiological analyses combining sufficient credibility and friendliness to challenge the plate count. What these techniques will have in common is minimal and rapid sample preparation, large sample-volume capability, continuous computerized monitoring of the development of biochemical or other parameters pertinent to product quality, completely automated detection of course, but an interactive capability permitting the microbiologist to oversee the instrument's performance and make his own decisions if need be. These techniques will make it easy to feel close to the microorganisms as they do their varied thing and easy to feel in control of the output. The vanguard of these shimmering techniques is electrical impedance.

Like most "alternative" techniques, the electrical impedance method subsisted for many lean years without accumulating a noticeable following. But that has changed and impedance is currently gathering up an approval and acceptability quite unprecedented among the alternative methods. We may eventually acknowledge our debt to the impedance people for paving the way to all those computerized biochemical analyses we come to rely on in the year 2005.

Without the development of the digital computer this would not have been possible. But impedance merchants over the years have developed the necessary interactive systems, theoretical and statistical supports, and demonstrated applications and data bases to show convincingly that impedance instruments can be used both reliably and profitably in the right circumstances. One can sense the mounting respectability of impedance; traditional suspicions are dropping away as the technique, aided by an unusually conservative marketing policy, gains adherents. Perhaps more important for the future, like all metabolism-based techniques, impedance data can be reasoned (and even shown) to be better predictors of product shelf-life than are plate counts, since both microbial number and microbial activity are taken into account during the measurement (Firstenberg-Eden and Eden 1984). A count alone conveys very little information about the microbiological state of a sample, and the quicker the concept of "CFU/g" becomes phased out of quality specifications, the quicker we shall be able to enjoy instruments which really permit us to control food quality.

The wedge is in the door and I expect to see other metabolism-based techniques on the heels of impedance. I have written much about the technique of "sequential analysis" (of which impedance is but one embodiment) and its potential in determining the shelf life of a food or predicting the physiological effect it will have on consumers. It is possible in principle, as I have shown (Sharpe 1980), to use computers in developing instruments capable of yielding much more meaningful data about food quality than plate counts are capable of giving. As these proliferate the "count" will pass—if not into oblivion—at least into insignificance.

One attractive characteristic of all such methods will be the ability to handle and keep track of large numbers of samples. Without doubt some very rapid analyses will be developed, perhaps even techniques based on automated DNA hybridization or immunological procedures. But for many applications of food microbiology it is desirable to determine the ability of the organisms to bring about changes in the food or to affect the consumer. Here there must almost certainly be some period of incubation during which the organisms can multiply and exercise their biochemical power and have it monitored. Therefore, the most powerful analyses will be those based on computerized incubator/detector combinations. As such systems become more common and reliance on counts diminishes, they will become increasingly attractive. With large sample-handling capability it will become increasingly feasible to carry out microbiological examinations on products and manufacturing processes, and to hold or rotate stock according to the results. Thus, one of the consequences of the infiltration of electronics into food microbiology may be increased microbiological testing.

The laboratory robot is but one small relative of those systems of automata that are already changing approaches to design, manufacturing, and product handling. I describe above an immediate future in which rapid and voluminous microbiological sampling is possible. But this same pervading electronics could bring about almost the opposite change in food microbiological analysis. We may eventually find ourselves less concerned with the need to rapidly analyze foods and food manufacturing processes for microbiological contamination.

Leaving aside a more fundamental argument that the major contributions to food poisoning statistics occur after food has passed out of the manufacturer's control and into the caterer's or consumer's (Todd 1983), there is little doubt that product quality does not pivot on microbiological analysis but rather on the excellence of the manufacturing practice and degree of control exercised over those microbiologically significant parameters such as water activity, temperature, pH, etc.

In this we are just beginning to see the use of manufacturing systems featuring continuous monitoring of the microbiological variables and integrated computerized control, for example, retorting processes monitored by the computer through various transducers and capable of adjusting to compensate for normal process deviations, or systems which follow the product's time/temperature experiences (e.g., through bar chart temperature indicators) and adjust date stamping accordingly.

In a few years we shall undoubtedly see the majority of food manufacturing processes pass into the control of intelligent robot systems that—through their communication with a variety of sensors of microbiological parameters at all stages of the materials/production/distribution/retail chain; through their ability to monitor and control raw material shipments (perhaps even farm operations), sanitizing, cleaning schedules etc.; through their ability to apply expert knowledge bases to food manufacture; and through their ability to predict the microbiological performance of products and initiate corrective action if necessary—will result in food products that are generally superior to those of today.

We are entering the "Fifth Generation" of computers, the age of "artificial intelligence." Telemetry and transducery are already sufficiently developed to permit, by the time the new computers are with us, of factories which veritably sense and understand the processes going on within them. These machines will be accepted and installed very quickly by food manufacturing companies, not particularly for the benefit of any microbiological elegance they might endow on the process, but because—by minimizing personnel, waste, turnaround time, holding times, etc.—they will produce food more cheaply. Improvement of the microbiological performance of the product, through optimization of processing conditions at all stages (not just "Critical" Control Points) will come about simply as one of the positive cost/benefits sought in setting up the system.

One of the requirements for microbiological control this way is the painstaking establishment of data bases from which product quality (shelf life, toxicity, etc.) can be described mathematically in terms of multi-dimensional functions of the various important parameters (initial microbial load, biochemical activity, water, salt, pH, temperature, etc.). My impression is that many large companies are engaged in developing just this type of data base and math. Since such information is very product specific and valuable to the owner, it will remain very much a proprietary thing.

This progress of electronics into the realm of food microbiology is inevitable and must surely quicken even as the pace of development in electronics itself increases. Much further in the future (assuming that humans remain connected with food handling in any degree) I can see all manner of capabilities which, today, might be thought of as frivolous daydreams, for example, sentient intelligent packaging which, by constantly monitoring itself, is able to detect violations of its proper storage conditions and which is able to communicate this information to the consumer or to the computer that controls the functions of his home, or even to the manufacturer or the regulatory agency involved with that product.

Such developments would have great impact on the statistics of food poisoning. For would-be investors in microbiological instrumentation developments of this type might be seen to so greatly improve the microbiological quality of foods as to make conventional (including computerized sequential analysis) testing either unnecessary or impractical. Thus, depending on which type of system establishes itself first, the heavily automated laboratory analyzer might or might never become a popular reality.

One can take projections like this to very great lengths. There is just one further possibility of the electronics/communication revolution I should like to touch on, and you can pursue your own deductions of its implications.

We are assured that information will soon become another piped-in necessity, just like electricity, gas, etc. At present a multitude of regulatory agencies oversee the activities of food manufacturing companies and caterers. Some of these are empowered to and do make regular inspections of plant activities or maintenance, collecting data on thermal processes, water activities, and so on. Some only inspect when things go wrong. Whatever level it is carried out at, inspection is an expensive commodity. Many agencies cannot employ the inspectors they feel necessary for adequate surveillance, and the problem will certainly not improve in the forseeable future.

One can argue that, if such inspection is necessary, then much of the required information could be transferred more effectively and less expensively, simply by allowing the company's computer to communicate with its regulatory counterpart, either on demand or at regular intervals. There are, I know, strong arguments against the desirability of this. But it is also technically feasible, even today, and feasibilities have a way of becoming realities once the smallest wedge is emplaced.

For example, consider an inspector collecting pasteurizer temperature data. At present it may take days or weeks for the data to become an official part of regulatory records. What if the data were to be electronically transmitted straight to the regulatory computer every year? Who would argue against this? With suitable checks to prevent error, fraud, and other mischances it does not seem a practice that should occasion much difficulty.

What if the data were to be transmitted every month? Every day? Then why not have it on-line? What if the product were subsequently implicated in a food poisoning outbreak? Who then is to take the responsibility—manufacturer or regulatory agency? One can say that such on-line communication between regulator and regulatee is not acceptable. But there is only the finest of lines between each step.

At the least then, electronics will bring about some changes in our approach to microbiological quality of food. I suspect the changes it wreaks will be much more fundamental than other changes currently infiltrating analytical microbiology via the immunologists and recombinantists. The next twenty years should be quite interesting times for food microbiologists.

REFERENCES

AOAC. 1981. Official final action Spiral Plate method for bacterial count of foods or cosmetics. *J. Assoc. Off. Anal. Chem.* 64(2): 528–529.

AOAC. 1984. Official final action Hydrophobic Grid Membrane Filter method for detecting total coliforms, fecal coliforms and *E. coli* in foods. *J. Assoc. Off. Anal. Chem.* 68(2): 481.

AOAC. 1985. *Salmonella* detection in foods: Hydrophobic Grid Membrane Filter method: first action. *J. Assoc. Off. Anal. Chem.* 68(2): 405–407.

FIRSTENBERG-EDEN, R. and EDEN, G. 1984. *Impedance Microbiology*. Research Studies Press Ltd., Letchworth, UK.

SHARPE, A. N. 1980. *Food Microbiology: a Framework for the Future*. Thomas, Springfield, IL.

TODD, E. C. D. 1983. Foodborne disease in Canada—a 5-year summary. *J. Food Protect*. 46: 650–657.

Index